Clinical Research in Oral Health

Clinical Research in Oral Health

Edited by

William V. Giannobile, DDS, DMSc

Brian A. Burt, PhD, MPH, BDSc

Robert J. Genco, DDS, PhD

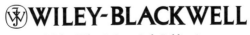

A John Wiley & Sons, Ltd., Publication

Blackwell Publishing was acquired by John Wiley & Sons in February 2007. Blackwell's publishing program has been merged with Wiley's global Scientific, Technical, and Medical business to form Wiley-Blackwell.

Editorial Office
2121 State Avenue, Ames, Iowa 50014-8300, USA

For details of our global editorial offices, for customer services, and for information about how to apply for permission to reuse the copyright material in this book, please see our website at www.wiley.com/wiley-blackwell.

Library of Congress Cataloging-in-Publication Data

Clinical research in oral health / [edited by] William V. Giannobile,
    Brian A. Burt, Robert J. Genco.
        p. ; cm.
    Includes bibliographical references and index.
    ISBN 978-0-8138-1529-9 (hardback : alk. paper)   1. Dentistry–Research.   I. Giannobile, William V.
II. Genco, Robert J.   III. Burt, Brian A.
    [DNLM: 1. Dental Research.   2. Oral Health. WU 20.5 C641 2010]
    RK80.C58 2010
    617.60072–dc22

                                                                                                          2009041419

A catalog record for this book is available from the U.S. Library of Congress.

Set in 10/12pt Times by Aptara® Inc., New Delhi, India
Printed in Singapore by Markono Print Media Pte Ltd

1   2010

Dedications

To my wife, Angela and son, Anthony for their love, patience, encouragement, and support

To my students who inspire and challenge me in my daily professional life

To my mentors who instilled in me a love for my career in clinical research

To my parents who made me believe in myself

– William Giannobile

To my wife Elizabeth, whose never-ending support is crucial to the production of this book. In addition, I salute all those dedicated research colleagues who have contributed so much to my research down the years.

– Brian A. Burt

My efforts in preparing this book are due in great part to the lessons I learned from my mentor, Dr. D. Walter Cohen; to the diligence and creativity of my clinical research colleagues; and to the enduring support of my wife, Frances.

– Robert Genco

Contents

Contributors

MAXWELL H. ANDERSON, DDS, MS, MEd, Director, Anderson Dental Consulting, Sequim, WA, USA

GARY C. ARMITAGE, DDS, MS, R. Earl Robinson Distinguished Professor, Division of Periodontology, Department of Orofacial Sciences, University of California, San Francisco, CA, USA

JAMES BADER, DDS, MPH, Research Professor, Operative Dentistry, The University of North Carolina at Chapel Hill, Chapel Hill, NC, USA

MICHAEL L. BARNETT, DDS, Oral Health Industry Consultant, Princeton, NJ, USA. Formerly: Senior Director of Dental Affairs and Technology Development for Warner-Lambert Company (later Pfizer Inc.)

EUGENIO D. BELTRÁN-AGUILAR, DMD, MPH, MS, DrPH, Senior Advisor on Epidemiology, Office of the Director, Division of Oral Health, NCCDPHP, Centers for Disease Control and Prevention, Atlanta, GA, USA

NORMAN S. BRAVEMAN, PhD, President, Braveman BioMed Consultants LLC, Rockville, MD, USA

BRIAN BURT, PhD, MPH, BDSc, Professor Emeritus, Epidemiology, Professor Emeritus, School of Dentistry, School of Public Health, University of Michigan, Ann Arbor, MI, USA

MARK CITRON, MS, VP Regulatory and Clinical Affairs, Tyrx Pharmaceuticals, Inc. Monmouth Junction, NJ, USA

RONALD G. CRAIG, DMD, PhD, PEARL Network Executive Management Team, NYU College of Dentistry, New York, NY, USA

MARY P. CULLINAN, BDS, MSc, FADI, Research Associate Professor, Discipline of Periodontics, Department of Oral Sciences and Sir John Walsh Research Institute Faculty of Dentistry, University of Otago, Dunedin, New Zealand

FREDERICK A. CURRO, DMD, PhD, PEARL Network Executive Management Team, NYU College of Dentistry, New York, NY, USA

DONALD J. DENUCCI, DDS, MS, Program Director, Practice-Based Research Networks, Center for Clinical Research, National Institute of Dental and Craniofacial Research, Bethesda, MD, USA

BRUCE A. DYE, DDS, MPH (CAPT USPHS), Dental Epidemiology Officer, Division of Health and Nutrition Examination Surveys, National Center for Health Statistics, Centers for Disease Control and Prevention, Hyattsville, MD, USA

JACK L. FERRACANE, PhD, Department of Restorative Dentistry, Oregon Health & Science University, Portland, OR, USA

KAY FULLER, RAC, IND/IDE Program Manager, Michigan Institute for Clinical and Health Research, Medical School, University of Michigan, Ann Arbor, MI, USA

ROBERT J. GENCO, DDS, PhD, SUNY Distinguished Professor, Departments of Oral Biology, Microbiology, and Immunology, Vice Provost, State University of New York at Buffalo, Amherst, NY, USA

WILLIAM V. GIANNOBILE, DDS, DMSc, Najjar Endowed Professor of Dentistry, Department of Periodontics and Oral Medicine, School of Dentistry, Professor, Department of Biomedical Engineering, College of Engineering, Director, Michigan Center for Oral Health Research, University of Michigan, Ann Arbor, MI, USA

GREGG H. GILBERT, DDS, MBA, Department of General Dental Sciences, School of Dentistry, University of Alabama at Birmingham, Birmingham, AL, USA

ANNE-MARIE GLENNY, PhD, Senior Lecturer in Evidence Based Oral Care, School of Dentistry, The University of Manchester, Manchester, England

LISA J.A. HEITZ-MAYFIELD, BDS, MDSc, Odont Dr, Professor, Centre for Rural and Remote Oral Health, The University of Western Australia, Western Australia, Australia

DOUGLAS W. HOLBOROW, BDS, FDSRCS, Faculty of Dentistry, Oral Sciences, University of Otago, Dunedin, New Zealand

THOMAS J. HILTON, DMD, MS, Alumni Centennial Professor in Operative Dentistry, Department of Restorative Dentistry, Oregon Health & Science University, Portland, OR, USA

PHILIPPE P. HUJOEL, DDS, PhD, Professor, Department of Dental Public Health Sciences, Adjunct Professor, Department of Epidemiology, School of Dentistry, University of Washington, Seattle, Washington, D.C., USA

AMID I. ISMAIL, BDS, MPH, MBA, DrPH, Office of the Dean, Temple University, School of Dental Medicine, Philadelphia, PA, USA

DARNELL KAIGLER JR., DDS, MS, PhD, Assistant Professor in Dentistry, Periodontics and Oral Medicine, Department of Periodontics and Oral Medicine, Michigan Center for Oral Health Research, School of Dentistry, Assistant Professor, Department of Biomedical Engineering, College of Engineering, University of Michigan, Ann Arbor, MI, USA

NIKLAUS P. LANG, DDS, MS, PhD, Professor of Implant Dentistry, University of Hong Kong, Hong Kong, SAR, People's Republic of China

BROOKE LATZKE, Clinical Research Associate, PRECEDENT Practice-based Research Network, University of Washington, Seattle, WA, USA

BRIAN G. LEROUX, PhD, Department of Biostatistics, University of Washington, Seattle, WA, USA

ANNE S. LINDBLAD, PhD, PEARL Senior Statistician, Executive Vice President, The EMMES Corporation, Rockville, MD, USA

SAMUEL E. LYNCH, DMD, DMSc, President and CEO, BioMimetic Therapeutics, Franklin, TN, USA

FRANCIS L. MACRINA, PhD, Edward Myers Professor of Dentistry and Vice President for Research, Virginia Commonwealth University, Richmond, VA, USA

MICHAEL C. MANZ, DDS, MPH, DrPH, Senior Research Associate in Health Sciences, Department of Cariology, Restorative Sciences, and Endodontics, University of Michigan School of Dentistry, Ann Arbor, MI, USA

ANDREA MATHEWS, RDH, BS, DPBRN Practice-based Research Network, Department of General Dental Sciences, School of Dentistry, University of Alabama at Birmingham, Birmingham, AL, USA

RUTH MCBRIDE, Axio Corporation, Scientific Director, Director Data Management Unit for NW PRECEDENT Dental Practice-based Research Network

BRYAN S. MICHALOWICZ, DDS, MS, Professor and Erwin Schaffer Chair in Periodontal Research, Division of Periodontology, Department of Developmental and Surgical Sciences, University of Minnesota, Minneapolis, MN, USA

JULES T. MITCHEL, MBA, PhD, President, Target Health Inc., New York, USA, Adjunct Professor, Department of Pharmacology & Toxicology, Ernest Mario School of Pharmacy, Rutgers University

SHEILA D. MOORE, CIP, Office of the Institutional Review Board, University of Alabama at Birmingham, Birmingham, AL, USA

HAL MORGENSTERN, PhD, Professor, Epidemiology and Environmental Health Sciences, Director, Graduate Summer Session in Epidemiology, School of Public Health, University of Michigan, Ann Arbor, MI, USA

IAN NEEDLEMAN, BDS, MSc, PhD, MRDRCS(Eng), FDSRCS(Eng), FFPH, FHEA, Professor of Restorative Dentistry and Evidence-Based Healthcare, Department of Clinical Research, Unit of Periodontology, Director, International Centre for Evidence-Based Oral Health (ICEBOH), UCL Eastman Dental Institute, University College London, London, England

RUSS PAGANO, PhD, VP Regulatory and Clinical Affairs, BioMimetic Therapeutics, Inc., Franklin, TN, USA

GLEN PARK, PharmD, Senior Director, Clinical and Regulatory Affairs, Target Health Inc., New York, USA

BRUCE L. PIHLSTROM, DDS, MS, Oral Health Clinical Research Consultant, Bethesda, MD, USA and Professor Emeritus, University of Minnesota, Formerly: Acting Director, Division of Extramural Clinical Research, NIDCR, Bethesda, MD, USA

DAN PIHLSTROM, DDS, Associate Director of Evidence Based Care & Oral Health Research, Permanente Dental Associates, Portland, OR, USA

D. BRAD RINDAL, DDS, Research Investigator, HealthPartners Dental Group & HealthPartners Research Foundation, Minneapolis, MN, USA

ELIZABETH B.D. RIPLEY, MD, MS, Professor of Medicine, Division of Nephrology, Virginia Commonwealth University, Richmond, VA, USA

JONATHAN A. SHIP, DMD (deceased), PEARL Network Executive Management Team, Director, Bluestone Center for Clinical Research, NYU College of Dentistry, New York, NY, USA

WOOSUNG SOHN, DDS, MS, PhD, DrPH, Assistant Professor of Dentistry, Department of Cariology, Restorative Sciences and Endodontics, School of Dentistry, Adjunct Assistant Professor of Epidemiology, School of Public Health, University of Michigan, Ann Arbor, MI, USA

ANITA H. SUNG, Clinical Research Associate, PEARL Network, NYU College of Dentistry, New York, NY, USA

VAN THOMPSON, DDS, PhD, PEARL Network Executive Management Team, NYU College of Dentistry, New York, NY, USA

DON VENA, Director, PEARL Network Coordinating Center, The EMMES Corporation, Rockville, MD, USA

O. DALE WILLIAMS, PhD, Division of Preventive Medicine, Department of Medicine, School of Medicine, University of Alabama at Birmingham, Birmingha AL, USA

LESLIE WISNER-LYNCH, DDS, DMSc, Sr. Director Applied Research, BioMimetic Therapeutics, Inc., Franklin, TN, USA

HELEN WORTHINGTON, CStat, PhD, Professor of Evidence Based Care and Coordinating Editor of the Cochrane, Oral Health Group, School of Dentistry, The University of Manchester, Manchester, England

Preface

Translational research is not only good science, but it is science that helps people. In creating this book, the editors (Drs. William V. Giannobile, Brian Burt, and Robert Genco) with the able assistance of an impressive collection of experts have created the essential dental investigators' handbook for translational research. This book presents the current best practices for conducting clinical research and will serve the needs of oral health investigators, trainees, and clinicians who seek to become better clinicians. The principles of the book are founded upon the profession's recognition of the central importance of evidence-based dentistry for clinical decision making. Dentistry has evolved beyond an apprenticeship "arts and craft" training model of disease management to a scientific model that includes lifelong learning and scientific evidence-based patient management and disease prevention. This book provides all the necessary tools that clinicians need to understand the underlying scientific basis for patient care. Understanding the scientific process is critical to be an effective dental health care provider in this postgenomic era and this book provides an excellent blueprint for transforming clinicians into clinical scientists.

Technically, the book is an impressive collection of topics presented by top leaders in the field. There are several unique aspects to this compilation that make the publication unprecedented. Special care has been applied to craft the presentation of the material as being specifically oriented to the needs of the dental investigator. Careful discussions of study design, biostatistical considerations, ethical and regulatory issues, grant writing and publication, data management, and data analysis are tailored for dental research and include many examples that make the information accessible to the reader and easily interpretable. Additional sections deal with the current national trends for dental research that include the utilization of practice-based networks and the adoption of new technologies to dental practice. Finally, the sections on publication and systematic reviews provide the tools needed for the clinician to interpret and apply the current scientific knowledge to the patient that is sitting in the chair. Thus, this book will provide important skills for not only the clinical scientist in training, but it will enrich the clinical scientist that is within every dental health care provider and enable better health care to emerge. In this manner, this book not only provides the reader with the skill set needed for conducting translational research, but it is a scientific blueprint that will enable each of us to be better clinicians to serve the health of the public.

Steven Offenbacher DDS, PhD, MMSc
OraPharma Distinguished Professor of Periodontal Medicine
Director, Center for Oral and Systemic Diseases
University of North Carolina-Chapel Hill
School of Dentistry
Chapel Hill, NC, USA

Acknowledgments

First, I would like to thank the authors of this textbook for their tireless, dedicated, and fruitful efforts in assembling this book. The editors believe it is a first of its kind book in the rapidly evolving area of clinical and translational research in the oral health arena.

I dedicated this book in part to my devoted mentors in clinical research including my coauthors Bob Genco and Brian Burt. Your insights and experience have greatly benefited this book's development and realization. I also appreciate the mentoring from my clinical research role models, Sig Socransky, Max Goodson, Anne Haffajee, Klaus Lang, Ron Nevins, and Sam Lynch. You each have played important parts in my clinical research career and its connection to clinical translation. Each of you serves as an important inspiration to me as well as to our field of oral health research.

I also acknowledge mentors in every sense of the word for their infectious excitement about scientific discovery including Don Siehr, George Riviere, Ray Williams, Charley Cobb, Chuck Stiles, Steve Goldstein, Dan Clauw, Martha Somerman, and Peter Polverini. You each serve as wonderful examples of inspiring and caring individuals in the future of science and innovation.

To my role models and mentors in the clinical care arena of my career—Alden Leib and Peter Billia. Both of you represent the best of what dentistry and patient care is all about.

I would like to acknowledge all of my colleagues in the Department of Periodontics and Oral Medicine University of Michigan. This group of individuals has greatly enriched my scientific life. I also greatly appreciate all of the clinical members of the Michigan Center for Oral Health Research and the Michigan Institute of Clinical and Health Research who have challenged me to best understand how teamwork is crucial in patient-related research.

I would like to thank Sophia Joyce of Wiley-Blackwell for approaching me to initiate this textbook. I have greatly appreciated your insights and support during the book's progress. I also appreciate the quality efforts on the planning and production of the text from Shelby Allen and the rest of the team at Wiley-Blackwell. Finally, I acknowledge Karen Gardner for her excellent attention to detail, tenacity, and dedication to our efforts in the assembly of the first edition of this textbook.

Will V. Giannobile
University of Michigan School of Dentistry
Ann Arbor, MI, USA

Clinical Research in Oral Health

1

Clinical and translational research: implications in the promotion of oral health

William V. Giannobile, DDS, DMSc

The field of clinical and translational research (CTR) has undergone tremendous growth and development over the last few years. Public pressure has helped bring CTR into focus as a high priority to drive basic science discovery to generate tangible advances to benefit society and oral health care. This trajectory of bringing "bench-to-bedside," or in the case of dentistry, "bench-to-chairside," research is important for development of the entire "translational continuum" (Figure 1.1). According to the National Cancer Institute Translational Research Working Group, translational research is defined as "research that transforms scientific discoveries arising from laboratory, clinical, or population studies into clinical applications to reduce the incidence, morbidity and mortality of disease" (National Cancer Institute, 2009). Translational research encompasses both the acquisition of new knowledge about oral disease prevention, preemption, and treatment, and the methodological research required to develop or improve research tools (Lenfant, 2003). In 2008, leaders within the organization "Agency for Healthcare Research and Quality (AHRQ)" (www.effectivehealthcare.ahrq.gov) described the need for three tiers of evidence translation: the first translating basic science into clinical efficacy data (T1), the second (T2) using patient-oriented outcomes and health services research to develop knowledge about clinical effectiveness, and the third (T3) using implementation research for continuous measurement and refinement of treatment implementation (Dougherty and Conway, 2008) (Table 1.1). Two critical areas of CTR that affect human oral health include (1) the process of applying discoveries generated during laboratory research and in preclinical studies to the development of trials in humans; and (2) research aimed at enhancing the adoption of best practices in the community (Zerhouni, 2007). Given that the majority of oral health care

The translational continuum for oral health research

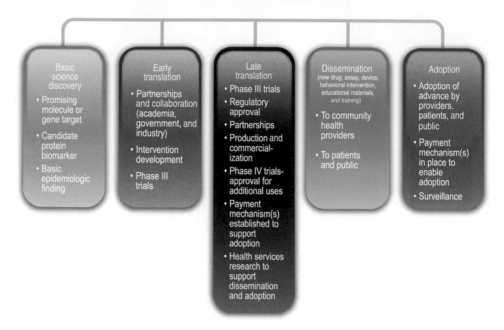

Figure 1.1 The translational continuum from basic science discovery to eventual adoption to dental practice. Adapted from National Cancer Institute, 2009.

Table 1.1   Examples of three translations required to improve the quality of oral health research.

Translational tier	Type of research	Product of research
T1	Clinical efficacy research	Proof that locally delivered antibiotics are beneficial when used adjunctively with scaling and root planing to reduce pocket depths
T2	Comparative-effectiveness and oral health services research	Establishment of 3-month recall intervals is beneficial to treat periodontal patients
T3	Implementation research	Identification of oral health screening strategies to diagnose oral cancer at earlier stages

practitioners such as dentists and dental hygienists are in private practice, there is a great need for the dissemination of new research findings into the oral health community from university, private, and hospital-based research entities (ADA News, 2007). Based on this large practice community available, there has been a widespread efforts in the utilization of practice-based research networks to better allow for clinical translation and to implement greater numbers of impactful "effectiveness" trials (see Chapter 14) (Curro et al., 2009). For the field of oral health research and dentistry, there have been renewed efforts in enhancing the efficiency of clinical trials for the promotion of global health (Barnett and Pihlstrom, 2004).

1.1   Challenges to the translation of clinical research to clinical practice

There is a great demand to bring cutting-edge therapeutics to patients in the face of ever increasing dental costs that drive the oral health care industry to seek collaboration with multiple entities to stimulate innovation (Melese et al., 2009). With the development of effective "business models" for new dental devices or biologics, one needs to consider a host of different supportive government, industrial, and academic agencies from the initial concept until the eventual product to affect oral health (see Figure 1.2). There is a multitude of

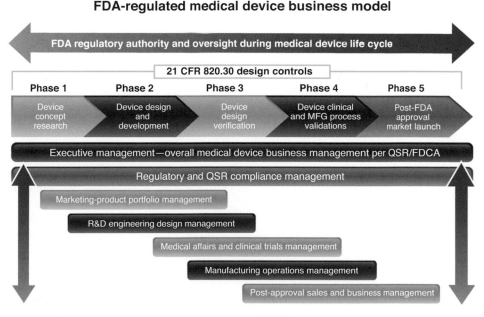

Figure 1.2 FDA/EMEA regulated dental device business model. Design controls are considered (phases 1–5) for the development of a new dental device considering a host of regulatory steps to gain approval of the prototype device.

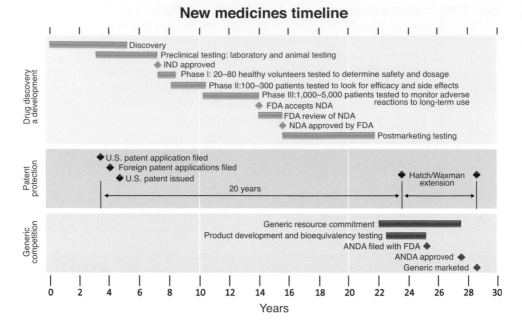

Figure 1.3 New medicines timeline. This trajectory demonstrates the steps required for the development of a new drug. FDA, Food and Drug Administration; NDA, new drug application; IND, investigational new drug; ANDA, abbreviated new drug application. Adapted from Pharmaceutical Research and Manufacturers of America (PhRMA website: www.phrma.org).

challenges to new drug or device development to affect patient health, and these trajectories typically take at least a decade or more due to technological, regulatory, and safety hurdles (Figure 1.3). Many cite the "art and science" of dentistry and its practice in oral health care delivery. Much is known about the science, but little in the proper application of the "art." The role of science in dental medicine is clear; however, what is less clear is the art on how dental innovations are implemented. The "art" part of medicine is "the combination of medical knowledge, intuition, and judgment" (Fauci et al., 2008). New approaches from the scientific standpoint demonstrate a high throughput of new knowledge as evidenced by the growth and expansion of dental and oral health-related research publications (see Chapters 17 and 18). However, moving this newly gained information from the research arena to clinical practice, making it relevant to oral health care providers and patients, requires true coupling of art and science and *clinical translation* (Lenfant, 2003). Improvements in health care delivery could be greatly impacted if investigators could better improve the translation of new knowledge to the clinical arena (Institute of Medicine of the National Academies, 2001; Berwick, 2003) (see also Chapters 15 and 16) (Text box 1.1). This becomes apparent about the implications of the translational aspects of bench-to-chairside translation given that the steps of basic science discovery to preclinical research and finally human studies are not necessarily successive steps, but are interdependent (Figure 1.4) (Willett, 2002).

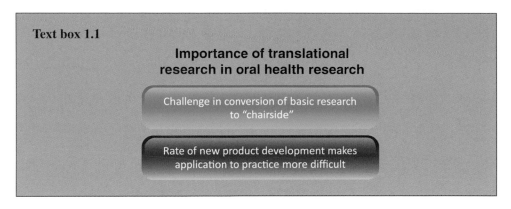

The ramifications of oral health research findings (such as the discovery of the values of fluoride in drinking by Dr. Frederick McKay and then the "translation" of this concept by GV Black) greatly transformed dentistry into a prevention-based profession, instead of the previous "reconstruction-only" type of one (Tabak, 2004). Dentistry has been involved in a myriad of advances from the bench-to-bedside in areas such as new dental biomaterials to reconstruct lost tooth structure, to the tissue engineering of lost periodontal support (Nakashima and Reddi, 2003). Dental implants are some of the most common osseous implants placed into the human body and have relied on years of research in oral and craniofacial health (Gotfredsen et al., 2008). Other areas such as oral cancer detection and prevention have not fared as well. Head and neck cancer is one of the more common cancers that afflicts Americans, and it has been estimated that more than 8,000 people in the United States will die from this cancer this year. Unfortunately, survival rates for patients have not significantly improved over the past 30 years, and as such, there is much work to do in this area (Michaud et al., 2008).

The framework for the emerging vision of CTR is well captured following the construction of the Clinical and Translational Science Award (CTSA) program by the National Institutes of Health (NIH) in 2006–2007 by then director, Dr. Elias Zerhouni. He proposed the framework for the new vision based on the 4Ps: *predictive, personalized, preemptive,*

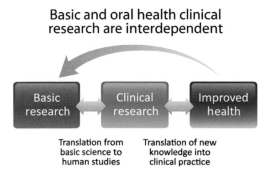

Figure 1.4 Interdependence of discovery and patient-oriented research in the generation of new knowledge.

and *participatory* medicine (Zerhouni, 2007). Clinical dental practice via this approach will advance more rapidly when we better understand the fundamental causes of oral diseases at their earliest molecular stages so that one can reliably predict how and when a disease will develop and in which patients; based on emerging data in the pharmacogenomics or the identification of the fact that specific patient populations are most responsive, a personalized medicine approach can be considered. These approaches will aid the dental practitioner in the identification of those patients who are responders and nonresponders to innovative dental drugs and devices for enhanced safety and clinical effectiveness. The use of metabolomics holds significant promise for improving disease diagnosis, prognosis, and disease management. Given the improvements in our abilities to prognosticate and identify patient risk factors and inherited genetic factors for disease, we can use a *preemptive* approach to deliver less invasive, more preventive, types of therapies or treatments. Finally, if the translation of clinical therapies is to have an impact on clinical practice and in patient care to enhance public trust, we need to encourage more active *participation* from patients and dental communities in shaping the future of dental medicine and global oral health.

1.2 Health technology assessments—identifying research priorities for oral health research

The use of health technology assessments (HTA) is a rich source of systematically generated information that have the potential to be used by granting agencies to support "researchable" questions that are relevant to decision makers and the public at large in the funding of clinical research (Scott et al., 2008). Traditionally, in order to receive Food and Drug Administration (FDA), European Medicines Agency (EMEA), or other international regulatory approvals (see Chapter 4), explanatory or mechanistic trials are most often utilized for new dental products (Tunis et al., 2003). These investigations recruit highly homogenous patient populations and determine how new drugs, devices, or biologics work under ideal conditions (efficacy trials; see Chapter 11). These types of clinical studies rarely satisfy all of the critical needs of health care decision makers at the policy level. In contrast to efficacy trials, pragmatic clinical trials assess the results of studies in "real-world" conditions whereby patients are exposed to a variety of environmental factors and comprise a heterogeneous racial/ethnic profile of individuals. These types of investigations can add to promote more generalized dental/oral health, since these are considered as effectiveness trials (see Chapters 12 and 13). The use of HTA results to identify research gaps can allow funding agencies to address the differences in research agenda priorities among different constituencies in the generation of clinical research programs (see Chapter 5). There are typically fewer research gaps than evidence gaps, since while it would be helpful to know the entire field (evidence gap), most of the time decision makers need to be satisfied and prioritize aspects within the evidence gap that would be most impactful to the field given time and resources available (see Chapter 18 and Figure 1.5). However, care must be given not to threaten personalized medicine and look at every targeted therapies for specific patient populations, as the broad strokes approach of comparative-effectiveness research can possibly marginalize such patient-specific therapeutics (Garber and Tunis, 2009).

Conceptual framework for the feedback loop involving oral health research gaps identified by health technology assessments

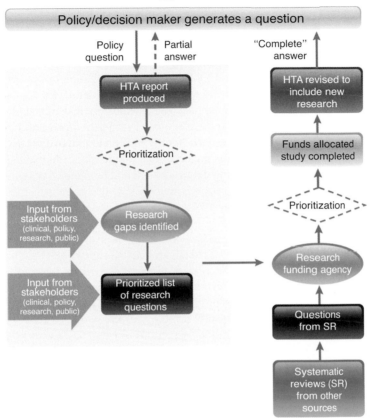

Figure 1.5 Flow diagram of the conceptual framework for the feedback loop involving research gaps identified by HTA (Scott et al., 2008).

1.3   Comparative-effectiveness research (CER)

CER is defined as "the generation and synthesis of evidence that compares the benefits and harms of alternative methods to prevent, diagnose, treat, and monitor a clinical condition or to improve the delivery of care." (IOM Report, 2009). The purpose of CER is to assist consumers, clinicians, purchasers, and policy makers to make informed decisions that will improve health care at both the individual and population levels. In June 2009, the Institutes of Medicine (IOM) published a report on CER as a way to identify what therapies work for which specific patients under discrete clinical situations (IOM Report, 2009). The U.S. Congress, in the American Reinvestment Act (ARRA) of 2009, appropriated $1.1 billion to support this nation's efforts to accelerate CER. Through the use of ARRA, the IOM developed national priorities for research questions to be addressed by CER and supported by ARRA funds. The IOM committee identified three report objectives: (1) to establish a working definition of CER; (2) to develop a priority list of research topics to be undertaken with ARRA funding using broad stakeholder input; and (3) to identify the necessary requirements to support a robust and sustainable CER enterprise (IOM Report, 2009). The use of the development of these important elements of CER will provide greater reality and application to innovations being developed for CTR. Given that many research studies (e.g., randomized controlled clinical trials) utilize homogenous patient populations (i.e., research participants that have been recruited to fulfill stringent inclusion and exclusion criteria), the use of CER could be a valuable arena to further the development of personalized medicine. Examples of CER may be the utilization of systematic reviews of the literature that can be applied toward clinical practice guideline development (see also Chapter 18). The utilization of large established databases from research consortia or third party dental insurance companies may be resources to capture broad and heterogeneous patient populations that represent more of the "real-world" patients that oral health clinicians treat (see Chapters 6 and 16). Thus, the goal of CER is better decision making by patients and oral health care providers including dentists and dental hygienists. A key aspect of the clinical translation aspect of this approach is that CER will require effective methods to disseminate and promote these findings to better exploit their adoption into clinical practice.

In summary, CTR is revolutionizing the way that research is being envisioned and applied for the driving of innovations in oral health care delivery. By exploiting the many opportunities in academic, governmental, foundational, and private oral health care entities for the support of "transformative" patient-based research, we will enrich our understanding of the mechanisms of oral disease as well as cultivate novel approaches for the prevention and treatment of oral afflictions.

Acknowledgments

The author appreciates Mr. Chris Jung for his assistance with the figures. The concept for Figure 1.2 comes from Ms. Kay Fuller. This research was supported in part by NIH/NCRR UL1RR024986.

References

ADA News. 2007. Employment situation of dentists in private practice. 38:1.

Barnett ML, Pihlstrom BL. 2004. Methods for enhancing the efficiency of dental/oral health clinical trials: current status and future possibilities. *Journal of Dental Research* 83:744–750.

Berwick DM. 2003. Disseminating innovations in health care. *The Journal of the American Medical Association* 289:1969–1975.

Curro FA, Craig RG, Thompson VP. 2009. Practice-based research networks and their impact on dentistry: creating a pathway for change in the profession. *Compendium of Continuing Education in Dentistry* 30:184–187.

Dougherty D, Conway PH. 2008. The "3T's" road map to transform US health care: the "how" of high-quality care. *The Journal of the American Medical Association* 299:2319–2321.

Fauci AS, Braunwald E, Kasper DL, Hauser SL, Longo DL, Jameson JL, Loscalzo J. 2008 *Harrison's Principles of Internal Medicine*. New York: McGraw-Hill Publishing.

Garber AM, Tunis SR. 2009. Does comparative-effectiveness research threaten personalized medicine? *New England Journal of Medicine* 360:1925–1927.

Gotfredsen K, Carlsson GE, Jokstad A, Arvidson Fyrberg K, Berge M, Bergendal B, Bergendal T, Ellingsen JE, Gunne J, Hofgren M, Holm B, Isidor F, Karlsson S, Klemetti E, Lang NP, Lindh T, Midtbo M, Molin M, Narhi T, Nilner K, Owall B, Pjetursson B, Saxegaard E, Schou S, Stokholm R, Thilander B, Tomasi C, Wennerberg A. 2008. Implants and/or teeth: consensus statements and recommendations. *Journal of Oral Rehabilitation* 35 (Suppl. 1):2–8.

Institute of Medicine of the National Academies. 2001. *Crossing the Quality Chasm: A New Health System for the 21st Century*. Washington, D.C.: The National Academies Press.

Institute of Medicine of the National Academies. 2009. *Initial National Priorities for Comparative Effectiveness Research*. Washington, D.C.: The National Academies Press, p. 220.

Lenfant C. 2003. Shattuck lecture—clinical research to clinical practice—lost in translation? *New England Journal of Medicine* 349:868–874.

Melese T, Lin SM, Chang JL, Cohen NH. 2009. Open innovation networks between academia and industry: an imperative for breakthrough therapies. *Nature Medicine* 15:502–507.

Michaud DS, Liu Y, Meyer M, Giovannucci E, Joshipura K. 2008. Periodontal disease, tooth loss, and cancer risk in male health professionals: a prospective cohort study. *Lancet Oncology* 9:550–558.

Nakashima M, Reddi AH. 2003. The application of bone morphogenetic proteins to dental tissue engineering. *Nature Biotechnology* 21:1025–1032.

National Cancer Institute. 2009. *Translational Research Working Group Definition of Translational Research*. Available online at http://www.cancer.gov/TRWG-definition-and-TR-continuum. Accessed on September 9, 2009.

Scott NA, Moga C, Harstall C, Magnan J. 2008. Using health technology assessment to identify research gaps: an unexploited resource for increasing the value of clinical research. *Healthc Policy* 3:e109–e127.

Tabak LA. 2004. Dentistry on the road(map). *Journal of the American Dental Association* 135:1362, 1364, 1366.

Tunis SR, Stryer DB, Clancy CM. 2003. Practical clinical trials: increasing the value of clinical research for decision making in clinical and health policy. *The Journal of the American Medical Association* 290:1624–1632.

Willett WC. 2002. Balancing life-style and genomics research for disease prevention. *Science* 296:695–698.

Zerhouni EA. 2007. Translational research: moving discovery to practice. *Clinical Pharmacology and Therapeutics* 81:126–128.

2

Ethics in oral health research

Elizabeth B.D. Ripley, MD, MS, **and**
Francis L. Macrina, PhD

2.1   Introduction

Over the past three decades, there have been widespread development and implementation of codes and policies concerning the conduct of scientific research. For example, policies on authorship and publication practices have been implemented by publishers and scientific societies. Further, federal agencies have implemented regulations and guidance that address the identification, disclosure, and management of conflicts of interest. These and other guidance and policy documents dealing with various aspects of scientific investigation have heightened the awareness of the importance of the responsible conduct of research (RCR). The education of trainees and scientists now frequently includes instruction in RCR. Such curricula may even be required by federal funding agencies or by training institutions themselves.

Human subjects experimentation is unique in this context. Arguably, no single area of scientific endeavor is more codified in terms of the acceptable practices of experimentation. Present-day codification of human experimentation dates back over six decades with the publication of the Nuremberg Code in 1947, a document that emanated from the war criminal trials at the end of World War II. The Nuremberg Code is one of several international guideline documents that has helped to shape and define the ethically appropriate use of human subjects in medical and behavioral research. In the United States, federal laws governing human subjects research date back to the National Research Act of 1974. Revision and expansion of these original regulations have continued since that time, and the Federal Code relating to human subjects research (45 CFR 46) is now comprised of four major components. A separate law governing human subjects research exists under the aegis of the U.S. Food and Drug Administration.

The codes governing human subject research deal with both the normative practice and ethical decision making that accompany such activity. When considering clinical research generally, and oral health clinical research specifically, there are a variety of levels of ethics that come into play. Clinical researchers represent a highly differentiated subset of scientific professionals in whom proper scientific conduct represents only a portion of their responsibility. Perhaps more importantly, the ethical responsibility to research subjects must be upheld. The potential harm from clinical research may be high. For example, procedures and interventions performed during the course of clinical research may endanger these subjects. Common examples are the administration of experimental drugs or the performance of surgical procedures, both of which may cause harm, or even precipitate a life-threatening event. Thus, when these procedures are being performed for research purposes, enormous responsibility is created that commands strict adherence to regulations and ethical principles.

This chapter centers on the ethical and normative behavior in clinical research that is informed by an evolving body of literature, policies, and laws. This narrative is guided by the conviction that an appreciation of the historical background of human subjects' research will help researchers understand the necessity and purpose of the policies and regulations that govern clinical research involving human subjects. Chapter 3 will further discuss the applications of these principles to both individuals and institutions. In this chapter, we will review central elements of this paradigm ranging from the ethical tenets of globally accepted standards to the operation of the review process required for performing clinical research with human subjects.

2.2   Ethical foundations

The ethical tenets and formal regulations that govern research on humans trace their roots to what has come to be called the Nuremberg Code (The Nuremberg Code, 1949). This code was developed during the American military tribunal proceedings (1946–1947) against Nazi physicians, scientists, and administrators for war crimes and crimes against humanity. The deeds carried out by the defendants, although sometimes referred to as "experimentation," were infamous atrocities that amounted to nothing more than torture and killing. In this vein, the "human subjects" were, in reality, victims. The original Code was submitted by American doctors to provide standards with which to judge those who had perpetrated the atrocities in the name of research. The first iteration of the Code contained six points but these ultimately evolved into ten principles intended to guide human experimentation. The guilty verdicts against the defendants reiterated almost all of ten principles of the Code.

The Nuremberg Code opens with the strong affirmation that human participation in medical experimentation be voluntary. It further states that consent be required and that it be free from any form of coercion or force. Full disclosure of the experiment's purpose, its duration, its conduct, and its dangers must be made. And all of these responsibilities rest squarely with the individual(s) who initiates, directs, or otherwise conducts the trial. The remaining nine Nuremberg principles focus on issues that also continue to be held to this day and have provided the substrate for other seminal guiding documents pertaining to human experimentation. Included in these are that the conduct of experimentation must yield benefit to society; be based on justification that invokes a knowledge of the disease or problem under study, and on the results of animal experimentation; not result in unnecessary pain and suffering; must not be considered if death or disablement are possible based on a priori reasons; should not involve a degree of risk that exceeds the humanitarian importance of the problem; should be carried out in adequate facilities conducive to safety and prevention of harm or death, and by scientifically qualified persons; may be stopped by the voluntary withdrawal of the human subject; must be stopped by the scientist in charge if judgment indicates continuation is likely to result in harm or death. The Nuremberg Code is also discussed in greater detail in Chapter 3 on institutional responsibilities related to clinical research.

Another international code relating to ethical principles for medical research involving human subjects was written under the authority of the World Medical Association (WMA). The 1964 WMA meeting that gave birth to the original document was held in Helsinki, Finland, and the document has been called the Declaration of Helsinki to commemorate that event (World Medical Association, 1964). The Helsinki Declaration has been updated at least once during every decade since its inception. It essentially embraces the tenets of the Nuremberg Code, but is more expansive and precise in its language. The most recent update of the Declaration occurred in 2008. Although it is primarily addressed to physicians, all participants in medical research are urged to adopt the principles. It is divided into three sections. The first is an introduction with general statements regarding research, the applicability of the principles and the responsibility of the investigators. The second section contains basic principles for all medical research. It states 20 basic principles for medical research covering areas from study design to publication with a strong emphasis on risk assessment and informed consent. The third part lists five additional principles that apply to the conduct of medical research when it is combined with medical care. Individuals who conduct medical research are strongly advised to read these principles.

Both the Nuremberg Code and the Declaration of Helsinki represent international guidelines for the conduct of human subjects research and they provided the prevailing standard in the 1950s and 1960s. Despite these documents and their expected impact, a study published in 1966 by Henry Beecher revealed serious ethical transgressions involving human subjects in 22 published studies (Beecher, 1966). These studies ranged in scope from failure to obtain informed consent to inappropriate use of vulnerable research populations. Moreover, in the early 1970s, the public press disclosed an ongoing U.S. Public Health Service funded project. The aim of the study was to determine the untreated course of syphilis in African-American males. In the 1940s, when penicillin became available, the research subjects were not informed about this therapy even though it could have been used to cure their infection. Regretfully, the study was allowed to continue for almost three more decades, and it was 1973 before the U.S. government took steps to provide treatment to the surviving research subjects (U.S. Department of Health Education and Welfare, 1973). The 1960s in the United States bore witness to other scandalous examples of ethically inappropriate human subjects' research. One example of egregious ethical lapse involved experiments carried out at the Willowbrook Home for retarded children on Staten Island. In that work, institutionalized subjects were allowed to contract hepatitis in order to study the natural course of the disease. Another was a study at the Brooklyn Jewish Chronic Disease Hospital that involved elderly patients who were injected with live cancer cells without their consent in order to see if the cells would be immunologically rejected (Katz, 1972).

In the wake of these and other offensive incidents, the U.S. Congress passed the National Research Act (PL 93–348) in 1974. This Act mandated the creation and implementation of Institutional Review Boards to review and approve human subjects' research (see below). Moreover, it established the National Commission for the Protection of Human Subjects of Biomedical and Biobehavioral Research. In response to its charge, this group set out to write guiding principles for the use of human subjects in clinical research. A number of reports ensued over time, which culminated in the Belmont Report published in 1979 (National Commission for the Protection of Human Subjects of Biomedical and Behavioral Research, 1979).

The Belmont Report posits three ethical principles. The first is respect for persons. It holds that individuals must be treated as autonomous agents. Furthermore, it says that those whose autonomy has been compromised are entitled to protection depending on the potential for harm and the possibility of benefit from participation. Implicit in such respect is the informed consent process. Respect as described in the Belmont Report also means that the subject has grasped and understands the implications of the study as they apply to him or her. The third facet of respect involves that of voluntary participation. Subjects agree to participate in the research wholly of their free will and without any outside influence or coercion. They also enter the participation knowing that they can withdraw from the study at any time without losing rights to which they are entitled as part of the study.

The second Belmont Report principle is beneficence. This principle embraces the obligation to provide protection from harm. Before research can be approved and conducted, the analysis of risks and benefit should be done. Researchers are obligated to minimize risk and to maximize benefit. Only a favorable risk–benefit ratio can justify approval of the research. Harm that might be incurred during the course of research is considered in the broadest context to include that which is physical, psychological, social, or legal. Potential harm as well as anticipated benefits from the research must be disclosed during the informed consent process.

The third Belmont Report principle is justice. This principle requires that both the benefits and burdens of the research be distributed in a fair and equitable manner. Justice mandates that selection of subjects not be based on availability or on ease of manipulation. Further, according to the principle of justice, advantages coming from research should not accrue only to those who can afford them, and such research should not unduly involve subjects who are not likely to get benefit from its application.

In summary, there are overlapping principles covered in the Nuremberg Code, the Declaration of Helsinki, and the Belmont Report. Together, they weave a fabric of guidance that provides the ethical foundations for the RCR with human subjects. These principles are also discussed in Chapter 3 on institutional responsibilities of research.

2.3   Is it human subjects research?

Before determining which ethical principles and regulations may apply to the research, it is important to determine if the planned study is indeed human subjects research. The U.S. Code of Federal Regulations (2005) provides definitions for both research (45 CFR 46.102d) and human subjects (45 CFR 46.102f). Quoting from this law:

> Research means a systematic investigation, including research development, testing and evaluation, designed to develop or contribute to generalizable knowledge. Activities which meet this definition constitute research for purposes of this policy, whether or not they are conducted or supported under a program which is considered research for other purposes. For example, some demonstration and service programs may include research activities.

Human subject means a living individual about whom an investigator (whether professional or student) conducting research obtains

(1) data through intervention or interaction with the individual, or
(2) identifiable private information.

Intervention includes both physical procedures by which data are gathered (for example, venipuncture) and manipulations of the subject or the subject's environment that are performed for research purposes. Interaction includes communication or interpersonal contact between investigator and subject. Private information includes information about behavior that occurs in a context in which an individual can reasonably expect that no observation or recording is taking place, and information that has been provided for specific purposes by an individual and which the individual can reasonably expect will not be made public (for example, a medical record). Private information must be individually identifiable (i.e., the identity of the subject is or may readily be ascertained by the investigator or associated with the information) in order for obtaining the information to constitute research involving human subjects.

Thus, an interaction with or an intervention involving a living human being happening within the context of research experimentation must be in compliance with relevant statutes and policies. The U.S. federal regulations that come into play here are discussed in the next section of this chapter.

Figure 2.1 is a flow diagram that can be used to guide decisions when considering the use of human subjects in research.

2.4   Federal regulations

The ethical principles that govern human subjects research apply no matter where, with what populations, and how the research is being conducted. All researchers should assure that their research methods maintain these principles and maximize human subjects' protection. Beyond these ethical principles are standards and laws that govern research. Investigators and Institutional Review Boards (IRB) should be aware of federal, state, and local laws regulating research. There are two major federal regulations regarding clinical research: Department of Health and Human Services (DHHS, 2004) and the Food and Drug Administration (FDA). Although these are the two primary regulations, other departments and agencies may have additional regulations. For example, the Department of Education has specific regulations related to the use of student records and the involvement of students in research.

The DHHS regulation 45 CFR 46 has four subparts (Code of Federal Regulations, 2005). Subpart A is often referred to as The Common Rule or the Federal Policy for the Protection of Human Subjects. These regulations cover all research involving human subjects, which is conducted, supported, or otherwise subject to regulation by any federal department or agency. Although the Common Rule does contain regulations that have been approved by multiple government agencies, there are some differences between the federal regulations.

In addition to federal law, states have laws and regulations that impact research. These vary by state and include issues of consent, documentation, minority status, and who may act as a legally authorized representative. Because these vary, researchers must be aware of local rules and regulations, and where state law is more stringent than federal law, the state law takes precedence.

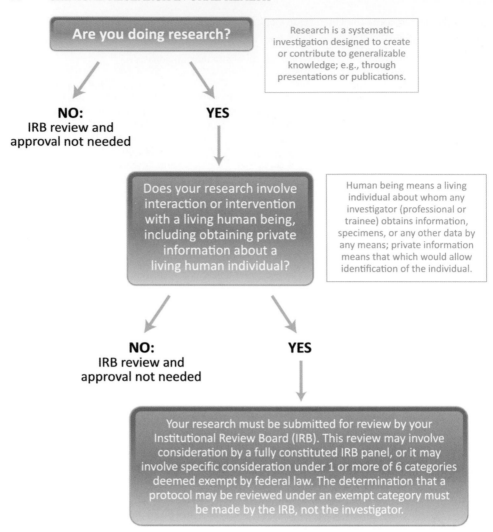

Figure 2.1 A simple decision tree for determining whether IRB review and approval are needed for your proposed work (modified from Macrina, 2005). Used with permission of ASM Press.

2.5   The Institutional and Ethical Review Board (IRB) for studies related to oral health

Like all human subjects research, oral health studies must follow the rules and regulations regarding research. Institutions that receive federal support in the United States are required to have an IRB to review human subjects' research. These panels are mandated by law (DHHS regulations 45 CFR 46) and fall under the jurisdiction of the Office of Human Research Protection, an arm of the Department of Health and Human Services. Researchers that conduct research at facilities that do not receive federal funds (e.g., a private health care practice) are not required to have an IRB; however, investigators are still under ethical requirements and should have their research reviewed by an objective person or panel to assure human subjects' protection is maximized. Editors and editorial boards are increasingly requiring affirmation of IRB approval for research being published in their journals.

IRBs may be institution specific or independent (both for profit and not for profit) review panels such as Western IRB or Chesapeake IRB. Institutions receiving federal funds decide whether to have their own panel or to contract with an independent panel, or both.

Although following these state and federal rules and regulations are required, this should not be the IRB's or investigators' primary mission. IRBs are charged with minimizing the risks to subjects. This begins with assuring that there is a valid scientific basis and that the methods are adequate to answer the scientific question. On the other hand, IRBs should not recommend altering the science unless it is to minimize participant risk. For placebo trials, participants should not be denied known beneficial care. Human subjects trials may involve multiple types of risk including physical, emotional, financial, employability, legal, and reputation. The IRB is charged with assessing these risks and evaluating the risk–benefit ratio. No risk to an individual is justified in the face of deficient or inappropriate research design.

Benefits should be considered both for the participant and the society resulting from the findings of the study. The IRB should not consider potential long-term benefits when deciding on the benefits of a study.

This risk determination is also critical in determining the type of review an IRB must make. Federal regulations (45 CFR 46.102(i)) define minimal risk as "the probability and magnitude of harm or discomfort anticipated in the research are not greater in and of themselves than those ordinarily encountered in daily life or during the performance of routine physical or psychological examinations or tests." The regulations do not specify if these are harms and discomfort that normal healthy individuals might experience versus participants with illness and disabilities. Most ethicists have leaned toward interpreting this as the risks and harms that the involved individuals encounter in daily life or when they have routine physical or psychological tests and examinations.

Unfortunately, there may not be adequate prior empiric data to guide IRBs in determining risk. Investigators should provide IRBs with current, accurate data on known risks. Potential risks should be quantitated to the extent possible. This is often easier in biomedical research than in social behavioral research. Although IRBs review all elements of a study, they are concerned with risks from the research, not those that would be present outside of the context of the research. For example, a study is correlating dental radiographic findings with prevalence of sickle cell anemia. If the radiographic films were obtained as part of the individual's routine dental care and correlated with a survey obtained after the visit, the risks of x-ray exposure would not be considered as a risk of the research.

Although the risk level should be decreased as much as possible for all studies, the determination of minimal risk is crucial in determining whether an entire IRB panel must review a study or whether the study is exempt or qualifies for expedited review. Studies must be minimal risk in order to be determined to be exempt or qualify for expedited review.

Exempt status of human subjects' research requires a determination by a designated individual at the institution. This is often an IRB member. Exempt does not imply that the study does not need review for this determination or that ethical guidelines for research do not need to be followed. The study is, however, exempt from the policies in Federal Regulations 45 CFR 46. For a study to qualify for exemption, all aspects of the study must fit completely within one or more of the categories. If a portion of the study does not qualify, then the entire study may not be exempted and must be reviewed either by expedited review or full panel. The paraphrased exempt categories and potential oral health research that may qualify under each category are given in Text box 2.1.

Text box 2.1   Exempt categories and examples of potential studies (DHHS regulations 45 CFR 46.101(b)).

1. Research conducted in established or commonly accepted educational settings involving normal educational practices such as (a) regular and special education instructional strategies, or (b) research on the effectiveness of or the comparison among instructional techniques, curricula, or classroom management methods. (Identifiers may be retained with appropriate protections.)
   Example: Comparison of the effectiveness of web-based versus classroom instruction on oral anatomy in dental school.

2. Research involving use of educational tests (cognitive, diagnostic, aptitude, achievement), survey or interview procedures, or observation of public behavior *unless* information obtained from these sources is recorded in such a manner that subjects can be identified (directly or through identifiers linked to the subjects), *and* disclosure of the subject's responses outside the research could reasonably place the subject at risk of criminal or civil liability or be damaging to his or her financial standing, employability, or reputation.
   Examples: (i) Analysis of deidentified aptitude tests results for dental school admission with performance on dental certification exams. (ii) National survey of oral surgeons to determine the rate of infection following tooth extraction and recommended treatment. (iii) Focus group discussion of individuals with recent dental implants.

3. Research involving the use of education tests (cognitive, diagnostic, aptitude, achievement), survey procedures, interview procedures, or observation of public behavior that is not exempt under exemption category (2) (above) of this section *if* (a) the human subjects are elected or appointed public officials or candidates for public office; *or* (b) federal statutes require, without exception, that the confidentiality of the personally identifiable information will be maintained throughout the research and thereafter. Children *may not* be involved in this research.
   Examples: (i) Survey of recent dental school graduates to determine the impact of dental supply company advertising on purchase of specific supplies. (ii) National survey of state governors to determine their attitudes and initiatives regarding state funding for dental care.

4. Research involving the collection or study of existing data, documents, records, pathological specimens, or diagnostic specimens, (a) *if* these sources are publicly available, or (b) *if* the information is recorded by the investigator in such a manner that subjects cannot be identified, directly or through identifiers linked to the subjects. (Identifiers *may* be retained for research related to (a) above. However, identifiers *may not* be retained for research relevant to (b) above.)

Examples: (i) Retrospective review of medical records of patients admitted to a general medicine service to determine the rate and extent of oral exams recorded during admission physicals. Would need to be recorded in a deidentified manner. (ii) Retrospective review of office records to determine the outcome of dental care in HIV-positive patients. Would need to be recorded in a deidentified manner. (iii) Review of deidentified pathology specimens to determine the presence of Stromal cell-derived factor-1 and CXCR4.

5. Research and demonstration projects that are conducted by or subject to approval of (federal) department or agency heads, and that are designed to study, evaluate, or otherwise examine (a) public benefit or service programs; (b) procedures for obtaining benefits or services under these programs; (c) possible changes or alternatives to those programs or procedures; or (d) possible changes in methods or levels of payments for benefits or services under those programs. (Identifiers may be retained with appropriate protections.)
Examples: (i) Study by Medicare to determine rate and racial differences in oral surgery in Medicare enrollees. (ii) Use Medicare billing information and ICD 9 codes to determine the rate of oral cancer in patients receiving dialysis.

6. Tests and food quality evaluation and consumer studies (a) if wholesome food without additives is consumed, or (b) if a food is consumed that contains a food ingredient at or below the level and for a use found to be safe, or agricultural chemical or environmental contaminant at or below the level found to be safe by the FDA or approved by the Environmental Protection Agency (EPA) or the Food Safety and Inspection Service of the U.S. Department of Agriculture (USDA). (Identifiers may be retained. This is the only exempt category that can be utilized for FDA-regulated research.)
Example: (i) Consumer study of college students to determine taste preferences for a variety of toothpastes.

The next more rigorous type of review is an expedited review although this is somewhat of a misnomer. It does not refer to the speed of the review, but the ability of the study to be reviewed by a single designated member of the IRB panel. Like exempt categories, the research must be minimal risk and all aspects of a protocol must fit within one or more expedited categories to be reviewed in this manner. Not all institutions allow expedited review. Paraphrased expedited categories with examples of research that may fit into that category are shown in Text box 2.2.

Text box 2.2   Expedited categories with examples (DHHS 45 CFR 46).

1. Clinical studies of drugs and medical devices only when condition (a) or (b) is met.
   (a) Research on drugs for which an investigational new drug application (21 CFR Part 312) is not required. (*Note*: Research on marketed drugs that significantly

increases the risks or decreases the acceptability of the risks associated with the use of the product is not eligible for expedited review.) *or* (b) Research on medical devices for which (i) an investigational device exemption application (21 CFR Part 812) is not required, or (ii) the medical device is cleared/approved for marketing and the medical device is being used in accordance with its cleared/approved labeling.

Examples: (i) Comparison of bacterial endocarditis occurrence with the two leading antibiotic regimens. (ii) Review of dental implant results to assess for indicators of successful outcome.

2. Collection of blood samples by finger stick, heel stick, ear stick, or venipuncture as follows: (a) from healthy, nonpregnant adults who weigh at least 110 pounds. For these subjects, the amounts drawn may not exceed 550 mL in an 8-week period and collection may not occur more frequently than two times per week; or (b) from other adults and children, considering the age, weight, and health of the subjects, the collection procedure, the amount of blood to be collected, and the frequency with which it will be collected. For these subjects, the amount drawn may not exceed the lesser of 50 or 3 mL/kg in an 8-week period and collection may not occur more frequently than 2 times per week.

Example: (i) Measurement of CRP levels before and after treatment for gingivitis. Requires 10 mL of blood drawn twice over a 3-month period.

3. Prospective collection of biological specimens for research purposes by noninvasive means. Examples: (a) hair and nail clippings in a nondisfiguring manner; (b) deciduous teeth at time of exfoliation or if routine patient care indicates a need for extraction; (c) permanent teeth if routine patient care indicates a need for extraction; (d) excreta and external secretions (including sweat); (e) uncannulated saliva collected either in an unstimulated fashion or stimulated by chewing gumbase or wax or by applying a dilute citric solution to the tongue; (f) placenta removed at delivery; (g) amniotic fluid obtained at the time of rupture of the membrane prior to or during labor; (h) supra- and subgingival dental plaque and calculus, provided the collection procedure is not more invasive than routine prophylactic scaling of the teeth and the process is accomplished in accordance with accepted prophylactic techniques; (i) mucosal and skin cells collected by buccal scraping or swab, skin swab, or mouth washings; (j) sputum collected after saline mist nebulization.

Examples: (i) Salivary cortisol levels before and after dental cleaning. (ii) Measurement of calcium content in permanent teeth extracted as part of routine care in patients with hyperpartathyroidism. (iii) Collection of buccal brushings for DNA samples to evaluate for candidate genes for development of squamous cell carcinoma of the oral pharynx.

4. Collection of data through noninvasive procedures (not involving general anesthesia or sedation) routinely employed in clinical practice, excluding procedures involving x-rays or microwaves. *Note*: Where medical devices are employed, they must be cleared/approved for marketing. (Studies intended to evaluate the safety

and effectiveness of the medical device are not generally eligible for expedited review, including studies of cleared medical devices for new indications.) Examples: (a) physical sensors that are applied either to the surface of the body or at a distance and do not involve input of significant amounts of energy into the subject or an invasion of the subject's privacy; (b) weighing or testing sensory acuity; (c) magnetic resonance imaging; (d) electrocardiography, electroencephalography, thermography, detection of naturally occurring radioactivity, electroretinography, ultrasound, diagnostic infrared imaging, Doppler blood flow, and echocardiography; (e) moderate exercise, muscular strength testing, body composition assessment, and flexibility testing where appropriate given the age, weight, and health of the individual.

Example: Analysis of measurements of blood pressure and heart rate using an automated blood pressure monitor every 10 minutes during tooth extraction, a comparison between routine local anesthesia and routine local anesthesia with hypnosis.

5. Research involving materials (data, documents, records, or specimens) that have been collected, or will be collected solely for nonresearch purposes (e.g., medical treatment or diagnosis). *Note*: Some research in this category may be exempt from the HHS regulations for the protection of human subjects. 45 CFR 46.101(b)(4). (This listing refers only to research that is not exempt.)

Example: (i) Prospective review of dental records to determine the outcome of standard treatment of oral ulcers in HIV-positive patients. (ii) Review of medical records and pathology samples of patients with parotid tumors to determine predictors of malignancy.

6. Collection of data from voice, video, digital, or image recordings made for research purposes.

Example: Video evaluation of paraplegic participants' ability to provide oral self-care and improvement with adaptive toothbrushes.

7. Research on individual or group characteristics or behavior (including, but not limited to, research on perception, cognition, motivation, identity, language, communication, cultural beliefs or practices, and social behavior) or research employing survey, interview, oral history, focus group, program evaluation, human factors evaluation, or quality assurance methodologies. *Note*: Some research in this category may be exempt from the HHS regulations for the protection of human subjects. (45 CFR 46.101(b)(2) and (b)(3). This listing refers only to research that is not exempt.)

Examples: (i) Survey of children in a Headstart program to determine knowledge about dental care. (ii) Focus group of multiple ethnic groups to determine attitudes and practices about oral health.

8. Continuing review of research previously approved by the convened IRB as follows: (a) where (i) the research is permanently closed to the enrollment of new subjects; (ii) all subjects have completed all research-related interventions; and (iii) the research remains active only for long-term follow-up of subjects; or

(b) where no subjects have been enrolled and no additional risks have been identified; or (c) where the remaining research activities are limited to data analysis.
Example: (i) A study of patients who received two different chemotherapy treatments for breast cancer to determine incidence and type of oral pathology occurring after treatment. This study was previously approved by a full IRB panel.
The participants have completed all treatments and are now being followed for
3 months to determine outcomes. (ii) A study of three dental implants has been
completed, the data has been collected and the statisticians are analyzing the
data.

9. Continuing review of research, not conducted under an investigational new drug
application or investigational device exemption where categories two (2) through
eight (8) do not apply but the IRB has determined and documented at a convened
meeting that the research involves no greater than minimal risk and no additional
risks have been identified.

All human subjects research that does not fit the exempt or expedited categories must
be reviewed by the entire panel. This is the most rigorous review. IRB panels by design are
made of diverse individuals. This allows for review and discussion from varied backgrounds
and expertise. IRB panels are required to have a minimum of five members who cannot have
the same profession and at least one member whose primary work is nonscientific (e.g.,
lawyer or clergy). There must also be at least one member not affiliated with the institution
(this individual's family also cannot have an institutional affiliation). The nonaffiliated
member may also be the nonscientist.

Figure 2.2 shows the general process for a full board review. At the meeting, panel
members will discuss the protocol, review the science, and the human subjects protection
issues and assure that federal, state, and institutional regulations are followed. After the
discussion, the panel will vote to approve the study as submitted, request scripted changes
(specific wording changes to the consent/assent or protocol), or table the study to allow
the reviewers and investigator to clarify or modify the protocol, consent, or documents. A
study may not begin until the study is approved by the panel.

Investigators should plan for, and IRB should review for equitable subject selection.
This requires both inclusion of all populations that could benefit from the study while
maintaining the scientific integrity of the study and not unduly subjecting populations to
research where their benefits may be low and their risks high. Examples would include
limiting enrollment into potentially beneficial treatment trials for oral cancer to elite upper
class clinics while focusing on enrollment of indigent or institutionalized patients in a
physiologic nontherapeutic study.

All trials require safety monitoring but the level of monitoring should be commensurate
with the level of risk of the study. All studies should have a data safety monitoring plan
that outlines who, when, what, and how protocol adherence, participant safety, and data
management will be monitored. For simple, low-risk studies, the investigator may be
responsible for safety monitoring (DSMB). Higher risk studies may require the development
of a data safety monitoring board. This board is made up of people external to the study
group, and to avoid conflict of interest, it is usually independent of the sponsor of the study.

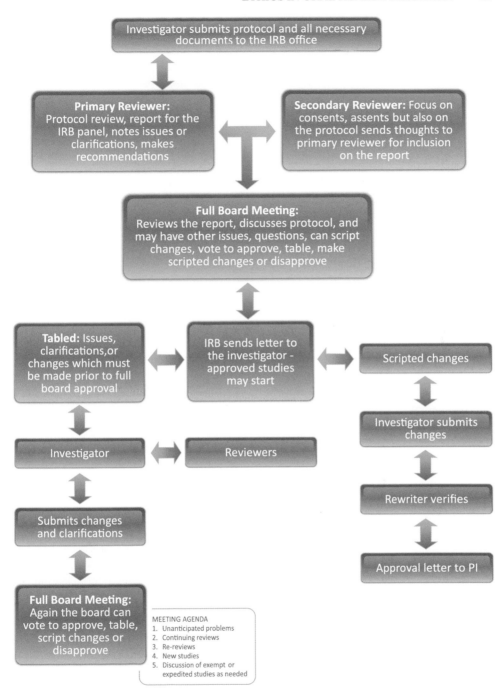

Investigator submits protocol and all necessary documents to the IRB office

Primary Reviewer: Protocol review, report for the IRB panel, notes issues or clarifications, makes recommendations

Secondary Reviewer: Focus on consents, assents but also on the protocol sends thoughts to primary reviewer for inclusion on the report

Full Board Meeting: Reviews the report, discusses protocol, and may have other issues, questions, can script changes, vote to approve, table, make scripted changes or disapprove

Tabled: Issues, clarifications, or changes which must be made prior to full board approval

IRB sends letter to the investigator - approved studies may start

Scripted changes

Investigator

Reviewers

Investigator submits changes

Submits changes and clarifications

Rewriter verifies

Approval letter to PI

Full Board Meeting: Again the board can vote to approve, table, script changes or disapprove

MEETING AGENDA
1. Unanticipated problems
2. Continuing reviews
3. Re-reviews
4. New studies
5. Discussion of exempt or expedited studies as needed

Figure 2.2 The IRB review process for full board studies. All arrows denote places for communication.

In order to maintain objectivity in reviewing the study, members of the board must not have a financial conflict or have scientific recognition in the form of publications or promotions from the results. Members of the board should be specifically selected for each study. They must have relevant expertise for clinical, statistical, and study design, and may include an ethicist or patient advocate. This board reviews the study prior to initiation, receives adverse event or unanticipated event reports during the trial, and may do interim analysis to determine if the study should continue and if possible reports from the DSMB should be provided to the IRB for continuing review.

Each IRB has policies and procedures that they follow. It is imperative that investigators know and follow these policies and procedures. These policies and procedures include when the IRB meets, required investigator human subjects training, forms, and other information that must be included with a protocol submission and the number of copies. Prior to submission of a protocol, investigators new to the process should contact the IRB to learn these policies and procedures. Studies must be reviewed at least annually for continuing review, and serious and unanticipated events and protocol amendments must be submitted according to these policies and procedures. Although every IRB may have their own procedures, Text box 2.3 gives ideas to improve investigator's IRB review experience and to speed up the review process.

Text box 2.3   Tips for working with your IRB.

Submission:

1. Use the right forms and submit the correct number of copies—IRBs often update forms. Make sure you have the most recent version.

2. Make sure you submit all documents including protocol, questionnaires, instruments, consent/assent, investigator CV, and advertisements.

3. Find out when the IRB panel meets and when the deadline for submission for the next meeting is so that your protocol is not delayed to the following meeting.

4. Think ahead—do not save the IRB submission for the last task before starting the study. If you have a deadline to start the study, begin the IRB process ASAP.

Protocol issues:

1. Think about human subject's issues as you write the protocol. Are you minimizing risk, inconvenience, and maximizing confidentiality and benefit? IRB members can be excellent resources for methods that can work for recruitment, retention, and confidentiality.

2. Make sure the hypothesis, specific aims, and background are clear and specific enough to allow the science to be assessed.

3. Provide as much information regarding risk and benefit as possible, especially if this is a new or modified procedure, questionnaire, or treatment.

4. Review the methods for clarity and consistency with the consent/assent.

5. A sample size calculation or at least justification should be present and at least a basic analysis plan.

6. If appropriate, discuss how collaborators will be trained regarding human subjects' protection and confidentiality.

7. Although IRBs are not focused on grammatical, spelling, and formatting issues, a well-written protocol, consent/assent does provide a level of comfort.

Consent/assent/parental permission:

1. Make sure that required sections are not missing from the consent or parental permission, and if sections are excluded, request a waiver of these sections or waiver of documentation of consent.

2. If a request is being made to waive or modify consent/assent/parental permission, this must be requested and justification given.

3. Make sure the consent/assent is at the appropriate reading level and language for the population.

4. If enrolling participants with potentially limited capacity to give consent, discuss how understanding of the methods, risks, and benefits are going to be assessed.

Communication:

1. Find an IRB resource to discuss questions and potential issues prior to submission.

2. If you anticipate that your protocol or portions of the procedures may concern the IRB panel, contact them ahead and provide as much information as possible. Many IRB panels will allow investigators to be present when the protocol is discussed in panel to provide clarifications or discuss acceptable changes.

3. Many IRB panel submissions and communications are becoming electronic. Whether communication is electronic, paper, or telephone, be sure to answer questions in a timely manner. If you do not seem in a hurry to get the protocol approved, they may not be either.

Questions or problems:

1. Establish a working relationship with your IRB. Know who to contact if problems or questions arise.

2.6 Informed consent

Informed consent is fundamental to ethical research with human subjects. Although an IRB approves an informed consent document as part of the protocol, in reality, informed consent is an ongoing interaction and process between investigator and the research participant. It provides an individual, or their legally authorized representative, the necessary information to make an informed, thoughtful, and voluntary decision to participate. Exempt studies do not require informed consent; although when appropriate, participants should be aware of the study. Other than exempt research, there are few exceptions to the requirement that research may not begin until the investigator has obtained legally informed consent. This informed consent must be obtained from the subject or the subject's legally authorized representative prior to participation. The purpose of obtaining informed consent is to provide information on the study's purpose, duration, experimental procedures, alternatives, risks, and benefits to the participants. This requires that the information be provided in a language that they can understand and in terms that they comprehend. Participants should be given sufficient opportunity to consider whether or not to participate, and coercion and undue influence must be minimized. The informed consent must not include exculpatory language that would require the participant to waive or appear to waive any of their legal rights, or release the investigator, sponsor, or institution from liability for negligence. It should delineate any costs to participation, and if portions of the study are gathering data from standard clinical care, which will be charged to the participant or their insurance, this must be outlined in the consent.

Each individual enrolled in the study must give informed consent. This may require more than one consent for a study. For example, a study of the genetic determinants of oral squamous cell cancer requires a history, oral exam, and DNA sample from as many family members as possible and a medical record review, with additional questionnaires and blood work for the index case. A consent with the information for the index case would provide the information about the study and his or her involvement including permission to contact family members. Consent for the family members would provide general information about the study and their involvement.

There are eight required elements of informed consent. Some of these elements may not apply to a particular research study. This is often true for low-risk studies but all elements that add to the participants understanding should be included. Text box 2.4 shows the required elements for the consent and additional elements.

Text box 2.4   Required elements of consent and additional elements (DHHS regulations 45 CFR 46 and FDA 21 CFR 50).

Required:

- A statement that the study involves research, an explanation of the purposes of the research and the expected duration of the subject's participation, a description of the procedures to be followed, and identification of any procedures that are experimental.

- A description of any reasonably foreseeable risks or discomforts to the subject.

- A description of any benefits to the subject or to others that may reasonably be expected from the research.

- A disclosure of appropriate alternative procedures or courses of treatment, if any, that might be advantageous to the subject.

- A statement describing the extent, if any, to which confidentiality of records identifying the subject will be maintained (and the possibility that the FDA may inspect the records—if the research is FDA regulated).

- For research involving more than minimal risk, an explanation as to whether any compensation and any medical treatments are available if injury occurs, and, if so, what they consist of, or where further information may be obtained.

- An explanation of whom to contact for answers to pertinent questions about the research and research subjects' rights, and whom to contact in the event of a research-related injury to the subject.

- A statement that participation is voluntary, refusal to participate will involve no penalty or loss of benefits to which the subject is otherwise entitled and the subject may discontinue participation at any time without penalty or loss of benefits to which the subject is otherwise entitled.

Additional elements that may be applicable and add to the participants understanding of the study are as follows:

- A statement that the particular treatment or procedure may involve risks to the subject (or to the embryo or fetus, if the subject is or may become pregnant), which are currently unforeseeable.

- Anticipated circumstances under which the subject's participation may be terminated by the investigator without regard to the subject's consent.

- Any additional costs to the subject that may result from participation in the research.

- The consequences of a subject's decision to withdraw from the research and procedures for orderly termination of participation by the subject.

- A statement that significant new findings developed during the course of the research that may relate to the subject's willingness to continue participation will be provided to the subject.

- The approximate number of subjects involved in the study.

The written consent may need to be read to individuals with low literacy. It is important that these individuals be provided the same information and be able to ask questions so that they can understand the procedures, risks, and benefits. Participants with low English proficiency must also be provided the information in a language that they can understand. It is important that these individuals be included in appropriate research and not excluded out of convenience. If inclusion is anticipated, then the consent should be translated into the appropriate language. When an unanticipated participant is eligible for enrollment, then a translator should be found that can translate the consent and assist with the participants understanding. It is critical that the ability of the participant to communicate with the research team is maintained throughout the study. Especially for more than minimal risk studies, this includes the ability of the participant to be able to reach and communicate with the investigator 24 hours a day.

Research in emergency settings where consent cannot be obtained requires additional safeguards and review. This type of research is rare and only justifiable after considerable institutional and community review.

If the research includes developing a registry of individuals to be invited to participate in future research, or for their data or specimens to be used, the participants must give consent for maintaining their identifying and contact information. Studies that collect DNA require special consent. Participants should be given the option of either limiting DNA use to the current study or allowing for inclusion in future studies. Use in future studies should be either by giving future consent or obtaining consent for unrestricted use at the time of collection.

There are instances where a waiver or alteration in the consent process can be approved by the IRB. For FDA-regulated research, consent may be waived only in emergency situations. For DHHS-regulated research, the IRB may approve a consent procedure, which does not include, or which alters some or all of the elements of informed consent. There are two categories for this waiver of consent. Federal Regulation 45 CFR 46.116(c) allows for waiver if the research is a demonstration project approved by state or local government officials and is designed to study, evaluate, or examine public benefit of service programs, procedures for obtaining benefits, alternatives to those procedures or programs, and possible changes to the method or level of payment for benefits, and the research could not practicably be carried out without waiver or alteration. Practicably implies feasibility not convenience. The second category of waiver (45 CFR 46.116(d)) is for minimal risk research where the waiver or alteration would not adversely affect the rights and welfare of the subjects; the research could not practicably be carried out without it, and whenever possible, subjects will be provided with additional pertinent information after participation.

2.7   Vulnerable populations

All participants should be treated ethically; however, several groups of participants are considered to be vulnerable. Any participant who cannot make a voluntary decision to participate or is unable to understand the research, especially the procedures and risks, may be vulnerable. Traditionally, and by federal regulations, these groups are children, pregnant women (fetuses and neonates), and prisoners. These three categories have additional federal regulations for their inclusion in research.

2.7.1   Children

For many areas of research, the inclusion of children in research is necessary, beneficial, and always requires additional safeguards. The definition of a minor varies by state; for instance, in Virginia, the age is younger than 18 or not legally emancipated (a legal determination that the minor is independent from parents or guardian and able to make legal decisions for themselves). The federal regulations for human subject protection do not specify an age.

In order for children to participate, the legally authorized representative must give informed permission for the child to participate. For minimal risk research or for greater than minimal risk research with the potential for direct benefit to the child, the IRB may determine if one or two parent(s) or guardian(s) signature are required. For greater than minimal risk research with no direct benefit, two signatures are required unless one parent is deceased, unknown, incompetent, not reasonably available, or not a custodial parent. While parents or legally authorized representatives give parental permission, children are not able to give legal consent. However, when possible, it is best to obtain the agreement of the child to participate. This agreement is called an assent and contains the information in terms and details that the child can understand. How much a child can understand varies both by age, maturity, and psychological status. Studies enrolling a wide age of children may require several assents with increasing amounts of information for the older children. If it is determined that the child cannot comprehend even a limited assent, the assent can be waived. Studies that enroll children and follow them to adulthood will require initial assent and then obtaining consent from the participant when they become an adult.

For treatment trials where the research offers potential important health benefits to the child, it is disingenuous to offer assent to the child unless their refusal will be honored. In these cases, the child should be informed of the study and allowed as much information as they request rather than requiring assent. Specific criteria and plans for this should be included in the protocol and approved by the IRB.

2.7.2   Pregnant women, human fetuses, and neonates

All nonexempt research regardless of funding source that is subject to federal regulation and allows for the inclusion of data on pregnant women, human fetuses, and/or neonates is subject to 45CFR 46 subpart B. The investigator must provide the necessary information and provisions for inclusion of these vulnerable individuals. Each of these groups has specific requirements. The regulations require both preclinical trials and a specific assessment of risks and benefits to both the mother and the fetus. Investigators and IRB must review the study and consent to assure that these specific regulations are met.

2.7.3   Prisoners

Prisoners require additional protections because they have decreased autonomy and are subject to many potential coercions. DHHS regulations define prisoner as:

> any individual involuntarily confined or detained in a penal institution. The term is intended to encompass individuals sentenced to such an institution under a criminal or civil statute, individuals detained in other facilities by virtue of statutes or commitment procedures which provide alternatives to criminal prosecution or incarceration in a penal institution, and individuals detained pending arraignment, trial, or sentencing.

IRB review for these protocols must include a prisoner representative on the panel. If a research project is underway that was not intended to include prisoners but has a research participant become incarcerated or meet the definition of prisoner, immediate action must be taken. The IRB must be notified, and unless there is direct benefit to the participant, all research activities must stop until the IRB can review the protocol with the prisoner guidelines and must not resume until all the requirements are met. When research is planned with prisoners, the IRB should be consulted early to assure that processes that are required for approval can be accomplished.

There are five categories that are acceptable for prisoner research. These are listed in Text box 2.5. Categories 1, 2, and 5 must be minimal risk and no more than inconvenience to the subject. The definition of minimal risk for prisoner research differs from the definition for other individuals. The prisoner minimal risk is defined as "the probability and magnitude of physical or psychological harm that is normally encountered in the daily lives, or in the routine medical, dental, or psychological examination of healthy persons." Categories 3 and 4 may require prior approval by the Secretary after consultation with appropriate experts including experts in penology, medicine, ethics, and be posted in the Federal Register.

Text box 2.5   Acceptable categories for prisoner research.

1. The study of the possible causes, effects, and processes of incarceration, and of criminal behavior, provided that the study presents no more than minimal risk and no more than inconvenience to the prisoner.

2. The study of prisons as institutional structures or the study of prisoners as incarcerated persons provided no more than minimal risk and no more than inconvenience.

3. Research on conditions particularly affecting prisoners as a class (e.g., vaccine trials and other research on hepatitis, or research on social and psychological problems such as alcoholism, drug addiction, and sexual assaults).

4. Research involving practices, both innovative and accepted, which have the intent and reasonable probability of improving the health or well-being of the subject.

5. Epidemiological research defined as "public health research that focuses on a particular condition or disease in order to either describe its prevalence or incidence by identifying all cases, including prisoner cases, or study potential risk factor associations, where the human subjects may include prisoners in the study population but not exclusively as a target group."

2.7.4   Individuals with impaired decision-making capacity

Research may at times involve individuals with limited decision-making capacity. Limited decision-making capacity covers a broad spectrum. It may be temporary such as after a shock or trauma or permanent and may be variable in an individual. Impaired capacity can be seen in individuals with particular illnesses such as neurologic, psychiatric, or substance abuse problems; however, it is not limited to these groups. It should also not be assumed that these groups of individuals are incapable of making informed consent to participate. This assessment may be able to be determined by the procedures involved in the study or may require individual assessment of the capacity of the participant. Just as there are reasons to do research with children, there are some research questions that can only be answered by research that involves persons with impaired decision-making capacity.

Unlike research involving children, prisoners, pregnant women, and fetuses, no additional Department of Health and Human Services regulations specifically govern research involving persons who are cognitively impaired. Investigators should plan for their participation, especially how competence and understanding will be assessed; the method for enrollment and retention and the IRB should give careful scrutiny to these plans.

This group of participants may have the greatest risk for being unable to distinguish between clinical care and research. This "therapeutic misconception" can be confusing for both the participant and their families. It is critical that the consent process clearly outlines the research aspects of the study and the role of the investigator rather than clinician. The ability of individuals to provide consent should be assessed including the ability to answer questions about the study as well as the ability to appreciate the risks, benefits, and alternatives to participation. Legally authorized representatives will need to consent for individuals unable to give their own consent. The decision to participate should reflect the views of the impaired individual. When their opinion is not known, the best interest of the individual should be used to decide. Similar to enrolling children, care should be made that the risks are not assumed by the impaired individual while benefits are accrued by the representative. An assent process similar to children's assent can allow a decisionally impaired individual to be given as much information as they are able to comprehend and be allowed to agree to participate with their approval. As with children, the acceptability of the person's refusal to participate in therapeutic trials should be determined prior to requesting assent.

2.8 Privacy, confidentiality, and HIPAA

The rights of patients to have their private health information protected have been legally established in Health Insurance Portability and Accountability Act (HIPAA) in 1996 (Privacy Rule, 1996). This law covers not only classically considered medical information (e.g., diagnosis and test results) but also personal information such as date of birth, social security number, address including zip code, and phone number. Investigators working in a HIPAA-covered entity must follow these rules. Information on the impact of HIPAA on research can be obtained online from DHHS (Privacy Rule, 1996).

Beyond the law though, there is an ethical imperative to protect the confidentiality of the participant. This requires collecting the minimal amount of information required and protecting the data. Participants' identification should be limited as much as possible throughout the study, for example, using a participant number rather than names or initials. Data files should be password protected, and when possible, encrypted especially during transport either via the internet or on removable media. When the information being obtained is highly sensitive, particularly if it could adversely affect a participant's reputation, insurability, financial standing, or employability, a certificate of confidentiality can be obtained from the National Institutes of Health (NIH Guide, 2002). These certificates protect identifiable research information from forced disclosure but do not limit the participants' voluntary release of information. The certificate allows research staff to refuse to disclose identifying information in any civil, criminal, administrative, or legislative proceedings. Protecting the confidentiality of participants is not only a matter of law but also of respect (a Belmont principle).

2.9 Oral health clinical research

The regulations that apply to the use of human subjects in research are broadly applicable across health care disciplines. The ethical foundations, federal regulations, principles of informed consent, and the protection of vulnerable populations apply in the same manner to health care scientists, from oncologists to orthodontists. The application of the principles of respect, beneficence, and justice is the same for the research patient populations of such disparate researchers. In 1979, the Council on Dental Research articulated guidance with special relevance to research populations involved in dental research (Council on Dental Research, 1979). These "Guidelines for the Use of Human Subjects in Dental Research" were published as approved by the American Dental Association, the American Association for Dental Research, and the American Association of Dental Schools. The guidelines present three categories of clinical research in humans. The first involves research aimed at diagnosis, control, or treatment of a disease or condition. The second involves research aimed at prevention of a disease or condition. And the third category encompasses research not directly concerned with either of the first two categories. Examples of such research include behavioral studies and plaque or saliva sampling.

In the case of research on diagnosis, control, or treatment, the guidance document states that the clinical investigator is obligated to ensure subjects with a disease or condition receive or are referred for treatment. Placebo-treated groups are usually not appropriate if the disease or condition is not reversible. Allowing patients to develop gingivitis may be acceptable, owing to its reversal by appropriate oral hygienic treatment. Allowing the development of periodontitis including loss of alveolar bone is not acceptable owing to its natural irreversibility. Commentary on such research extends also to the use of new or experimental therapeutic measures, stating that their use is appropriate only when evidence indicates they are likely to be at least as effective as existing modalities. Also, existing methods or agents should be considered as positive controls in experimental protocols. Next, the relationship of dependence between the clinical investigator and the research subject should never be exploited in soliciting consent and participation in such research. Finally, the prime importance of informed consent is asserted.

With regard to research on preventative measures, the guidance document reminds investigators that they are responsible for the rights and welfare of participants in such studies that are often done using groups of students in schools or in adult subjects outside of a controlled clinical setting. Investigators are also obligated to inform subjects in prevention experiments of their existing oral diseases or conditions. In such cases, even if the subjects cannot be appropriately treated, they have the right to be informed of diseases or conditions that may affect their health, and should be encouraged by the investigator to seek appropriate treatment. Depriving subjects in control groups from beneficial treatment should be carefully weighed and the use of alternative designs used when feasible; for example, comparison to historical baselines or to reference populations. Significant study findings should be conveyed, as appropriate, to subjects, family members, institutional, and health officials.

Concerning research other than for treatment or prevention, the guidance document notes that such research does not usually result in therapeutic benefits or have specific value to subjects. Accordingly, such research should be well-grounded scientifically and be expected to contribute knowledge for the good of society. The importance of confidentiality is emphasized, especially in studies where information of a personal nature is being collected (e.g., education or income). Finally, the use of procedures that run the risk of causing serious harm to subjects is not justified in clinical research. In this vein, the Council of Dental Research has affirmed the universal applicability of U.S. Public Health Service and FDA regulations to human subjects in dental research (Council on Dental Research, 1985).

Several articles have been published on ethical issues in dental research. Gillett points out that dentistry is a Hippocratic profession and is therefore committed to ongoing research into the causes and treatments of disease. He discusses the various pressures, often competing, placed on biomedical sciences (Gillett, 1994). Harrison (2005) reviewed a number of published orthodontic clinical trials to see if they complied with the requirements of the Declaration of Helsinki. She found several areas lacking including the statement that the study had received ethical approval and if consent had been obtained. The Journal of the American Dental Association has also published several articles on research ethics including topics of industry support, publication, and conducting ethical research (Bornfeld, 2007; Dunn, 2007; Glick, 2007).

In summary, the Council of Dental Research has provided guidance of specific applicability of the regulations to dental clinical researchers, and the role of the dentist in conducting and publishing ethical human subjects research is being defined.

2.10   Conclusion

As Gillett (1994) points out, dental and oral health professionals have an obligation to promote research. For the investigator, this requires knowledge of rules, regulations, and guidelines for conducting ethical research. The conduct of research involving human subjects carries with it the highest level of responsibility. The community of oral health researchers are vested with this responsibility in the conduct and translation of this research for the betterment of oral and systemic health. This level of responsibility must be continually visible to the profession and to the public. Only in this way can investigators earn and maintain the required trust needed to advance the human experimentation enterprise.

References

Beecher HK. 1966. Ethics and clinical research. *New England Journal of Medicine* 274: 1354–1360.
Bornfeld M. 2007. Industry support questioned. *Journal of the American Dental Association* 138: 150.
Council on Dental Research. 1979. Guidelines for the use of human subjects in dental research. *Journal of the American Dental Association* 98: 86–88.
Council on Dental Research. 1985. Human subjects in dental research: coping with the regulations. *Journal of American Dental Association* 110: 243–246.
Dunn WJ. 2007. Ethical Research. *Journal of American Dental Association* 138: 1534–1535.
Gillett GR. 1994. Ethics and dental research. *Journal of Dental Research* 73 (11): 1766–1722.
Glick M. 2007. Ethical considerations in publishing research involving human subjects. *Journal of American Dental Association* 138: 1300–1302.
Harrison JE. 2005. Orthodontic clinical trials III: reporting of ethical issues associated with clinical trials published in three orthodontic journals between 1989 and 1998. *Journal of Orthodontics* 32: 115–121.
Katz, J. 1972. The Jewish chronic disease case. *Experimentation with Human Beings—The Authority of the Investigator, Subject, Professions, and State in the Human Experimentation Process*. New York: Russell Sage Foundation.
Macrina, FL. 2005. *Scientific Integrity. Text and Cases in Responsible Conduct of Research*. Washington, D.C.: ASM Press.

National Commission for the Protection of Human Subjects of Biomedical and Behavioral Research. 1979. *The Belmont Report: Ethical Principles and Guidelines for the Protection of Human Subjects of Research.* Washington, D.C.: U. S. Government Printing Office. Available online at http://www.hhs.gov/ohrp/ (USHHS Office for Human Research Protections). Accessed on February 3, 2009.

NIH Guide. 2002. *Certificates of Confidentiality.* Available online at http://grants.nih.gov/grants/policy/coc/. Accessed on May 26, 2008.

Privacy Rule. 1996. Information on HIPAA and Research can be found in Protecting Personal Health Information in Research: Understanding the HIPAA Privacy Rule and is available online at http://privacyruleandresearch.nih.gov/pr_02.asp. Accessed on May 26, 2008.

The Code of Federal Regulations, Title 45 Part 46. 2005. Protection of Human Subjects is available online at http://www.hhs.gov/ohrp/humansubjects/guidance/45cfr46.htm. Accessed on May 26, 2008.

The Nuremberg Code. 1949. *Trials of War Criminals Before the Nuremberg Military Tribunals Under Control Council Law No. 10*, Vol. 2. Washington, D.C.: U.S. Government Printing Office, pp. 181–182. Available online at USHHS Office for Human Research Protections: http://www.hhs.gov/ohrp/. Accessed on February 3, 2009.

U.S. Department of Health Education and Welfare. 1973. *Final Report of the Tuskegee Syphilis Study Ad Hoc Advisory Panel.* Washington, D.C. Available online at http://biotech.law.lsu.edu/cphl/history/reports/tuskegee/tuskegee.htm. Accessed on February 3, 2009.

U.S. Department of Health and Human Services. 2005. Public health service policies on research misconduct (42 CFR parts 50 and 93). *Federal Register* 70 (94): 28369–28400.

World Medical Association. 1964. *Declaration of Helsinki. Ethical Principles for Medical Research Involving Human Subjects.* Adopted by the 18th World Medical Assembly, Helsinki, Finland. (Last approved modification, 2008, WMA General Assembly). Available online at http://www.wma.net/e/policy/b3.htm. Accessed on February 3, 2009.

Additional Resources

The DHHS Office of Human Research Protection (OHRP) offers both specific rules and regulations as well as educational resources and opinions regarding human subjects research. The Office of Human Research Protection (OHRP) website is located at http://www.hhs.gov/ohrp/policy/. Accessed on May 26, 2008.

A Current Bibliographies in Medicine 99–2 for Ethical Issues in Research involving human participants contains 4650 citations including books, audiovisual materials and journal articles and it can be found at http://www.nlm.nih.gov/archive//20061214/pubs/cbm/hum_exp.html. Accessed on May 26, 2008.

3

Responsibilities of institutions and individuals in clinical research in the oral health sciences

Gary C. Armitage, DDS, MS

A major responsibility of institutions in which clinical research is being conducted is to ensure that its employees adhere to all regulations and policies associated with research involving human volunteers. This requires that the institution have an organizational structure that provides educational, business/financial, and oversight/enforcement activities associated with clinical research. Individuals who are engaged in clinical research activities must receive the training that allows them to understand and follow all of the governmental and institutional requirements. Such researchers must also have the willingness to ethically adhere to these requirements. The purpose of this chapter is to summarize the complex group of responsibilities of institutions and individuals associated with clinical research in the craniofacial sciences. For the most part, these responsibilities are not discipline specific since they are applicable to all forms of clinical research involving human subjects. This chapter complements and builds on ethical principles in clinical research, set forth in Chapter 2.

3.1   Governmental and institutional regulations, policies, and guidelines

3.1.1   Nuremberg Code

(See also Chapter 2 on Ethics in Oral Health Research.)

Modern clinical research is a demanding and complex activity that is usually conducted by a team of investigators in an appropriate setting such as a university. Virtually all of the governmental and institutional regulations, policies, rules, guidelines, and guidances are intended to minimize any harm to human subjects who volunteer for a study. Heightened awareness of the need for governmental and institutional oversight of research activities involving human subjects occurred after World War II when the atrocities performed by Nazi doctors in the name of medical research came to light during the Nuremberg trials of war criminals. Included in the proceedings of these trials were ten points that described the elements of conducting ethical research on human subjects. These points or characteristics of "permissible medical experiments" became known as the Nuremberg Code (OHSR, NIH, 1949). This code includes the following major items:

- Voluntary informed consent is absolutely essential.

- Experiment should yield results for the good of society that cannot be obtained by any other means.

- Experiment should be based on the results of previous animal studies.

- Experiment should avoid unnecessary mental or physical harm.

- Experiment should not be conducted if death or disabling injury is expected.

- Degree of risk should not exceed anticipated benefits.

- Experiment should be conducted under conditions and facilities that protect against the possibility of injury, disability, or death.

- Experiment should be conducted by scientifically qualified persons.

- Human subject should be at liberty to withdraw from the study.

- Scientist in charge of the study should stop the experiment if its continuation is likely to result in injury, disability, or death of the subject.

Another important international document that endorses and expands the ethical principles for medical research outlined in the Nuremberg Code is the Declaration of Helsinki (World Medical Association, 1964). Readers are referred to Chapter 2 for a discussion of this and other ethical considerations in oral health research (Ripley and Macrina, 2009).

The immediate impact of the Nuremberg Code on human research was negligible since most investigators believed that human research conducted in the United States followed high ethical standards. This opinion gradually began to change when it was pointed out, by highly respected medical scientists, that there were many examples of unethical human research being conducted in the United States and the world with the results published in major scientific journals (Beecher, 1966; Pappworth, 1967). As examples of unethical or questionable human research continued to accumulate and were brought to the attention of the public in the lay press, the U.S. Congress took action in an attempt to address the problem with legislation.

3.1.2   Belmont Report

An important landmark in the governmental oversight of clinical research was the signing into law of the National Research Act (Public Law 93-348) in 1974 (DHHS, 1974). This law amended "... the Public Health Service Act to establish a national program, of biomedical research fellowships, traineeships, and training to assure the continued excellence of biomedical research in the United States, and for other purposes." This law created the formation of the National Commission for the Protection of Human Subjects of Biomedical and Behavioral Research. This commission met on a regular basis from 1976 to 1979 in the Belmont Conference Center of the Smithsonian Institution. What emerged was the "Belmont Report" that summarizes the basic ethical principles and guidelines for the protection of subjects of research (DHHS, 1979). The Belmont Report is important because it emphasized three principles that are the foundation for the ethical protection of human subjects of research: (i) respect for persons, (ii) beneficence (i.e., minimize harms and maximize benefits), and (iii) justice (i.e., treat people fairly).

3.1.3   President's commission for the study of ethical problems in biomedical research

Another landmark in this area was the publication of the First Biennial Report on the Adequacy and Uniformity of Federal Rules and Policies, and Their Implementation for the Protection of Human Subjects in Biomedical and Behavioral Research; Report of the President's Commission for the Study of Ethical Problems in Medicine and Biomedical and Behavioral Research (Abram et al., 1982). This commission was formed in 1978 in response to numerous allegations in the lay press of clinical research being conducted without prior review and approval of Institutional Review Boards (IRB). In addition to alleged investigator fraud, falsification of data and other forms of scientific misconduct were examined by the commission. The nine major recommendations of this commission are summarized in Table 3.1. The recommendations focus on two main areas: (i) uniform application of federal laws and regulations across all governmental agencies for the protection of human subjects, and (ii) improvement in federal oversight and response to reports of investigator or institutional misconduct.

3.1.4   Federal policy for the protection of human subjects—"Common Rule"

As governmental oversight of federally funded clinical research continued to grow, the Office for Human Research Protections (OHRP) under the Department of Health and Human Services (DHHS) was formed. The OHRP is organized into three major divisions: (1) Compliance Oversight, (2) Education and Development, and (3) Policy and Assurances. In general, the OHRP is charged with promoting adherence to the Federal Policy for the Protection of Human Subjects (also known as the "Common Rule") (DHHS, 1991). This policy specifies the basic requirements for the protection of human subjects involved in

Table 3.1   Recommendations of the President's commission for the study of ethical problems in medicine and biomedical and behavioral research (Abram et al., 1982).

A. Recommendations for improving the adequacy and uniformity of federal laws and regulations for the protection of human subjects
  1. All federal agencies should adopt the Regulations of Health and Human Services (HHS) (45 CFR Part 46)[a]
  2. The Secretary, HHS, should establish an office to coordinate government-wide implementation of the regulations
  3. Each federal agency should apply one set of rules consistently to all its subunits and funding mechanisms
  4. Principal Investigator (PI) should be required to submit annual data on the number of subjects in their research and the number and nature of adverse effects
  5. The National Commission's recommendations on research involving children and the mentally disabled should be acted upon promptly[b]
  6. "Private" research organizations receiving federal appropriations should be required to follow regulations for the protection of human subjects
B. Recommendations for improving institutional and federal oversight of research and the response to reports of misconduct
  7. Institutions should be free to use offices other than IRB to respond to reports of misconduct and should have procedures for prompt reporting of the findings to the funding agency
  8. IRB should be required only to report to appropriate officials of their institution (rather than to the funding agency) when they learn of possible misconduct and to respond to the findings of those officials
  9. There should be government-wide procedures for disbarring grantees and contractors found guilty of serious misconduct, as well as a consolidated list of formal disbarments and suspensions actively shared with government agencies, professional societies, and licensing boards

[a]45 CFR 46, Code of Federal Regulations. Title 45 Public Welfare. Department of Health and Human Services. Part 46 Protection of Human Subjects (Revised: June 23, 2005). Available online at http://www.hhs.gov/ohrp/humansubjects/guidance/45cfr46.htm.
[b]National Commission for the Protection of Human Subjects of Biomedical and Behavioral Research, *Report and Recommendations: Research Involving Children*, U.S. Government Printing Office, Washington (1977); National Commission for the Protection of Human Subjects of Biomedical and Behavioral Research, *Report and Recommendations: Those Institutionalized as Mentally Infirm*, U.S. Government Printing Office, Washington, D.C. (1978).

research conducted or funded by any federal agency. Since most research institutions in the United States receive some federal funds to support clinical research activities, these institutions are required to provide "assurances" through the Division of Policy and Assurances of the OHRP that the applicable federal policies will be followed for all clinical research supported by federal funds. Over 10,000 universities, hospitals, and other research institutions in the United States have formal agreements or written assurances with the OHRP to comply with existing regulations for the protection of human research subjects. In addition, any institution that accepts federal funds to conduct human research outside of the United States is also required to provide similar assurances to the OHRP. An OHRP-approved assurance commits the entire institution to full compliance with DHHS regulations. This includes all institutional officials, IRB, research investigators, and employees involved in human research activities. In addition to following the "Common Rule," institutional assurances include compliance with all relevant DHHS regulations and policies dealing with such issues as the educational requirements for key research personnel, financial disclosure statements, conflict of interest, procedures to investigate allegations of scientific misconduct, and adherence to the HIPAA (Health Insurance Portability and Accountability Act) Privacy Rule.

The Division of Compliance Oversight of the OHRP evaluates all substantive written allegations of an institution's noncompliance with applicable federal policies and regulations governing the protection of human subjects in DHHS-sponsored research (Title 45, Part 46, *Code of Federal Regulations* (45 *CFR* 46)) (DHHS, 1991). OHRP procedures for possible noncompliance might involve for-cause and not-for-cause compliance oversight evaluations (OHRP Guidance, 2005). For-cause evaluations can be triggered by substantive complaints of noncompliance with DHHS regulations from research subjects or their family members, investigators, study coordinators, institutional officials, or any other credible source. In addition, publications that appear to have involved human research that is not in compliance with DHHS regulations might initiate an OHRP evaluation. Not-for-cause compliance oversight evaluations are conducted in the absence of substantive allegations or indications of noncompliance. These evaluations can be based on a number of items, but are not limited to, volume of DHHS-supported research, geographical location, continuing concerns from a previous for-cause OHRP evaluation, and audits by other regulatory agencies such as the Food and Drug Administration (OHRP Guidance, 2005).

The Division of Education and Development of the OHRP provides guidance to individuals and institutions involved in human subject research through national and regional conferences. It also develops and distributes resource materials that enhance the protection of human subjects. It acts as a center for information on state-of-the-art educational programs for investigators conducting human research and on ethical issues associated with biomedical and behavioral research (OHRP Education, 2008).

3.2   Educational responsibilities of institutions

In order to enhance the federal commitment to the protection of participants in human clinical studies, in 2000, the Secretary of the DHHS issued a directive requiring all key personnel involved in such studies to document that they have completed an educational program on the protection of human research subjects (NIH Guide Notice: NOT-OD-00-039, 2000). Key personnel are defined as individuals who are involved in the design and conduct of human subjects research. Although this educational requirement was specifically directed toward clinical research funded by the NIH and other governmental agencies, virtually all IRB have adopted the policy. IRB approval of clinical research studies, regardless of the funding source (e.g., industry) is contingent upon all key personnel meeting the NIH-mandated educational requirement.

The educational requirement can be met by several computer-based training modules including one recently released by the NIH Office of Extramural Research (OER) (NIH Guide Notice: NOT-OD-08-054, 2008). This online tutorial replaces a web-based training module developed by the National Cancer Institute. Also available is an excellent online course initiated by a group at the University of Miami. The course is called the Collaborative Institutional Training Initiative (CITI) Program that is currently used by over 715 institutions in dozens of countries (Braunschweiger and Goodman, 2007). One of the strengths of the CITI Program is its versatility since it has individual modules designed specifically for different groups of people involved in clinical research such as biomedical researchers, IRB members, those conducting social or behavioral research, bench scientists, institutional officials, and staff of health research protection programs (HRPP).

In fact, institutions where clinical research is carried out consider the online offerings such as the CITI Program as a minimum educational requirement. It is the policy of most research institutions (e.g., universities) to provide additional in-service training on the protection of human subjects and responsible conduct of research in multiple formats such as periodic seminars and workshops. It is an institutional responsibility to provide these educational opportunities and to ensure that employees engaged in clinical research take advantage of them.

3.2.1   HIPAA Privacy Rule

In addition to basic courses on the protection of human research subjects, institutions must also offer an educational program on the HIPAA Privacy Rule as it relates to clinical research. One portion of the rule specifies the conditions under which protected health information (PHI) may be used or disclosed in a research setting. PHI includes any individually identifiable health information that is often obtained, created, used, and/or disclosed during the course of clinical research. PHI of an individual includes items such as their medical/dental records, progress notes, list of current medications, radiographic reports, examination findings, and literally any other health or personal information that can be linked to that individual by name or identifier. The Privacy Rule uses the definition of research as it appears in DHHS regulations at 45 CFR 46.102(d)—"a systematic investigation, including research development, testing, evaluation, designed to develop or contribute to generalizable knowledge." (NIH, 2005). Therefore, any type of clinical research falls under this definition. Under the Privacy Rule, research subjects may give written authorization to investigators to use or disclose PHI for purposes of research. The authorization form usually specifies the types of PHI that will be used or disclosed. In addition, in its review of the study protocol, the IRB must agree that the types of PHI that will be used or disclosed is a necessary part of the investigation. Under the HIPAA Privacy Rule, it is also possible to use or disclose PHI *without* authorization of the research subject. However, this may only be done after IRB approval and when the following three criteria of the Privacy Rule are satisfied (NIH, 2005):

- Use or disclosure of PHI involves no more than minimal risk to the privacy of individuals, based on the presence of an adequate plan to (i) protect the identifiers from improper use or disclosure, (ii) destroy the identifiers after completion of the research if permitted by law, and (iii) provide assurances that the PHI will not be reused or disclosed to any person or entity, except as required by law.

- The research could not practicably be conducted without the waiver.

- The research could not practicably be conducted without access to and use of the PHI.

The HIPAA Privacy Rule is a complex piece of legislation that applies to all health care activities in which PHI is used and generated. Clinical research is only one of these activities. For a general overview of the HIPAA legislation as it applies to health care, readers are referred to a summary prepared by the Office for Civil Rights (OCR, 2003).

Many institutions offer educational programs dealing with other aspects of the complex human interactions that are encountered during the course of performing clinical research. Separate online courses for researchers on ethics, conflict-of-interest issues, and the prevention of sexual harassment are available at most universities.

3.3   Financial responsibilities of institutions

As part of the OHRP-approved institutional assurances, it is the responsibility of the institution to have in place the infrastructure and procedures to properly handle grant funds that are used to support clinical research activities. This requires that the institution have employees skilled in accounting procedures, preparation and justification of research budgets, preaward and postaward contracts/grants management, and all other financial activities associated with the business aspects of a clinical research program. The accounting procedures should be able to withstand the scrutiny of internal and external auditors. It is critically important that the institution make sure that funds provided by the contract or grant are used specifically for the intended research purpose. The institution must also ensure that clinical investigators provide a signed financial disclosure statement as required by the DHHS (DHHS, 2004). The 2004 guidance document dealing with this disclosure states that a conflicting financial interest is any "financial interest related to a research study that will, or may be reasonably expected to create a bias." (DHHS, 2004). The intent of this guidance is to ensure that any financial interests of an investigator are not in conflict with the basic principles stated in the Belmont Report—respect for persons, beneficence, and justice.

If the clinical research involves testing a drug, biological product, or device that is regulated by the Food and Drug Administration (FDA), a somewhat different guidance that interprets applicable provisions of FDA regulations should be followed (FDA, 2001). The basic financial disclosure requirements of the FDA state that clinical investigators must disclose any financial arrangements with the sponsor and steps have been taken to minimize the potential for bias. The FDA Guidance on Financial Disclosure by Clinical Investigators (FDA, 2001) lists "disclosable financial arrangements" as follows:

1. Compensation made to the investigator in which the value of compensation could be affected by the outcome.

2. A proprietary interest in the tested product, including, but not limited to, a patent, trademark, copyright, or licensing agreement.

3. Any equity interest in the sponsor of a covered study, that is, any ownership interest, stock options, or other financial interest whose value cannot be readily determined through reference to public prices.

4. Any equity interest in a publicly held company that exceeds $50,000 in value. This requirement applies to interests held during the time the clinical investigator is carrying out the study and for 1 year following completion of the study.

5. Significant payments of other sorts, which are payments that have a cumulative monetary value of $25,000 or more made by the sponsor of a covered study to the investigator or the investigator's institution to support activities of the investigator exclusive of the costs of conducting the clinical study or other clinical studies during the time the clinical investigator is carrying out the study and for 1 year following completion of the study.

3.4   Responsibilities of investigators for FDA-regulated clinical research

(See also Chapter 4 on regulatory aspects of clinical research.)

Section 21 of the Code of Federal Regulations (CFR) contains most of the regulations dealing with food and drugs. Part 312 of Section 21 deals with investigational new drug or device (IND) applications including regulations that delineate the individual responsibilities of clinical investigators (FDA, 2008). In general, the investigator is responsible for conducting the study in accordance with a signed investigator statement on "Form FDA 1572." This statement certifies that the study will be carried out following the IRB-approved protocol and all applicable regulations that deal with protecting the rights, safety, and welfare of human subjects. Form FDA 1572 documents the qualifications of the principal investigator (PI), address of the study site, address of the IRB, and study title. It includes the names of any subinvestigators who are supervised by the PI. The form also lists the commitments or responsibilities that the PI agrees to while conducting the clinical study. Part 312 of Section 21 of the CFR lists six major responsibilities of the PI:

1. **Control of the investigational drug or device (Part 312.61)**. This regulation requires that the drug or device be administered only under the personal supervision of the PI or by a subinvestigator supervised by the PI. The PI may not supply the investigational drug or device to any unauthorized person.

2. **Accurate record keeping and retention (Part 312.62).** The PI must maintain accurate records on the *disposition of the investigational drug or device* including dates, quantity administered, and use by subjects. Thorough *documentation of case histories* must be prepared and maintained. This includes accurate case-report forms, source documents (i.e., medical/dental charts or records), signed informed consent forms, and progress notes. Case history documents must be *retained for at least 2 years* following the date a marketing application is approved by the FDA for the indication for which the drug or device is being investigated. If the FDA does not approve the application, or if no application is filed by the study sponsor, the case histories still need to be retained for at least 2 years after the investigation is discontinued.

3. **Preparation of required reports (Part 312.64).** During the course of the study, the PI must provide the study sponsor with *progress and safety reports*. Adverse events caused by, or probably caused by, the drug or study intervention need to be promptly reported to the sponsor. Some IRB also require that they be notified of minor adverse effects. If serious adverse events (SAE) occur, for whatever reason, the IRB and the study sponsor must be notified immediately. The PI

is also required to provide the sponsor with a *final report* at the end of the study. Finally, if changes occur in the study-related *financial disclosure* statements filed at the start of the study, updated reports must be provided to the study sponsor during the course of the study and for 1 year following completion of the investigation.

4. **Assurance of required IRB approvals (Part 312.66).** This regulation requires that the PI assures that IRB approval is obtained for initial and continuing reviews of the proposed clinical study. Furthermore, once the study has started, the PI must obtain IRB approval prior to making any changes in the study protocol. The only exception to this requirement is when it becomes necessary to make immediate changes to eliminate unequivocal hazards to patient/subject safety.

5. **Cooperate with external auditors of study records (Part 312.68).** In situations where an FDA audit of the study records becomes necessary, the PI is required to facilitate examination of the appropriate study documents by a properly authorized officer or employee of the FDA.

6. **Proper handling of investigational drugs or devices (Part 312.69).** If the investigation drug falls under the Controlled Substances Act, the PI must take adequate precautions to prevent theft of the drug. Indeed, any investigational drug or device should be kept in well-constructed and securely locked storage cabinets. Access should only be granted to properly authorized study personnel.

3.5   Intellectual property and clinical research

(Also see Chapter 15 on technology transfer for life science innovations in academic institutions.)

3.5.1   Bayh–Dole Act of 1980 (Public Law 96-517)

One of the major outcomes of biomedical research is the generation of intellectual property in the form of inventions with considerable commercial or monetary value. In many cases, these inventions are developed by university scientists who are partially supported by research grants from governmental agencies such as the NIH. Prior to 1980, ownership of the rights to such inventions was unclear. Who should own the rights to the invention? Should it be the scientist, the university that employs the scientist, or the governmental agency that funded the research? Valid arguments can be made for each party, although the strongest case can be made for the governmental funding agency. Since many inventions developed under federal grants and contracts, and therefore technically owned by the federal government, were not being commercialized, Congress passed Public Law [P.L.] 96-517 that amended the existing patent and trademark laws. This amendment, also known as the Bayh–Dole Act of 1980, was designed to promote the transfer of federally funded technologies to public entities interested in commercial development of the inventions. The Act (P.L. 96-517) states, "It is the policy and objective of the Congress to use the patent system to promote the utilization of inventions arising from federally supported research or development; to encourage maximum participation of small business firms in

Federally sponsored research and development efforts; to promote collaboration between commercial concerns and nonprofit organizations, including universities; to ensure that inventions made by nonprofit organizations and small business firms are used to promote free competition and enterprise; to promote the commercialization and public availability of inventions made in the United States by United States industry and labor; to ensure that the Government obtains sufficient rights in federally supported inventions to meet the needs of the Government and protect against nonuse or unreasonable use of inventions; and to minimize the costs of administering policies in this area."

The impact of this legislation has been substantial since it accelerated the application of technological innovations to clinical practice. It also promoted the expansion and proliferation of offices of technology management, intellectual property, and industry/research development within the infrastructure of universities. Most research universities now consider it their responsibility to manage and protect the intellectual property developed by its scientists. Through a variety of complex licensing agreements, scientists, and the universities they work for, share in the revenue generated by patented technologies. The NIH has published a guidance on sponsored research agreements for institutions that are recipients of NIH grants and contracts (NIH, 1994). In this guidance, "recipients" includes for-profit organizations and nonprofit groups such as institutions of higher education and research institutes. In general, this guidance emphasizes the mandate of the Bayh–Dole Act that requires recipients to effectively and efficiently transfer technology to industry for commercial development. In doing so, it is the responsibility of the recipient institution or organization to make the research findings available to the public at large in a timely fashion. Other important responsibilities or requirements include protection of an investigator's academic freedom. This includes the investigator's freedom to (i) decide on what types of studies they wish to conduct, (ii) choose their own collaborators, (iii) publish results of the studies, and (iv) present their research findings at scientific meetings (NIH, 1994).

In an effort to document that NIH expenditures for basic research leading to the development of commercially valuable drugs or devices, Congress directed the DHHS to draft a plan to ensure that taxpayers' interests are protected (NIH, 2001). Under this plan, an important institutional/investigator responsibility is to report to the agency the name, trademark, or other appropriate identifiers of a therapeutic drug or device that embodies technology funded by the NIH once it is FDA approved and reaches the market. Reported information should include the following details: (i) NIH grants or contracts that led to the development of the drug or device, (ii) date of first disclosure to the government, (iii) the licensee, (iv) date of first commercial sale, and (v) product's commercial name (NIH, 2001).

3.6   Authorship

(Also see Chapter 17 on publication of research findings.)

In most situations, clinical research is a collaborative effort between many individuals with diverse skill sets. This is especially true of a multicenter clinical trial that usually involves research teams from several university medical centers. An important product that emerges from any type of clinical research is a refereed publication in a respected professional journal. Authorship of the publication can be a point of contention among the investigators unless the topic is dealt with well in advance of starting the study. The main issues to be decided are as follows:

- Who should write the paper?

- Who should be on the list of authors?

- What should be the sequence of authors on the list (i.e., first through last)?

- To which journal should the paper be submitted?

3.6.1   Who should write the paper?

With approval of the group, this decision is usually made by the senior investigator (i.e., the individual in overall charge of the project). There are no formal or fixed procedures to determine who actually writes the paper. In most cases, the senior author either writes the paper or delegates portions of the manuscript to other members of the investigative team. The final draft of the paper needs to be reviewed and approved by all of the coauthors listed on the manuscript. It is the responsibility of the senior author to determine that all coauthors consent to having their names placed on the list of authors. Most journals require that all listed authors sign a statement indicating that they have made a substantial contribution to the submitted paper and have read and approved of the final manuscript. In addition, all authors must disclose any commercial or financial interests that they may have in the content of the paper.

3.6.2   Who should be on the list of authors?

In general, all individuals who did some of the work or had substantive intellectual input into the project should be listed as authors. The names of individuals whose only contribution was to supply the financial resources to conduct the study are not customarily placed on the list of authors. Even the name of the director of a clinical research center or unit where the study was conducted should not be listed as an author unless the individual had some physical or intellectual involvement in the project. However, this opinion is not shared by all since some administrators insist on having their names placed on all manuscripts produced by their staff; a questionable practice at best. Under no circumstances should an individual's name be listed as an author without their knowledge or consent.

3.6.3   What should be the sequence of authors on the list?

In general, the sequence of names on the list of authors indicates the relative amount of work each individual contributed to the project. The first few authors are frequently those who had the idea for the project, did most of the work, and wrote the paper. The sequence of authors on the list of contributors is a reflection of who did most of the work. A frequent exception to this is the last author on the list. This place is often reserved for the senior or corresponding author in charge of the overall investigation. In academic life, sequence of authorship is important since university committees dealing with promotion and tenure often give considerable weight to first-author papers in the review of an individual's portfolio. Indeed, senior investigators, who already are tenured, often encourage junior clinical scientists to take on much of the paper-writing activity to become first authors, thereby enhancing their chances of academic advancement.

3.6.4   To which journal should the paper be submitted?

This group decision is often made after the study has been completed and the results analyzed. If the findings are of major importance and interest to the entire biomedical community, the manuscript is often submitted to a top-tier journal with a large general audience such as *Science, Nature, The Lancet*, and the *New England Journal of Medicine*. However, in most cases, the results of clinical research projects are of interest to a smaller audience and the decision is made to submit the paper to a specialty journal. As a general rule, most investigators prefer to publish their papers in rigorously refereed and highly prestigious journals with large readerships.

3.7   Scientific misconduct

3.7.1   Federal definition of scientific misconduct

Scientific misconduct can and does occur in clinical research. According to the Code of Federal Regulations (42 CFR Parts 50 and 93), ". . . research misconduct means fabrication, falsification, or plagiarism in proposing, performing, or reviewing research, or in reporting research results." (DHHS, 2005). It is the responsibility of institutions in which clinical research is being performed to have in place safeguards and procedures to minimize investigator wrongdoing. A report from the Institute of Medicine (IOM) states that individual investigators and institutions share in the responsibility to prevent scientific misconduct (IOM, 2002).

Falsified or fabricated research results do not have to be published to qualify for the federal definition of scientific misconduct. In addition to published material, the federal government considers reported research as follows:

- Data presented in manuscripts, theses, or lab reports as representing the results of experiments.

- Reports submitted to the Public Health Service (PHS) such as progress reports or preliminary data in grant applications.

- Abstracts, posters, oral presentations, and preliminary reports presented at scientific meetings; patent applications (ORI, 2007).

Although the federal definition of research misconduct is limited to plagiarism, fabrication/falsification of data, or other actions that seriously deviate from common practices in the scientific community (DHHS, 2005), some institutions use additional behaviors as evidence of scientific misconduct. These include items such as (1) a material failure to comply with governmental regulations, (2) unauthorized use of confidential information, and (3) retaliation or threat of retaliation against persons involved in the allegation or investigation of misconduct (ORI, 2000). Research institutions also need to have written procedures to effectively handle allegations of scientific misconduct. It is critically important that an investigator who has been accused of research misconduct be afforded legal due process in dealing with the allegations.

Under the assurances program that an extramural research institution provides to the OHRP, the institution promises to properly investigate all good faith allegations of scientific misconduct involving PHS-funded or PHS-regulated projects. PHS-funded or PHS-regulated projects include those from any of the following PHS agencies: National Institutes of Health (NIH), Center for Disease Control and Prevention, FDA, Substance Abuse and Mental Health Services Administration, Health Resources and Services Administration, Agency for Healthcare Research and Quality, Agency for Toxic Substances and Disease Registry, and the Indian Health Service (ORI, 2007). If the institution concludes that an investigation is warranted, it must report the alleged misconduct to the DHHS Office of Research Integrity (ORI). The ORI is the governmental unit that develops policies and regulations to prevent, detect, and investigate possible misconduct in PHS-funded or PHS-regulated studies. It monitors misconduct investigations carried out by extramural institutions to ensure that the inquiries are appropriately conducted.

The ORI does not have jurisdiction to review investigative issues surrounding an allegation of scientific misconduct for a study supported by non-PHS funds. Nor does the adoption of ORI policies by an institution for non-PHS issues extend the authority of the ORI to these matters. It can be argued that the indirect costs that an institution receives, as part of any PHS grant, to support its research infrastructure should place any research performed at that institution under ORI jurisdiction. However, it is the position of the ORI that this would extend the authority of the ORI beyond that which is granted by federal statutes and regulations (ORI, 2007). Nevertheless, most research institutions have developed procedures for handling scientific misconduct of all research, regardless of funding source, that comply with ORI policies.

3.7.2   Individual and institutional responsibilities for handling alleged scientific misconduct

It is the ethical responsibility of all members of the academic community to report to the proper institutional authorities any suspected research misconduct. At most institutions, the next procedural step is to confront the accused investigator with the allegations. If the investigator admits or confesses to the research misconduct, then a variety of penalties or sanctions can be levied depending on the severity and nature of the offense. Even in cases where a confession has been received, it is a good idea to fully investigate the extent and impact of the scientific misconduct and report the findings to the ORI if the study is PHS funded or PHS regulated. In most cases, receipt of a confession is an insufficient basis for closing a case (ORI, 2007).

Procedures for handling allegations of research misconduct may vary somewhat from institution to institution. However, the general procedural components include (1) notification of the accused, (2) investigation, (3) notification of appropriate authorities, (4) bring formal charges of misconduct based on investigation findings, (5) impose punishment or sanctions, (6) right of the accused to appeal, (7) formal hearing involving legal counsel on both sides, and (8) dismiss or uphold the sanctions depending on the results of the formal hearing.

If the accused denies the allegations and an initial investigation verifies that there is sufficient evidence to believe that some wrongdoing has occurred, a very detailed investigation is conducted. This may include confiscation of all research records of the accused including laboratory/office computers and interviews with study personnel. If the investigation confirms that scientific misconduct has occurred, the chief administrator of the institution may impose a variety of disciplinary actions including suspension without pay, dismissal, or the filing of a criminal complaint with law-enforcement authorities. At most of the universities, the accused has the right to appeal the charges and sanctions and request that a formal hearing be conducted. Overall, it is the ethical responsibility of the institution to thoroughly evaluate the allegations of scientific misconduct while at the same time protecting the legal rights of the accused.

It is important to remember that data generated using PHS funds are owned by the grantee institution, not the PI or research team that produced the data (ORI, 2007). The institution is the grantee and is legally accountable for how the funds are spent. This accountability includes verification that the data produced by the study are genuine. Most institutions in developing their research contracts with industrial sponsors of research include language stipulating that the data are freely supplied to the sponsor, but are owned by the institution.

Although conflicts of interest do not automatically lead to scientific misconduct, the chances of investigator wrongdoing are increased when competing interests are present (Bodenheimer, 2000).

3.8   Conflicts of interest (COI)

3.8.1   Different types of competing interests

In addition to the financial COI discussed above, competing interests can include conflicts between an investigator's personal interests and the best interests of a research subject (Rodwin, 1993). This might occur in cases where a marginally qualified subject is enrolled because of the eagerness of an investigator to meet an enrollment target. Clinical investigators who rapidly reach enrollment goals are often rewarded by increased praise from their peers as well as being sought-after investigators by industrial sponsors of clinical studies. In this example, an enhanced professional reputation is certainly among the personal interests of most investigators. Another type of conflict involves competing loyalties owed by an investigator to a third party, such as a study sponsor, and the well-being of a private patient (Rodwin, 1993). Health care providers who are also conducting a clinical study should not personally urge their private patients to volunteer for the study. Patients should never be recruited in this manner since they are likely to conclude that their doctor is advising them to enroll in the study. A subject's decision to enroll in a study should not be directly linked to the advice of their personal health care provider. Even if the health care provider believes that it would be in the best interests of their patient to enroll in the study, a personal invitation to join the study taints the informed consent process.

A longstanding debate among clinical researchers on COI issues continues to receive considerable attention in the biomedical literature. Individuals on one side of this debate have argued that COI issues are ubiquitous throughout academic life and it is not possible to eradicate all of them (Korn, 2000). Clear-cut financial conflicts are the easiest to identify and manage. However, there are many primarily nonfinancial pressures that have the potential to increase competing interests. Important among these are, "…the desire for faculty advancement, to compete successfully and repetitively for sponsored research funding, to receive accolades from professional peers and win prestigious research prizes, and to alleviate pain and suffering." (Korn, 2000). Some prominent clinical researchers strongly believe that the hunt for COI has gone too far and has harmed the public's interest in and support of research leading to biomedical innovations (Stossel, 2008).

Other investigators take the opposite position and advocate the continuation of a vigorous hunt for COI (Lee, 2008). The potential for a breach of trust in COI issues is probably at its greatest in the area of industry-sponsored clinical trials. However, the financial arrangements between industry and clinical researchers can be in other forms such as (1) service as paid consultants to companies whose products they study, (2) service on scientific advisory boards and speakers' bureaus, (3) agreeing to patent and royalty agreements, (4) allowing to have their names listed as authors on papers written by company ghostwriters, (5) promoting drugs or devices at company-sponsored symposia, and (6) acceptance of company-provided expensive gifts and trips (Angell, 2000). Particularly troublesome is finding of a systematic review showing that industry sponsorship of studies affects the outcome of the investigations (Lexchin et al., 2003). Outcomes favorable to the sponsor's product suggest that some systematic bias may occur in studies supported by industry.

It is clear that both sides to this debate have valid points and the issues will not be resolved anytime soon. In recent decades, many therapeutic innovations can be directly linked to research funds supplied by the biotechnology and pharmaceutical industries to university-based investigators (Montaner et al., 2001). The downside of this trend is an increase in the real or perceived conflict of interest of investigators who accept industrial support. Part of the controversy surrounding the overall relationship between health care professions and industry is the widespread practice of manufacturers and companies of providing free products and training on how to use their products. Some have urged that all academic medical centers endorse policies that eliminate, "... common practices related to small gifts, pharmaceutical samples, continuing medical education, funds for physician travel, speakers bureaus, ghostwriting, and consulting and research contracts." (Brennan et al., 2006). Many medical schools including Yale University and Stanford University "... have passed rules restricting gifts, free lunches and money that often flows freely from pharmaceutical companies, medical device manufacturers and other industry sources to doctors, researchers and students." (Check, 2007).

3.9   Concluding remarks

In the past 60 years, a complex array of governmental and institutional regulations, policies, and guidelines have evolved that directly deal with the protection of people who volunteer to be subjects for clinical research studies. Institutional responsibilities, in which clinical research is being conducted, include provision of educational opportunities for investigators, an infrastructure capable of dealing with the business/financial aspects of clinical research, and oversight/enforcement procedures. Individual investigators have the responsibility to obtain the training required to become ethical clinician/scientists who are committed to following governmental and institutional requirements for conducting research on human volunteers. It is important to remember that most of the existing regulations and policies in this area were developed in response to documented problems and abuse of human research subjects. In the future, it is likely that federal and other governmental oversight for clinical research involving humans will increase in complexity. Therefore, it is critically important that institutions and investigators alike stay abreast of new developments as this field continues to evolve.

References

Abram MB, Fox RC, Garcia-Palmieri M, Graham FK, Jonsen AR, Krim M, Medearis DN Jr., Motulsky AG, Scitovsky AA, Walker CJ, Williams CA. 1982. Protection of human subjects: First biennial report on the adequacy and uniformity of federal rules and policies, and their implementation for the protection of human subjects in biomedical and behavioral research; report of the President's commission for the study of ethical problems in medicine and biomedical and behavioral research. *Federal Register* 47(60):13272–13305.

Angell M. 2000. Is academic medicine for sale? *New England Journal of Medicine* 342(20): 1516–1518.

Beecher HK. 1966. Ethics and clinical research. *New England Journal of Medicine* 274(24):367–372.

Bodenheimer T. 2000. Uneasy alliance—clinical investigators and the pharmaceutical industry. *New England Journal of Medicine* 342(20):1539–1544.

Braunschweiger P, Goodman KW. 2007. The CITI program: an international online resource for education in human subjects protection and the responsible conduct of research. *Academic Medicine* 82(9):861–864.

Brennan TA, Rothman DJ, Blank L, Blumenthal D, Chimonas SC, Cohen JJ, Goldman J, Kassirer JP, Kimball H, Naughton J, Smelser N. 2006. Health industry practices that create conflicts of interest. A policy proposal for academic medical centers. *Journal of the American Medical Association* 295(4):429–433.

Check E. 2007. California campuses resist industry restrictions. *Nature* 448(7152):394–395.

DHHS. 1974. Protection of human subjects. *Federal Register* 39(105):18914–18920.

DHHS. 1979. *The Belmont Report. Ethical principles and guidelines for the protection of human subjects of research. The National Commission for the Protection of Human Subjects of Biomedical & Behavioral Research*. Available online at http://www.hhs.gov/ohrp/humansubjects/guidance/belmont/htm. Accessed on March 3, 2008.

DHHS. 1991. Federal policy for the protection of human subjects; notices and rules. 45 CFR Part 46. *Federal Register* 56(117):28003–28032.

DHHS. 2004. *Financial Relationships and Interests in Research Involving Human Subjects: Guidance for Human Subject Protection*. Final guidance document. Available online at http://www.hhs.gov/ohrp/humansubjects/finreltn/fguid.pdf. Accessed on March 3, 2008.

DHHS. 2005. Public health service policies on research misconduct. 45 CFR Parts 50 and 93; RIN 0940-AA04. *Federal Register* 70(94):28370–28400.

FDA. 2001. *Guidance. Financial Disclosure by Clinical Investigators*. Available online at http://www.fda.gov/oc/guidance/financialdis.html. Accessed on March 1, 2008.

FDA. 2008. *Federal Regulations for Clinical Investigators*. Last updated: February 4, 2008. Available online at http://www.fda.gov/cder/about/smallbiz/CFR.htm. Accessed on February 25, 2008.

IOM (Institute of Medicine). 2002. *Integrity in Scientific Research: Creating an Environment that Promotes Responsible Conduct*. Washington, D.C.: The National Academies Press, p. 202.

Korn D. 2000. Conflicts of interest in biomedical research. *Journal of the American Medical Association* 284(17):2234–2237.

Lee K. 2008. Has the hunt for conflicts of interest gone too far? No. *British Medical Journal* 336(7642):477.

Lexchin J, Bero LA, Djulbegovic B, Clark O. 2003. Pharmaceutical industry sponsorship and research outcome and quality: systematic review. *British Medical Journal* 326(7400):1167–1170.

Montaner JSG, O'Shaughnessy MV, Schechter MT. 2001. Industry-sponsored clinical research: a double-edged sword. *The Lancet* 358:1893–1895.

NIH. 1994. Developing sponsored research agreements. Considerations for recipients of NIH research grants and contracts. *Federal Register* 59(215):55674–55679.

NIH. 2001. *NIH Response to the Conference Report Request for a Plan to Ensure Taxpayers' Interests are Protected*. Available online at http://ott.od.nih.gov/policy/policy_protect_text.html. Accessed on March 2, 2008.

NIH. 2005. *Clinical Research and the HIPAA Privacy Rule*. Available online at http://privacyruleandresearch.nih.gov/healthservicesprivacy.asp. Accessed on March 15, 2008.

NIH Guide Notice. NOT-OD-00-039. 2000. *Required education in the protection of human research participants*. Available online at http://grants.nih.gov/grants/guide/notice-files/NOT-OD-00-039.html. Accessed on March 5, 2008.

NIH Guide Notice. NOT-OD-08-054. 2008. *Guidance on NIH Office of Extramural Research (OER) On-Line Tutorial Protecting Human Research Participants (PHRP)*. Available online at http://grants.nih.gov/grants/guide/notice-files/NOT-OD-08-054.html. Accessed on March 5, 2008.

OCR (Office for Civil Rights). 2003. *OCR Privacy Brief. Summary of the HIPAA Privacy Rule*. Available online at http://www.hhs.gov/ocr/privacysummary.pdf. Accessed on March 21, 2008.

OHRP Education. 2008. *Division of Education and Development*. Available online at http://www.hhs.gov/education/. Accessed on March 15, 2008.

OHRP Guidance. 2005. *OHRP's Compliance Oversight Procedures for Evaluating Institutions*. October 19, 2005. Available online at http://www.hhs.gov/ohrp/compliance/. Accessed on March 3, 2008.

OHSR, NIH. 1949. (Office of Human Subjects Research, National Institutes of Health). Regulations and ethical guidelines. Directives for human experimentation. Nuremberg Code. Available online at http://ohsr.od.nih.gov/guidelines/nuremberg.html. Accessed on March 7, 2008.

ORI (Office of Research Integrity). 2000. *Final Report. Analysis of Institutional Policies for Responding to Allegations of Scientific Misconduct*. Task Order #4. Contract No. 282-98-0008. Available online at http://ori.dhhs.gov/documents/institutional_policies.pdf. Accessed on March 24, 2008.

ORI (Office of Research Integrity). 2007. *Handling Misconduct—Inquiry Issues. ORI Responses to Issues Arising from Inquiries and Investigations*. Available online at http://ori.dhhs.gov/misconduct/inquiry_issues.shtml. Accessed on March 24, 2008.

Pappworth MH. 1967. *Human Guinea Pigs: Experimentation on Man*. London: Routledge & Kegan Paul.

P.L. 96-517. 1980. *The Patent and Trademark Amendments of 1980 (Bayh–Dole)*. Available online at http://history.nih.gov/01docs/historical/documents/PL96-517.pdf. Accessed on March 10, 2008.

Ripley E, Macrina FL. 2009. Ethics in oral health research (Chapter 2). In: Giannobile WV, Burt BA, Genco RJ (eds). *Principles of Clinical Oral Health Research*. New York: Blackwell Publishing Co.

Rodwin MA. 1993. *Medicine, Money, and Morals: Physician's Conflict of Interest*. New York: Oxford University Press.

Stossel TP. 2008. Has the hunt for conflicts of interest gone too far? Yes. *British Medical Journal* 336(7642):476.

World Medical Association. 1964. *Declaration of Helsinki. Ethical Principles for Medical Research Involving Human Subjects*. Adopted by the 18th World Medical Assembly, Helsinki, Finland. (Last approved modification, 2004, WMA General Assembly, Tokyo).

4

Regulatory process for the evaluation of dental drugs, devices, and biologics

Darnell Kaigler Jr., DDS, MS, PhD, **Kay Fuller,** RAC, **and William V. Giannobile,** DDS, DMSc

It is without question that the age of "Information and Technology" has enabled and produced more advances in the medical and dental profession than during any other period in history. In dentistry, the rapid rate at which discoveries are made and products developed makes it increasingly difficult to appropriately evaluate and monitor these products and technologies. However, the need for cautious and critical oversight is greater than ever to ensure that the best interest and safety of the consumers (dentists) and beneficiaries (patients) are upheld. One of the most significant challenges regarding the conduct of dental research aimed at development of new therapies or therapeutics lies in understanding and navigating through the appropriate regulatory review and approval mechanisms. Worldwide, each country has a regulatory process through which products are tested and evaluated prior to widespread distribution and use; yet, from country to country, there exist vast differences not only in these processes, but also in the organizational structures of the governing bodies that establish them and how they are ultimately enforced. Clinical testing of new dental products and treatments requires approval from the U.S. Food and Drug Administration (FDA), European Medicines Agency (EMEA), or other international regulatory agencies prior to clinical study initiation. The clinical studies are utilized to gain sound scientific evidence that the new product or therapy is deemed safe and effective. Assuming safety and efficacy criteria are met, additional approval from the FDA is required prior to the product/therapy being placed on the market for commercial widespread use and distribution in clinical practice. Without the appropriate understanding of the mechanisms for obtaining FDA approval, this process can take a significant amount of time and create a high level of frustration to those who embark upon it. In the United States and abroad, it is of paramount importance to understand and follow the regulations and guidelines set forth by the appropriate regulatory agency for obtaining approval for use of new products, and in most cases, there are significant ramifications associated with deviation from these regulations. This chapter provides a general overview of the function and oversight of the U.S. FDA as well as other international agencies such as the EMEA regarding the mechanisms for approval of new products and therapies. The chapter will also discuss the regulatory approval process specific to dental and oral-related products.

4.1   Mission of FDA

The federal regulatory agency that has evolved into the U.S. FDA had its conception just a little over a century ago. In the late nineteenth century and early twentieth century, the competitive culture of the agricultural industry bred a climate for widespread packaging and distribution of food products that were tainted with improper ingredients and additives. These products, termed "adulterated," ranged from "watered down" milk to spoiled canned goods (Hart, 1952). This practice spurred an initiative for a centralized governing body that would help to ensure consistency in the manufacturing of produce and quality of the final product. In 1906, led by the efforts of Harvey W. Wiley, this movement culminated in the Pure Food and Drugs Act, which was signed into law by Theodore Roosevelt (Hart, 1952). This Act was originally set in place to give the federal government regulatory authority over food and drugs. Over the next 100 years, the emergence of more innovative food manufacturing processes, new medical devices and technologies, and an array of novel medications for treatment and cure of disease led to the expansion of this Act into very detailed regulations and guidelines, now overseen by over 10,000 employees who collectively comprise what is currently known as the FDA. A timeline highlighting key events and medical advances during this time is shown in Table 4.1.

The FDA is the branch of the U.S. Department of Health and Human Services whose primary mission is to protect "the public health by assuring the safety, efficacy, and security of human and veterinary drugs, biological products, medical devices, our nation's food supply, cosmetics, and products that emit radiation." It is also responsible for "advancing the public health by helping to speed innovations that make medicines and foods more effective, safer, and more affordable." Finally, it serves to help the "public get the accurate, science-based information they need to use medicines and foods to improve their health" (FDA, 2008). Its jurisdiction covers all food, drug, and medical device manufacturing agencies and research entities whose products are intended for consumption or therapeutic use in humans and animals. The FDA is empowered to develop rules and guidelines that govern the food, drug, device, and cosmetic industry, and when these regulations are not met, it has the authority to mandate action against the offending party (FDA, 2008). The FDA's organizational structure is very intricate and its regulatory categorization scheme is stratified into a very specific format, as highlighted in Figure 4.1. The "Code of Federal Regulations" (CFR, 2009) is the codification of the general and permanent rules published in the *Federal Register* by the Executive departments and agencies of the federal government. It is divided into 50 *titles*, which represent broad areas subject to regulation. Each title is further divided into *chapters*, which generally bear the name of the issuing agency. Each of these chapters is subcategorized into *parts* that cover specific regulatory areas and large

Table 4.1   Timeline: Chronology of Key Regulatory Events in Evolution of FDA.
Adapted from http://www.fda.gov/cder/about/history/time1.htm.

1820	Eleven physicians meet in Washington, D.C., to establish the U.S. Pharmacopeia, the first compendium of standard drugs for the United States
1846	Publication of Lewis Caleb Beck's *Adulteration of Various Substances Used in Medicine and the Arts* helps document problems in the drug supply
1906	The original Food and Drugs Act is passed. It prohibits interstate commerce in misbranded and adulterated foods and drugs. The Meat Inspection Act is passed the same day
1914	The Harrison Narcotic Act imposes upper limits on the amount of opium, opium-derived products, and cocaine allowed in products available to the public; requires prescriptions for products exceeding the allowable limit of narcotics; and mandates increased record-keeping for physicians and pharmacists that dispense narcotics. A separate law dealing with marijuana would be enacted in 1937
1937	Elixir sulfanilamide, containing the poisonous solvent diethylene glycol, kills 107 persons, many of whom are children, dramatizing the need to establish drug safety before marketing and to enact the pending food and drug law
1938	The Federal Food, Drug, and Cosmetic Act of 1938 is passed by Congress (replacing the 1906 Food and Drugs Act), containing new provisions: <ul><li>Requiring new drugs to be shown safe before marketing; this starts a new system of drug regulation</li><li>Providing that safe tolerances be set for unavoidable poisonous substances</li><li>Authorizing standards of identity, quality, and fill-of-container for foods</li><li>Authorizing factory inspections</li><li>Adding the remedy of court injunctions to the previous penalties of seizures and prosecutions</li></ul>
1951	Durham–Humphrey Amendment defines the kinds of drugs that cannot be used safely without medical supervision and restricts their sale to prescription by a licensed practitioner
1962	Kefauver–Harris Drug Amendments are passed to ensure drug efficacy and greater drug safety. For the first time, drug manufacturers are required to prove to FDA the effectiveness of their products before marketing them
1970	FDA requires the first patient package insert: oral contraceptives must contain information for the patient about specific risks and benefits
1982	Merger of the Bureau of Drugs and the Bureau of Biologics to form the National Center for Drugs and Biologics (NCDB) to streamline FDA's approval procedures in drugs and biologics and to increase the public's assurance of the safety and effectiveness of the drug supply
1983	Orphan Drug Act passed, enabling FDA to promote research and marketing of drugs needed for treating rare diseases
1987	Due to the increasing number of NDA, the Center for Drugs and Biologics was split into the Center for Drug Evaluation and Research and the CBER

(Continued)

Table 4.1   Timeline: Chronology of Key Regulatory Events in Evolution of FDA. Adapted from http://www.fda.gov/cder/about/history/time1.htm. (*Continued*)

1997	FDA Modernization Act reauthorizes the Prescription Drug User Fee Act of 1992 and mandates the most wide-ranging reforms in agency practices since 1938. Provisions include measures to accelerate review of devices, advertising unapproved uses of approved drugs and devices, health claims for foods in agreement with published data by a reputable public health source, and development of good guidance practices for agency decision making *First FDA approval of toothpaste (Colgate Total$^{®}$) to help prevent gingivitis, plaque, and cavities*
2002	Development of the Office of Combination Products, which facilitates and coordinates review of products that could be considered a combination of at least two of the following: drug, biologic, or device
2005	GEM 21S$^{®}$ becomes the first FDA-approved dental product incorporating a purified recombinant growth factor, PDGF
2007	INFUSE$^{®}$ bone graft becomes first FDA-approved bone morphogenetic protein product for sinus floor elevation and alveolar ridge repair

parts may be even further broken down into *subparts*. All of the parts are finally organized in sections and a representative breakdown of the classification of a dental implant is shown to highlight this classification scheme (Figure 4.2, Table 4.2).

4.2   FDA nomenclature

The FDA utilizes many terms and acronyms that are used to denote everything from various branches of the FDA to the products that it regulates. Many of these terms are misnomers or used inappropriately, which often leads to confusion among those who are not affiliated with the FDA or have had limited to no experience working with the agency. Thus, in order to provide clarity on some important terms and abbreviations, a list of definitions of several of these key terms is provided in Table 4.3.

4.3   Different pathways to approval

Dental products regulated by the FDA have various routes they must take in order to successfully navigate through the FDA approval process and ultimately reach the market. Depending on the type of product under consideration, it must go through one of a few different mechanisms for approval. The formal mechanisms of approval for drugs, devices, biologics, and combination products are described in detail below, and general overview schematics of the processes for drugs, biologics, and devices are included (Figure 4.3).

4.3.1   Drugs

On average, it takes about 12 years and over $350 million to move a new drug through the drug development life cycle, which includes discovery, preclinical development,

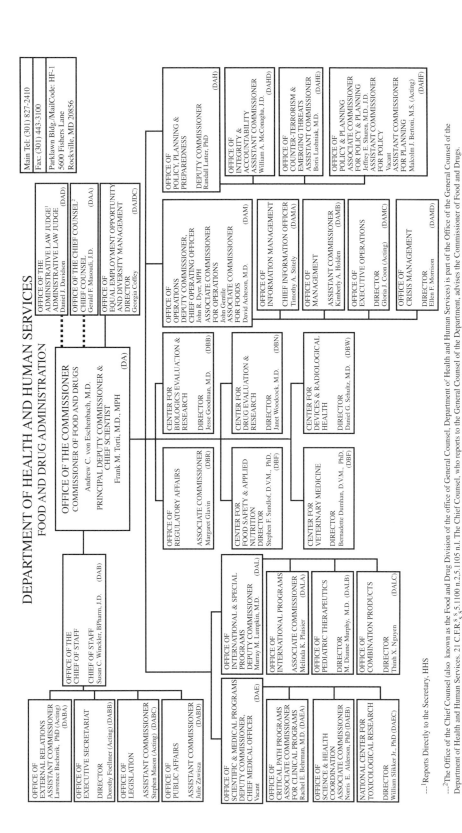

Figure 4.1 Organizational structure of FDA. Adapted from http://www.fda.gov/oc/orgcharts/orgchart.htm.

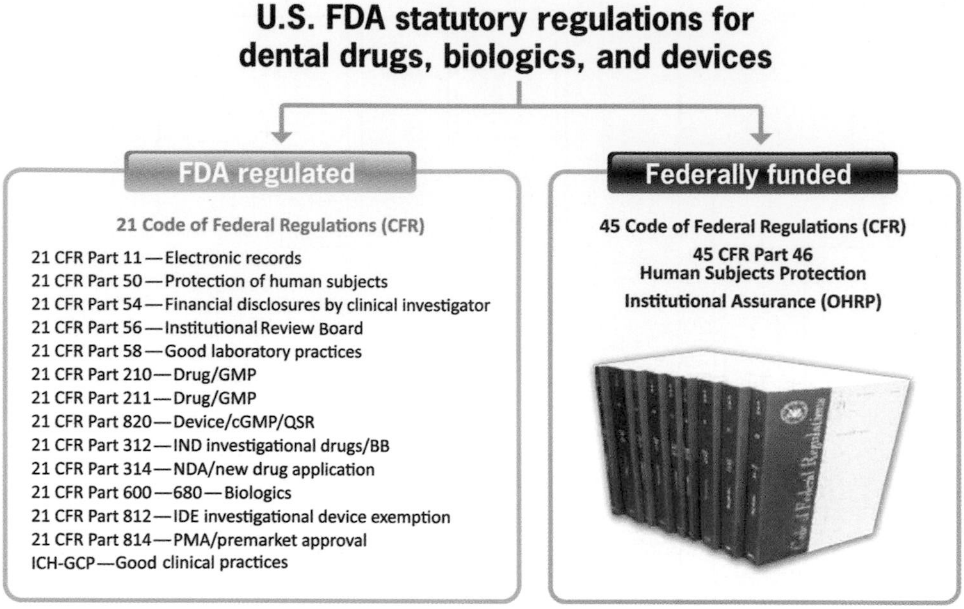

U.S. FDA statutory regulations for dental drugs, biologics, and devices

Figure 4.2 U.S. FDA statutory regulations for dental drugs, biologics, and devices. FDA-regulated and federally funded regulations are highlighted.

Table 4.2   Classification of endosseous dental implants.

(21CFR872.3640)
TITLE 21—FOOD AND DRUGS
CHAPTER I—FOOD AND DRUG ADMINISTRATION
DEPARTMENT OF HEALTH AND HUMAN SERVICES
SUBCHAPTER H—MEDICAL DEVICES

Part 872—Dental Devices
Subpart D—Prosthetic Devices
Sec. 872.3640 Endosseous Dental Implant.

(a)   *Identification.* An endosseous dental implant is a device made of a material such as titanium or titanium alloy, that is intended to be surgically placed in the bone of the upper or lower jaw arches to provide support for prosthetic devices, such as artificial teeth, in order to restore a patient's chewing function

(b)   *Classification.* (1) Class II (special controls). The device is classified as Class II if it is a root-form endosseous dental implant. The root-form endosseous dental implant is characterized by four geometrically distinct types: basket, screw, solid cylinder, and hollow cylinder. The guidance document entitled "Class II Special Controls Guidance Document: Root-Form Endosseous Dental Implants and Endosseous Dental Implant Abutments" will serve as the special control (see 872.1(e) for the availability of this guidance document)

(c)   Class III (premarket approval). The device is classified as Class III if it is a blade-form endosseous dental implant

---

Table 4.3   Nomenclature of FDA branches, classification of FDA products, and clinical trial definitions.

CFR	The codification of the general and permanent rules published in the *Federal Register* by the executive departments and agencies of the federal government
CDER	Center for Drug Evaluation and Research
CBER	Center for Biologics Evaluation and Research
CVM	Center for Veterinary Research
Biologic	Product made or derived from a living organism
Device	An instrument, apparatus, implement, machine, contrivance, implant, *in vitro* reagent, or other similar or related article, including a component part, or accessory that is:

- recognized in the official National Formulary, or the U.S. Pharmacopoeia, or any supplement to them

- intended for use in the diagnosis of disease or other conditions, or in the cure, mitigation, treatment, or prevention of disease, in man or other animals

- intended to affect the structure or any function of the body of man or other animals, and which does not achieve any of its primary intended purposes through chemical action within or on the body of man or other animals and which is not dependent upon being metabolized for the achievement of any of its primary intended purposes

Device classification

- **Class I (general controls)**: Devices subject to the least regulatory control; they present minimal potential for harm to the user and are often simpler in design than Class II or III devices; *dental examples*: manual toothbrush, dental floss, gutta percha, dental chair and accessories, articulation paper, dental surgical handpiece and accessories, dental diamond instrument

- **Class II (special controls):** Devices for which general controls alone are insufficient to ensure safety and effectiveness, and existing methods are available to ensure such assurances. Special controls may include special labeling requirements, mandatory performance standards, and postmarket surveillance; *dental examples*: temporary crown and bridge resin, dental bone grafting material devices (i.e., hydroxyapatite, tricalcium phosphate), ultrasonic scalers

- **Class III (premarket approval/510k)**: Most stringent regulatory category; devices for which insufficient information exists to ensure safety and efficacy; premarket approval is required in order to ensure safety and efficacy; *dental examples*: dental bone grafting materials that contain a drug that is a therapeutic biologic (i.e., bone morphogenetic proteins (BMP)), total temporomandibular joint prosthesis, mandibular condyle prosthesis

(Continued)

Table 4.3   Nomenclature of FDA branches, classification of FDA products, and clinical trial definitions. (*Continued*)

Drug	Articles intended for use in the diagnosis, cure, mitigation, treatment, or prevention of disease; and articles (other than food) intended to affect the structure or any function of the body of man or other animals
Combination product	
(1)	A product comprised of two or more regulated components, that is, drug/device, biologic/device, drug/biologic, or drug/device/biologic, that are physically, chemically, or otherwise combined or mixed and produced as a single entity
(2)	Two or more separate products packaged together in a single package or as a unit and comprised of drug and device products, device and biological products, or biological and drug products
(3)	A drug, device, or biological product packaged separately that according to its investigational plan or proposed labeling is intended for use only with an approved individually specified drug, device, or biological product where both are required to achieve the intended use, indication, or effect, and where upon approval of the proposed product, the labeling of the approved product would need to be changed, for example, to reflect a change in intended use, dosage form, strength, route of administration, or significant change in dose
(4)	Any investigational drug, device, or biological product packaged separately that according to its proposed labeling is for use only with another individually specified investigational drug, device, or biological product where both are required to achieve the intended use, indication, or effect
Phase I trial	First stage of testing in human subjects; normally, a small (20–80) group of healthy volunteers selected to assess the safety, tolerability, pharmacokinetics, and pharmacodynamics of a drug (see Chapter 11)
Phase II trial	Designed to assess how well the drug works, as well as to continue phase I safety assessments in a larger group (20–300) of volunteers and patients (see Chapter 11)
Phase III trial	Randomized controlled multicenter trials on large patient groups (300–3,000 or more depending upon the disease/medical condition studied) aimed at being the definitive assessment of how effective the drug is, in comparison with current "gold standard" treatment (see Chapter 12)
Phase IV trial	*Postmarketing Surveillance Trial* involving the safety surveillance and ongoing technical support of a drug after it receives permission to be sold (see Chapter 13 on postmarketing surveillance)
IND	Investigational new drug application
IDE	Investigational device exemption
NDA	New drug application
510(k)	Submission to the FDA to demonstrate that the device to be marketed is substantially equivalent to a legally marketed device [21 807.92(a)(3)] that is not subject to a PMA
Off-label	Prescribed or used in a way for a condition not covered by the original FDA cleared or approved intended use and labeling

SIMPLIFIED CLINICAL RESEARCH PROCESS

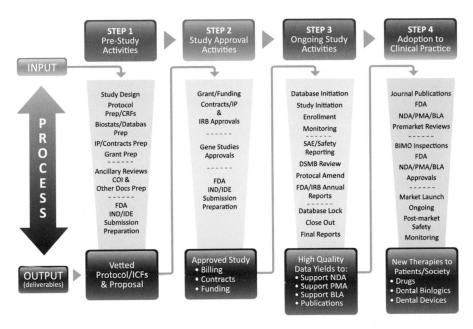

Figure 4.3 Steps involved in clinical research development through the regulatory paths. CRF, case report form; IRB, Institutional Review Board; IP, intellectual property; SAE, serious adverse event; NDA, new drug application; PMA, postmarket approval; BLA, biological license application; COI, conflict of interest; IND, investigational new drug; IDE, investigational device exemption; IP, intellectual property; FDA, Food and Drug Administration.

manufacturing, clinical trials, and eventual regulatory review and approval so that the drug may be legally placed on the market for the health care consumer (see also Figure 1.3). Testing in the laboratory and animal (preclinical) phase can take 3–4 years prior to applying to the FDA to gain permission to initiate human clinical trials. Only 1 out of every 1,000 compounds that undergoes this initial phase of testing will ever reach the human testing phase of development (CDER, 2008). The FDA approves proposals for testing new drugs in humans via the investigational new drug (IND) submission process. The IND regulations are included in Chapter 21 CFR 312. Clinical trials designed to evaluate drugs involve three distinct phases: phase I—designed for establishing dosage safety of the drug (about 1–2 years); phase II—designed to gain preliminary data relative to the efficacy of the drug (2–3 years); phase III—often designed to be multicentered, randomized, and controlled in order to definitively determine efficacy of the drug (3–5 years). The steps involved in the approval of an IND are highlighted in Figure 4.4.

Following phase III clinical trial testing and demonstration of the investigational drug's efficacy, the pharmaceutical manufacturing company will then submit a new drug application (NDA) to the FDA for approval per the regulatory requirements noted in 21 CFR 314—a key section of the NDA application includes the data gained from the clinical trials

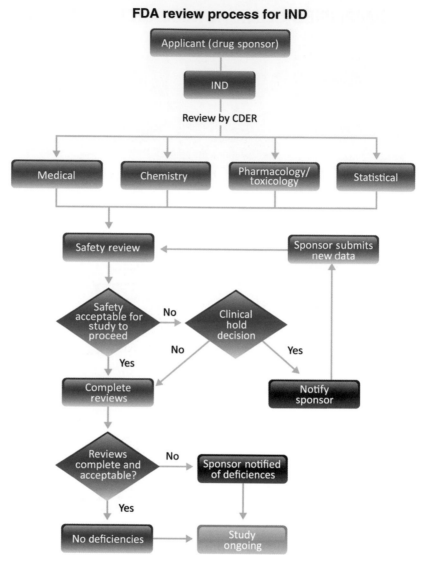

Figure 4.4 Steps involved in the approval of an investigational new drug (IND). Adapted from CDER, Center for Drug Evaluation and Research (www.fda.gov/cder/).

to show sound scientific evidence of the drug is safe and effective according to its labeled intended use. The process for FDA review and approval can be lengthy, often taking more than 2 years, including the time it takes for the FDA to review the initial NDA application (often a submission that contains more than 100,000 pages) and any revisions or resubmissions that are generally requested to address issues and/or deficiencies regarding the initial application (CDER, 2008) (Figure 4.5). Once final FDA NDA approval is obtained, the drug then becomes available for doctors to prescribe; however, communication with the FDA does not end at this point as continual reporting of adverse events and findings from

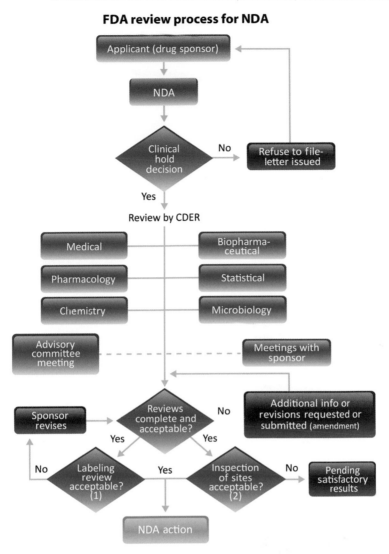

FDA review process for NDA

Figure 4.5 Steps involved in the approval of a new drug application (NDA). Adapted from CDER, Center for Drug Evaluation and Research (www.fda.gov/cder/).

ongoing clinical experiences occur for the life of the drug to ensure its continued safe use in humans. The "life cycle" of development for a new drug is summarized in Figure 4.6.

4.3.2 Devices

The initial step in the approval process for a device is to determine whether or not the product is actually a medical device. While this may seem rather intuitive for some devices such as dental handpieces and articulators, there are other types of "devices" that are not commonly considered in that context (i.e., dental cements, sutures, bone graft material). To eliminate

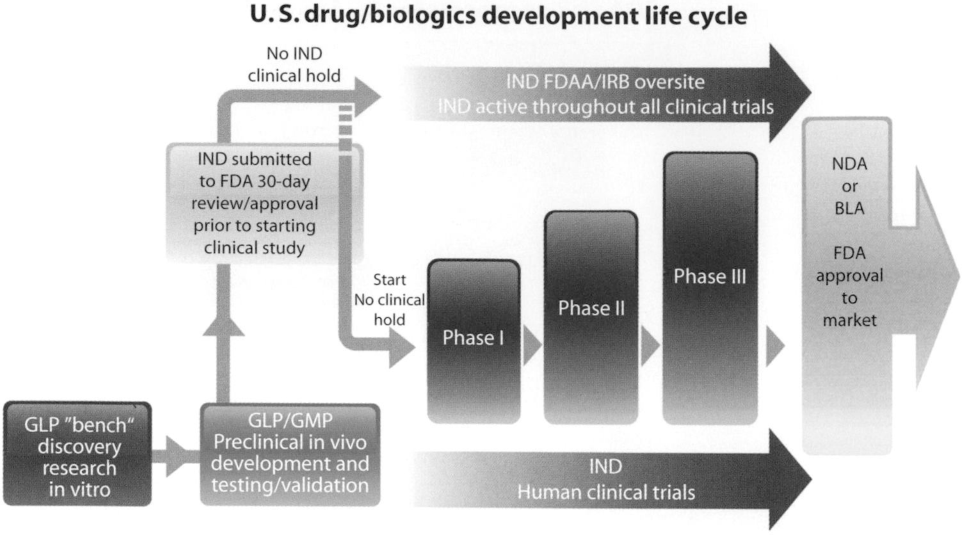

U. S. drug/biologics development life cycle

No IND
clinical hold

IND FDAA/IRB oversite
IND active throughout all clinical trials

IND submitted
to FDA 30-day
review/approval
prior to starting
clinical study

NDA
or
BLA

Start
No clinical
hold

Phase III

FDA
approval
to
market

Phase II

Phase I

GLP "bench"
discovery
research
in vitro

GLP/GMP
Preclinical in vivo
development and
testing/validation

IND
Human clinical trials

Figure 4.6 U.S. Dental Drug/Biologics Life Cycle. Steps involved in the development of a new drug or device. GLP, good laboratory practice; GMP, good manufacturing practice; IND, investigational new drug; NDA, new drug application; BLA, biological license application; FDA, Food and Drug Administration.

confusion, the FDA has very specific definitions regarding what constitutes or is considered a medical device (section 201(h) of the FD&C Act) (CDRH, 2008b)—refer to Table 4.3 for definition. The FDA has established descriptions of roughly 1,700 different "generic" types of devices, and organized them into 16 medical specialties, referred to as panels. These panels (parts) are listed below and a section (subpart) of the "dental" devices panel is shown below (Table 4.4). Each of these "generic" types of devices, described in depth within the appropriate classification panel, is assigned to one of three regulatory classes (CDRH, 2008a). In the United States, medical devices are classified based on a risk profile schema. The "class" of a device is determined by the level of regulatory oversight necessary to assure safety and efficacy of the device. In general, the higher levels of classification (II and III) demand more documentation from the manufacturers upon submitting their premarket review submissions to the FDA. Thus, once it has been determined that the product is a device, it must then be determined the FDA classification of your device into one of three possible risk-based classes. The three classes are described above in the list of definitions: *Class I*—"general controls" (with or without exemptions) (i.e., dental burs, facebows, and preformed crowns); *Class II*—special controls (with or without exemptions) (i.e., cavity varnish, acrylic denture teeth, impression materials); and *Class III*—premarket approval (i.e., dental implants) (Figure 4.7). Unless the product is deemed exempt from the FDA premarket review, the classification of the device will determine the FDA regulatory review process by which the manufacturer has to proceed in order to legally place the product into commercialization. Once it is determined which regulatory review pathway is required, it is then necessary to prepare a premarketing application that includes all relevant data and pertinent information regarding the device's intended use, development processes, manufacturing methods for assuring high quality, labeling, and instructions for

Table 4.4   Panels of medical devices and subpart E of dental device panel/parts.

CFR Title 21—Food and Drugs: Parts 862–892

862	Clinical chemistry and clinical toxicology devices
864	Hematology and pathology devices
866	Immunology and microbiology devices
868	Anesthesiology devices
870	Cardiovascular devices
872	Dental devices
874	Ear, nose, and throat devices
876	Gastroenterology–urology devices
878	General and plastic surgery devices
880	General hospital and personal use devices
882	Neurological devices
884	Obstetrical and gynecological devices
886	Ophthalmic devices
888	Orthopedic devices
890	Physical medicine devices
892	Radiology devices

Subpart E—surgical devices
    Section 872.4120—Bone cutting instrument and accessories
    Section 872.4130—Intraoral dental drill
    Section 872.4200—Dental handpieces and accessories
    Section 872.4465—Gas-powered jet injector
    Section 872.4475—Spring-powered jet injector
    Section 872.4535—Dental diamond instrument
    Section 872.4565—Dental hand instrument
    Section 872.4600—Intraoral ligature and wire lock
    Section 872.4620—Fiber optic dental light
    Section 872.4630—Dental operating light
    Section 872.4730—Dental injecting needle
    Section 872.4760—Bone plate
    Section 872.4840—Rotary scaler
    Section 872.4850—Ultrasonic scaler
    Section 872.4880—Intraosseous fixation screw or wire
    Section 872.4920—Dental electrosurgical unit and accessories

use. For medium-risk Class II devices, the manufacturer is required to submit a Premarket Notification to the FDA. The Premarket Notification is more commonly known as the 510(k) submission. The majority of dental devices on the U.S. market are Class II devices and entered the marketplace via the FDA 510(k) review and clearance process. An essential component of the 510(k) application is the product's preclinical performance data. Such data are required to provide scientific evidence that the Class II device is "substantially equivalent" (SE) to a similar device legally marketed in the United States. The majority of Class II devices do not require clinical trial data to gain FDA 510(k) clearance to enter

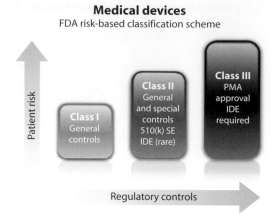

Figure 4.7 Medical device risk classification scheme. IDE, investigational device exemption; PMA, postmarket approval; cGMP, current good manufacturing practice.

the U.S. market. This important point distinguishes the Class II device regulatory pathway from the higher risk Class III device's more stringent regulatory path burden. For Class III devices, the manufacturer must submit a Premarket Approval (PMA) application for FDA review and approval prior to placing the Class III device into U.S. commercialization. Because Class III devices are by definition those devices that support or sustain human life and present a significant potential for causing severe injury or illness should the device fail, the manufacturer is obligated to show clinical trial data that demonstrates the device is "safe and effective" when utilized as intended (Figure 4.8). This stringent regulatory requirement helps the FDA and the manufacturers ensure high-risk devices do not enter the marketplace until they have been carefully tested in a controlled clinical trial setting. Additional information regarding clinical trial submissions will be discussed later in this chapter. Once submitted, the FDA's Center for Devices and Radiological Health is responsible for determining whether or not the device is suitable for marketing and use in the Unites States. The developmental "life cycle" for devices that require an IDE is summarized in Figure 4.9.

4.3.3   Biologics

In recent years, there has been a significant increase in the therapeutic need and demand for more "biologic" approaches to treatment of dental and craniofacial diseases and conditions. This trend has resulted in substantial rises in "biologic" product sales, with global sales expected to reach $105 billion in 2010 (Belsey et al., 2006). Individuals or companies who manufacture biologics are required to hold a license for introduction into interstate commerce. The process for licensure of biologic products is very similar to that for drug approval and this process is handled by the FDA's Center for Biologics Evaluation and Research (CBER) (Kelleher, 2007). Following initial laboratory testing and the appropriate preclinical studies, safety and effectiveness of a biologic are evaluated in human clinical trials (beginning with phase I) under the governance of an IND application. If the findings

U.S. FDA premarket submission content and review process for new dental devices

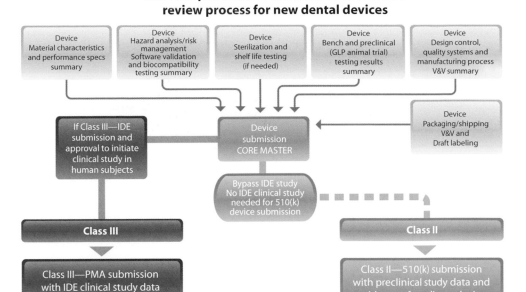

Figure 4.8 Premarket submission process for new dental devices. IDE, investigational device exemption; PMA, postmarket approval; V & V, validation and verification summary.

of the clinical studies demonstrate that the product is safe and effective for its intended use, the data are submitted to CBER as part of a biologics license application for review and approval for marketing. Following approval, the biologic is subject to lot release meaning that the manufacturer is required to perform certain tests on each lot of the product before it is released for distribution. In addition to quality control tests performed by the manufacturer, CBER may perform its own tests to help ensure the safety, purity, potency, and effectiveness of products prior to their release for distribution.

4.3.4 Combination products

With the advent of fields such as tissue engineering and biomimetics, dentistry has seen an increase in cutting-edge technologies that have the potential to incorporate biologics with devices, devices with drugs, and drugs with biologics. A good example of such a product is Gem21S® (Osteohealth Co., Shirley, NY), which combines a drug (platelet-derived growth factor BB, PDGF-BB) with a device (β-tricalcium phosphate) to create a product used in periodontal and bone regenerative procedures (Nevins et al., 2005). To address

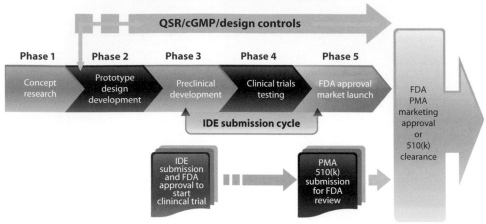

Figure 4.9 Medical and dental device developmental life cycle for devices that require an IDE. IDE, investigational device exemption; PMA, postmarket approval; QSR, quality system regulation; FDA, Food and Drug Administration.

these types of products, the FDA developed the Office of Combination Products (OCP) in 2002. Though this branch of the FDA has broad responsibilities covering the regulatory process for combination products, the primary oversight of these products remains with one of three product regulatory centers: CDER, CBER, or CDRH (OCP, 2008). OCP responsibilities include assignment of a combination product for review and jurisdiction to one of the three centers, insurance of timeliness and consistency of premarket review, assessing appropriateness of postmarket regulation, serving as a liaison between the three centers regarding overlap of jurisdiction of a product if necessary, and update and review regulations regarding combination products. Thus, the OCP is not directly involved in the initial review of the product, but plays an integral role in determining where and how timely it is reviewed.

Because of the complexity associated with how to define many combination devices based upon potentially different applications, the OCP helps the manufacturer define the product's "primary mode of action" or "most important therapeutic action" (2004). Based upon this designation, the product is then given the most appropriate assignment. If this designation does not provide sufficient clarity to properly assign to the appropriate center due to the product having dual independent modes of action, the OCP will then evaluate which center has the "best" expertise to handle review of the product. Once a formal request is made by the applicant for "jurisdictional assignment" to one of the three centers, the OCP has 60 days to determine the most appropriate center for review of the application. Once assigned, the approval process for these combination products then follows the regulatory pathway set forth by the respective center. In instances when approval for different functions of a combination product is needed, dual assignment is necessary and independent reviews of different aspects of the combination product are conducted by the designated centers. For these products, the OCP carries forth the critical function of coordinating correspondence and communication between the centers and the applicant (Kramer, 2008).

4.3.5   Reasons for disapproval of FDA-regulated products

There are a number of reasons that prevent an FDA-regulated product from gaining FDA approval for use in a clinical study or sale in the U.S. market. The primary challenge is preparing and compiling the appropriate and compliant documentation for inclusion in the initial and subsequent applications submitted for FDA review. Though seemingly trivial, this can be a significant challenge and, if done incorrectly, can delay or prevent the clinical study initiation and subsequent successful new product market introductions.

4.3.6   Clinical trials related submission

The FDA regulations specify the information required for proposed clinical trial submissions for investigational drugs and biologics. These detailed requirements are found in 21 CFR 312. Similarly, the requirements for investigational device clinical trials are included in the investigational device exemption (IDE) regulations (21 CFR 812).

In the case of IND or IDE clinical trial submissions, the agency is tasked with reviewing the submission content to ensure the investigational drug, biologic or dental device will be "considered reasonably safe to proceed" into human testing. The FDA conducts a thorough, scientific review of preclinical test results, previous human studies (if any), and product manufacturing information to ensure the product was prepared under current good manufacturing practice (cGMP) conditions.

Certainly, some of the most important information the FDA scrutinize during an IND or IDE review are the clinical study related sections of the submission. The proposed study design and protocol, informed consent forms and data collection forms (CRF) are the essential elements of a clinical trial. Since the creation of the Nuremburg Code (1947), the World Medical Association's adoption of the Declaration of Helsinki (1964), and the International Conference on Harmonization Good Clinical Practice (ICH-GCP) guidelines (1996), numerous regulations have been codified in the United States to protect humans involved in clinical research (also see Chapter 3 on institutional policies related to clinical research regulation).

Significant delays can occur if the agency receives a submission that lacks the statutory content requirements. If deficiencies are significant, the agency may even refuse to review the submission and return it to the applicant.

Some of the most common reasons IND and IDE applications get delayed during the FDA review/approval cycle include those summarized in Table 4.5.

4.3.7   Product premarketing approval submissions

Product premarketing applications such as the NDA (21 CFR 314), BLA (21 CFR 601), and PMA (21 CFR 814) submissions require clinical trial data to demonstrate the product's safety and efficacy. Thus, the aforementioned elements that can delay or prevent a clinical trial from succeeding can have a tremendous impact on whether or not a premarket submission will gain ultimate FDA approval.

Table 4.5   FDA clinical trial submissions: common deficiencies.

IND—drug or biologic clinical trial	
Subject population	• Number of proposed subjects unreasonable • Inadequate inclusion/exclusion criteria
Starting dose/dose regimen	• Insufficient data to justify proposed starting dose/dosing escalation plan • Investigational agent administration risk inadequately described
CMC/cGMP	• Inadequate chemical analysis or descriptions • Investigational agent manufacturing info/documentation inadequate
Safety monitoring	• Adverse event reporting methods/procedures inadequate or absent • Subject treatment discontinuation criteria (stopping rules) absent/unreasonable • Expected adverse events poorly described or absent • Subject long-term follow-up absent or inadequately described

IDE—dental or medical device clinical trial	
IDE not required	• Only significant risk (SR) devices require FDA IDE approval: FDA will refuse to accept IDE application if clinical trial involves a nonsignificant risk (NSR) device
Device development	• Device developed under inadequate design control methods and documentation requirements per the quality system regulation (QSR/cGMP)
Preclinical testing	• *In vitro* (bench) and/or *in vivo* (animal) testing conducted under non-GLP compliant conditions • Inadequate: materials biocompatibility, sterilization validation and/or device performance testing
Study protocol	• Indications for use poorly conceived or absent • Primary/secondary study end points inadequate or confusing • Study design inadequately addresses primary study end points
Risk analysis	• Risk–benefit analysis inadequate or absent • Definitions of adverse events and reporting procedures inadequate or absent
Monitoring	• Study monitoring plan inadequate or absent

4.4   Approved and nonapproved dental-related products

In dentistry, most of the drugs, materials, devices, and biologics routinely used in everyday practice have gone through one of the aforementioned FDA regulatory review processes. This section will highlight some of these products and their regulatory pathways to market entry.

4.4.1   Dental drugs

Systemic medications used for dental-related procedures to manage pain and infections have undergone traditional FDA approval mechanisms, as their use is not limited to the scope of dentistry. However, in recent years, there has been interest in the adjunctive use of systemic medications to treat oral problems such as periodontal diseases. As an example, antimicrobials in the tetracycline family (doxycycline) administered at low doses have been studied in the treatment of periodontal disease (Golub et al., 2001). Initially used off-label, 20 mg doxycycline hyclate (Periostat®, Galderma, Fort Worth, TX) gained FDA approval (2005) for this indication. The effectiveness in the subantimicrobial use of doxycycline is attributed to its ability to modulate the "host response." In doing so, it decreases metalloproteinase enzyme activity, which is a necessary step in the process of periodontal tissue destruction and ultimately bone loss (Golub et al., 1997).

Dentistry has also seen the emergence of locally delivered agents, primarily antibiotics, whose use is limited for localized indications. The most widespread group of these products is locally delivered antimicrobials (Hanes and Purvis, 2003), again for the treatment of periodontal disease. The first of this classification of products to enter the market was Actisite® (ALZA Corp., Palo Alto, CA) approved by the FDA in 1994. Actisite® is comprised of an ethylene/vinyl acetate copolymer containing 12.7 mg tetracycline. It was indicated as an adjunct to scaling and root planing for reduction in periodontal pocket depth.

Oral dentrifices and rinses have also developed over the years and been FDA approved. In 1997, due to its active ingredient triclosan, Colgate's Total® (Colgate-Palmolive, Piscataway, NJ) toothpaste was credited as the first FDA-approved toothpaste to help prevent gingivitis, plaque, and cavities. As it relates to over-the-counter (OTC) oral health aids, another regulatory system is in place that provides oversight for these products. The American Dental Association's (ADA) Council on Scientific Affairs evaluates and disseminates information regarding the safety, efficacy, proper use, and promotional claims of dental therapeutic agents, their adjuncts and dental cosmetic agents used by the public or profession (ADA, 2008). In addition to therapeutic agents such as toothpaste and mouth rinses, the council also determines the safety and effectiveness of materials, instruments, and equipment offered to the profession. Products may be evaluated upon the request of a distributor, manufacturer, or the initiative of the council. The council also works closely with other regulatory and professional agencies in its review of products and only FDA-approved products are eligible to apply for the ADA Seal. Once a product is reviewed by the council, it is determined whether or not it will be granted the "ADA Seal of Acceptance." This seal signifies to consumers that the product has met the council's criteria with respect to safety, efficacy, composition, labeling, packaging, and advertising. Once accepted, a product is continually monitored, and if it is determined at any time that a product no longer meets the standards set forth by the council, it has the sole discretion to withdraw the ADA Seal of Acceptance from the product.

4.4.2   Dental devices and biologics

The use of appropriate materials and devices has historically been a significant component of the practice of dentistry and thus knowledge of materials science and biomaterials has always been a rich component of dental research. In the areas of restorative dentistry and prosthetics, all materials ranging from dental amalgams to ceramic restorations have undergone significant modifications in their compositions and structure, and these have been regulated by the FDA. One of the most long-standing restorative materials, dental amalgam, was first introduced into dentistry in the nineteenth century as a restorative material to treat dental caries. Amalgam is comprised of liquid mercury and a powder containing silver, tin, copper, zinc, and other metal. Because of the mercury component and the potential for release of mercury vapor during placement, removal, and even normal function, questions regarding its toxic effects have surfaced throughout the history of its use. The ADA, established in 1859 (long before the FDA was established), has never prohibited its use, and thus when the FDA emerged, its use was "grandfathered" in and has never been subject to the same processes of review in order to gain "FDA approval" as newer products (FDI Policy Statement/WHO Consensus Statement, 1997). As is the case with most dental restorative and prosthetic materials, amalgams meet the definition of medical devices and regulated by the Food Drug and Cosmetic Act Medical Device Amendments of 1976. As with other medical devices, the FDA's Center for Devices and Radiological Health (CDRH) oversees the marketing authorization reviews and other regulatory oversight activities. Over the past 10–15 years, the increased number of claims citing amalgam to have negative health effects coupled with the improvements in the material properties of other restorative materials has caused the dental patient population to seek more esthetic solutions to their restorative needs. As a result, patients are deferring the use of amalgam, and many dentists no longer present it as a treatment option for dental caries. Some individuals and community groups (i.e., Moms Against Mercury) have even made efforts to enact legislation to eliminate the use of dental amalgams (Kincade, 2008). In response to the increasing "weight" of these external pressures, the FDA has been looking more closely at the health effects resulting from dental amalgam use and has established a web page on its use, issuing a statement that "no valid scientific evidence has shown that amalgams cause harm to patients with dental restorations, except in the case of allergy" (FDA, 2006). However, the FDA plans to modify its current stance on amalgam use and this may include a reclassification (currently classified as Class II). A redefining or reclassification of amalgams could have dramatic influences on clinical practice in that this could mean that amalgam packaging would require new warning labels or that patients would need to provide special consent for its use. The amalgam issue is not unique to the Unites States and, in 2008, caused Norway to be the first country to place a ban on its use (Miller, 2008). Sweden followed suit just a few months later and many other countries are now contemplating similar moves.

4.4.3   Dental and oral implant devices

Because of the enormous growth in implant dentistry over the past 20 years, the FDA has paid considerable attention to the ever-growing number of implant systems made available.

Because implants are "implanted into the body," they were originally categorized as Class III devices and subject to the PMA process, the most stringent of the approval standards. In order to be approved through this process, a minimum of two clinical studies lasting 3 years are required with at least 50 subjects in each study. Due to the rigorous nature of these guidelines, in the "early days" of implant dentistry in the late 1980s and early 1990s, most manufacturers had been able to circumvent this process and market their implants based on "substantial equivalence" to devices that were marketed before 1976 (Medical Device Amendments were enacted). Devices marketed prior to 1976, called "preamendment devices," are not subject to modifications in their method of distribution unless specifically called for by the FDA (Eckert, 1995). Later, however, the FDA reclassified root-form endosseous dental implants and endosseous dental implant abutments from Class III to Class II (special controls). Dental implants are still subject to 510(k) approval (Premarket Notification), yet this process is less rigorous than that for PMA and does not require data from clinical studies with the device. If the device does not otherwise meet the definitions of a Class III device, the manufacturer can seek regulatory approval through a petition seeking to reclassify it to Class I or Class II, and this petition must demonstrate that the new device is SE to one that is currently marketed legally. Instead, these 510(k) applications must include a comprehensive report about the safety and effectiveness of the preexisting device (predicate device) to which the new device is being compared (Health Canada, 2008), as well as accounts of unfavorable or adverse events associated with the "predicate" device (Parr et al., 1992).

Though dental implant systems offer a highly predictable and effective solution to missing teeth, more "biologic" therapeutic replacements of missing tissues and teeth are on the frontier; yet, most of the ones that have reached the marketplace to date have been classified as "devices," though they are assuredly more "biologic" than dental metals, ceramics, and resins. Most of the bone grafting regenerative products, including allograft and alloplast materials, are considered Class II devices. Products that incorporate growth factors, such as GEM21S (PDGF) and INFUSE® (Medtronic, Minneapolis, MN; BMP-2) (Fiorellini et al., 2005), are also considered devices, but due to the inclusion of growth factors, these products were required to undergo the PMA process. Newer products on the horizon, including those that would employ gene and cell therapy approaches, would most likely fall into the classification of biologics, the same designation given to the skin allograft product Alloderm® (LifeCell Corp., Blanchburg, NJ).

4.5   Regulatory processes in Canada, Europe, and other countries

Because many drugs and devices are developed and manufactured in countries outside the United States, the FDA evaluates all premarket data and information regarding these products as part of its approval process for these products. Though most other countries do not have national regulatory agencies as large as the FDA, many do have well-defined regulatory guidelines and approval processes that are similar to those used by the FDA. In neighboring Canada, *Health Canada* is the federal department charged with the responsibility of protecting Canadians through regulating and facilitating the provision of health-related products distributed throughout the country, including foods, pharmaceuticals, medical devices, and biologics (Health Canada, 2008). Many of their approval processes mirror those used by the FDA of the United States. In Europe, manufacturers in the European Union (EU) and abroad must meet CE marking requirements in order to market and distribute their products in Europe. The CE marking (an acronym for the French "Conformite Europeenne"—European Conformity) certifies that a product has met EU health, safety, and environmental requirements set out in European Directives to ensure consumer safety (European Union, 2008). A directive is a legislative act of the EU that requires member states of the EU to achieve a particular result without dictating how that result will be achieved. Thus, some leeway is given on how to achieve this desired outcome; yet, if this outcome is not achieved or if there is lack of compliance with the requirements of the directive, the European Commission may initiate legal action in the European Court of Justice. CE marking provides product access to 27 countries with a consumer base of over 500 million people. Unlike the FDA, there is no list of all products that are subject to this process; thus, manufacturers must determine if a product requires CE marking. Other countries including those in Asia, Africa, and the Middle East have stringent guidelines. Yet, because many of these places do not have guidelines that are as stringent as those in the United States, important ethical issues must be considered regarding the conduct of "high-risk" research with highly innovative, but still premature therapies (i.e., gene therapy, stem cells). Because some of the populations within these regions are desperate for treatments and cures for disease, they can be considered "vulnerable populations" for studies involving these types of therapies.

4.6   Summary

In conclusion, there is a long history of dentistry's involvement in the development of innovations for new devices for oral reconstructive therapies ranging from tooth restorative materials to oral implants, and more recently, growth factors for tissue engineering. Having an adequate understanding of the regulatory processes involved in the approval of new devices, drugs, and biologics is critical for the end-user clinician to have available new technologies for the dental office setting. Regulatory agencies such as the FDA and the EMEA have led the way to work with researchers and clinicians to streamline these processes to accelerate and heighten safety of new therapies. As discussed throughout this text, the bench-to-chairside application of oral health innovations requires concerted efforts of collaborative teams to allow these new therapies to be fully realized. Once the new technologies enter the clinic, the continued process of surveillance (Chapter 13) and chairside-clinical practice (Chapter 16) will dictate the utilization and impact of these new innovations on dental patients in practice communities.

References

ADA. 2008. *About the ADA Seal of Acceptance: Guidelines for Participation*. Available online at http://www.ada.org/ada/seal/guidelines.asp. Accessed on May 30, 2009.
Belsey MJ, Harris LM, Das RR, Chertkow J. 2006. Biosimilars: initial excitement gives way to reality. *Nature Reviews Drug Discovery* 5:535–536.

CDER. 2008. *New Drug Approval Process*. Available online at http://www.drugs.com/fda-approval-process.html. Accessed on May 30, 2009.

CDRH. 2008a. *Classify Your Medical Device*. FDA. Available online at http://www.fda.gov/cdrh/devadvice/313.html. Accessed on May 30, 2009.

CDRH. 2008b. *Is the Product a Medical Device? Medical Device Definition*. Available online at http://www.fda.gov/cdrh/devadvice/312.html. Accessed on May 30, 2009.

Code of Federal Regulations. 2009. In: Federal (ed.). Government Printing Office. Available online at http://www.fda.gov/oc/orgcharts/orgchart.html. Accessed on May 30, 2009.

Eckert SE. 1995. Food and Drug Administration requirements for dental implants. *Journal of Prosthetic Dentistry* 74:162–168.

European Union. 2008. *CE Marking—Program Overview*. Available online at http://www.export.gov/cemark/CE. Accessed on May 30, 2009.

FDA. 2006. *Joint Meeting of the Dental Products Panel (CDRH) and the Peripheral and Central Nervous System Drugs Advisory Committee (CDER)*. Meeting on September 6–7, 2006. Gaithersburg, MD.

FDA U.S. 2008. *FDA. What We Do?* Available online at http://www.fda.gov/opacom/morechoices/mission.html. Accessed on May 22, 2009.

FDI Policy Statement/WHO Consensus Statement on Dental Amalgam. 1997. Accessed on March 8, 2007.

Fiorellini JP, Howell TH, Cochran D, Malmquist J, Lilly LC, Spagnoli D, Toljanic J, Jones A, Nevins M. 2005. Randomized study evaluating recombinant human bone morphogenetic protein-2 for extraction socket augmentation. *Journal of Periodontology* 76:605–613.

Golub LM, Mcnamara TF, Ryan ME, Kohut B, Blieden T, Payonk G, Sipos T, Baron HJ. 2001. Adjunctive treatment with subantimicrobial doses of doxycycline: effects on gingival fluid collagenase activity and attachment loss in adult periodontitis. *Journal of Clinical Periodontology* 28:146–156.

Golub LM, Lee HM, Greenwald RA, Ryan ME, Sorsa T, Salo T, Giannobile WV. 1997. A matrix metalloproteinase inhibitor reduces bone-type collagen degradation fragments and specific collagenases in GCF during adult periodontitis. *Inflammation Research* 46:310–319.

Hanes PJ, Purvis JP. 2003. Local anti-infective therapy: pharmacological agents. A systematic review. *Annals of Periodontology* 8:79–98.

Hart FL. 1952. A history of adulteration of food before 1906. *Food Drug Cosmetics Law Journal* 7:5.

Health Canada. 2008. *About Health Canada*. Available online at http://www.hc-sc.gc.ca/ahc-asc/activit/index-eng.php. Accessed on May 29, 2009.

Kelleher KR. 2007. *FDA Approval of Generic Biologics: Finding a Regulatory Pathway*. Michigan *Telecommunications and Technology Law Review* 14:245–264.

Kincade K. 2008. *FDA Revises Its Position on Dental Amalgams*. Available online at http://acedental.blogspot.com/2008/06/fda-revises-its-position-on-dental.html. Accessed on May 29, 2009.

Kramer MD. 2008. *FDA's Office of Combination Products: Roles, Progress, and Challenges*. FDA. Available online at http://www.fda.gov/oc/combination/jmdr2005.html. Accessed on November 8, 2008.

Miller A. 2008. *Norway Becomes First Country to Ban Amalgam*. Available online at http://www.naturalnews.com/022943.html. Accessed on May 30, 2009.

Nevins M, Giannobile WV, Mcguire MK, Kao RT, Mellonig JT, Hinrichs JE, Mcallister BS, Murphy KS, Mcclain PK, Nevins ML, Paquette DW, Han TJ, Reddy MS, Lavin PT, Genco RJ, Lynch SE. 2005. Platelet-derived growth factor stimulates bone fill and rate of attachment level gain:

results of a large multicenter randomized controlled trial. *Journal of Periodontology* 76:2205–2215.

OCP. 2008. Overview of the office of combination products. Available online at http://www.fda.gov/oc/combination/overview.html. Accessed on May 29, 2009.

Parr R, Kohler A, Clark G, Barcome A. 1992. *A Premarket Notification 510(k); Regulatory Requirements for Medical Devices*. August edn. Washington, D.C.: U.S. Government Printing Office.

5

Clinical and translational research grantsmanship: funding opportunities and obtaining research support

Bruce L. Pihlstrom, DDS, MS, **and**
Michael L. Barnett, DDS

5.1   Introduction and chapter overview

Clinical research is defined as a research that is conducted with human subjects (or on material of human origin such as tissues, specimens, and cognitive phenomena) in which a researcher directly interacts with human subjects, but it does not include *in vitro* studies using human tissues not linked to a living individual (NIH Office of Extramural Research, 2008b). There are many definitions of translational research, but for the purpose of this chapter, it is defined as a research that moves findings from basic research to clinical applications for the diagnosis, treatment, and/or prevention of human disease (see also Chapter 1 on clinical and translational research).

Assuming that the cost of a research project has been realistically estimated, a source of funding must be identified. Funding is generally available to answer important research questions, but one must be willing to actively seek support through grants and contracts, accept criticism, modify research plans when necessary, work collaboratively with others, and above all, be persistent.

Investigators should be aware of potential funding sources and the procedures for obtaining financial support from government, industry, or foundations. Researchers must be realistic in their funding expectations, have research goals that are aligned with those of the funding agency, and be willing to accept the terms and conditions of the funding source. The goal of this chapter is to assist investigators in obtaining funding for their research by (1) identifying funding sources and opportunities; (2) reviewing grant-writing basics; and (3) describing the oversight required by sponsoring agencies or industry.

5.2 Funding sources and opportunities

There are three main sources of funding for research: government, industry, and foundations. Government generally supports research that has broad implications for public health and clinical practice while industry supports research to gain government approval for marketing devices or drugs, to support advertising claims, or to obtain endorsements such as the American Dental Association's Seal of Acceptance. Foundation support is usually limited to research that meets the foundation's specific goals and will not be covered in this chapter. Investigators interested in pursuing foundation funding should contact foundations that specifically target their area of research, for example, the American Dental Association Foundation (American Dental Association Foundation, 2008).

5.2.1 Government support for oral health research

The main source of government funding for oral health research worldwide is U.S. National Institutes of Health (NIH) (U.S. National Institutes of Health Homepage, 2008), specifically the National Institute of Dental and Craniofacial Research (NIDCR) (National Institute of Dental and Craniofacial Research Homepage, 2008). While the bulk of its research funding is targeted to U.S. investigators, the NIH supports research in other countries if resources such as investigator expertise, instrumentation, or patient populations are not available in the United States and if the findings are applicable to people living in the United States. Because it is the primary source for oral health research funding in the world and because there is considerable variation in funding and application procedures among other countries, NIH funding opportunities will be emphasized in this chapter. Investigators who are interested in obtaining government funding from other countries should consult public health agencies in those countries for funding opportunities and application procedures.

Research funding may also be available from U.S. agencies such as the Agency for Healthcare Research and Quality (AHRQ) (Agency for Healthcare Research and Quality (AHRQ) Homepage, 2008). In general, oral health research funding from U.S. government agencies other than the NIH is quite limited and is aimed at specific research areas. For example, AHRQ funding is targeted to improve quality, safety, efficiency, and effectiveness of health care. Prior to making application to the U.S. government for oral health research, the specific agency website and program staff should be consulted regarding funding availability.

5.2.2 United States National Institutes of Health (NIH)

The NIH is composed of 27 institutes and centers and is an agency of the U.S. Department of Health and Human Service. It is administratively headquartered in Bethesda, Maryland, and annually invests over $28 billion in medical research (2009). About 80% of NIH funding is awarded through a competitive review process to more than 325,000 researchers at over

3,000 universities, medical and dental schools, and other research institutions in every U.S. state and around the world. About 10% of the NIH's budget supports research by nearly 6,000 scientists in its own laboratories. For an overview of NIH activities, the reader is referred to the NIH website (U.S. National Institutes of Health Homepage, 2008).

5.2.2.1 National Institute of Dental and Craniofacial Research (NIDCR)

The mission of the NIDCR (National Institute of Dental and Craniofacial Research Homepage, 2008) is "to improve oral, dental, and craniofacial health through research, research training, and dissemination of health information." With a 2009 annual budget of approximately $400 million, much of its mission is accomplished by conducting and funding basic and clinical research and by funding research training and career development programs.

Funding mechanisms   The NIDCR supports research through a variety of funding mechanisms under the broad categories of grants, contracts, and cooperative agreements. Table 5.1 lists definitions of common NIH terms. Additional definitions can be found at the NIH Office of Extramural Grants glossary website (NIH Office of Extramural Research, 2008b).

The purpose of an NIH grant can be determined by its letter prefix: research grants have an "R" prefix, training grants have a "T" prefix, and fellowship awards have an "F" prefix. Table 5.2 outlines five common research grant mechanisms supported by the NIDCR. The "Gold Standard" NIH funding award is the Research Project Grant, commonly referred to as a "R01" grant. The R01 grant provides funding for health-related research; it can be investigator initiated or can be awarded in response to a program announcement (PA) or a request for application (RFA) issued by NIH institutes or centers. Other common forms of grant support are the R03 mechanism for small grants and the R21 mechanism for exploratory grants. The cooperative agreement, or "U" award mechanism, is usually used for larger grants and clinical trials where substantial oversight by NIH and/or NIDCR program officials is needed.

Small Business Technology Transfer (STTR) and Small Business Innovation Research (SBIR) grants are also available from the U.S. government NIH, Centers for Disease Control (CDC), and the Food and Drug Administration (FDA) to stimulate STTR, the commercialization of innovative technologies, and to encourage participation by socially and economically disadvantaged small business and women-owned businesses (NIH Office of Extramural Research Small Business Research Funding Opportunities, 2008).

Identifying funding opportunities   All applications for U.S. government funding must be submitted in response to a Funding Opportunity Announcement (FOA) posted on the Grants.gov website (Grants.gov Homepage, 2008) or the websites of specific granting agencies. Oral health FOA can be found at three locations: (1) the Grants.gov website (Grants.gov Homepage, 2008), (2) the NIH Guide for Grants and Contracts (NIH Guide for Grants and Contracts, 2008), and (3) the NIDCR website (National Institute of Dental and Craniofacial Research Homepage, 2008).

Researchers may apply for NIH funding in response to two broad categories of FOA: (1) "Parent Funding Announcements" (NIH Office of Extramural Research PA, 2008) such as those listed in Table 5.2, and (2) solicitations for applications, such as NIDCR RFA or PA. Applications submitted in response to NIH Parent Announcements are unsolicited,

Table 5.1   Definitions of common NIH terms (see also http://grants.nih.gov/grants/glossary.htm).

Coinvestigator	An individual involved with the PI in the scientific development or execution of a project. The coinvestigator (collaborator) may be employed by, or be affiliated with, the applicant/grantee organization or another organization participating in the project under a consortium agreement. A coinvestigator typically devotes a specified percentage of time to the project and is considered "key personnel." The designation of a coinvestigator, if applicable, does not affect the PI's roles and responsibilities as specified in the NIH Grants Policy Statement (NIH GPS)
Contract	An award instrument establishing a binding legal procurement relationship between NIH and a recipient obligating the latter to furnish a product or service defined in detail by NIH and binding the institute to pay for it
Contracting officer	Government employee authorized to execute contractual agreements on behalf of the government
Cooperative agreement (U series)	A support mechanism used when there will be substantial federal scientific or programmatic involvement. Substantial involvement means that, after award, scientific or program staff will assist, guide, coordinate, or participate in project activities
Grant	Financial assistance mechanism providing money, property, or both to an eligible entity to carry out an approved project or activity. A grant is used whenever the NIH institute or center anticipates no substantial programmatic involvement with the recipient during performance of the financially assisted activities
Grantee	The organization or individual awarded a grant or cooperative agreement by NIH that is responsible and accountable for the use of the funds provided and for the performance of the grant-supported project or activities. The grantee is the entire legal entity even if a particular component is designated in the award document. The grantee is legally responsible and accountable to NIH for the performance and financial aspects of the grant-supported project or activity
Peer review	A system for evaluating research applications using reviewers who are the professional equals of the applicant
Principal investigator (PI)	An individual designated by the grantee to direct the project or activity being supported by the grant. He or she is responsible and accountable to the grantee and NIH for the proper conduct of the project or activity. Also known as Program Director or Project Director

(Continued)

Table 5.1   Definitions of common NIH terms (see also http://grants.nih.gov/grants/ glossary.htm). (*Continued*)

Priority score	A numerical rating of an application reflecting the scientific merit of the proposed research relative to stated evaluation criteria
Program	A coherent assembly of plans, project activities, and supporting resources contained within an administrative framework, the purpose of which is to implement an organization's mission or some specific program-related aspect of that mission.
Program official (PO)	The NIH official responsible for the programmatic, scientific, and/or technical aspects of a grant

investigator-initiated applications that are based on the ideas and research interests of investigators and aligned with the overall mission of the NIH institute to which the application is submitted. Over 80% of all grants funded by the NIH are submitted under Parent Funding Announcements as investigator-initiated applications.

Program Announcement for Grants   PA are solicitations for grant applications in specific research areas from one or more NIH institutes and centers (such as the NIDCR). PAs are developed in response to gaps in research needs identified by an analysis of institute research and in response to input from the research community and the public. PAs are published in Grants.gov (Grants.gov Homepage, 2008), in the NIH Guide for Grants and Contracts (NIH Guide for Grants and Contracts, 2008), and on the various NIH institute and center websites. In addition to describing the type of research being solicited, PAs include instructions and requirements for submission such as whether foreign applicants may apply. Applications submitted in response to a PA are reviewed by a study section, a panel of expert peer convened by the NIH Center for Scientific Review (CSR) (NIH Center for Scientific Review (CSR) Homepage, 2008).

Program Announcement With Institute Review (PAR) for Grants   A PAR is a funding announcement that is the same as a PA except that applications received in response to a PAR are peer reviewed by a panel of experts convened by the issuing NIH institute, for example, NIDCR. Institutes issue a PAR when special peer review expertise is needed that is not usually available in a CSR Study Section. For example, NIDCR phase III clinical trial applications are reviewed by a peer review panel, called a Special Review Group (SRG), convened by the NIDCR rather than by a study section convened by the NIH CSR.

Request for Applications for Grants (RFA)   In addition to issuing a PA or a PAR, NIH institutes such as the NIDCR often issue a RFA in areas of scientific priority identified by a NIH institute or center. A RFA differs from a PA and a PAR in that a specific amount of money is set-aside for funding applications in an RFA. For example, if the NIDCR wishes to solicit applications for clinical research aimed at reducing health disparities, it may issue

Table 5.2   Common NIH funding mechanisms (see also http://grants.nih.gov/grants/funding/funding_program.htm#RSeries).

Research Project Grant (R01)	• Most commonly used NIH grant mechanism • Often referred to as the "Gold Standard" NIH grant • Supports discrete, specified research project • No specific dollar limit unless specified in Funding Opportunities Announcement (FOA) • Advance permission required for $500 K or more (direct costs) in any year) • Generally awarded for 3–5 years • Can be investigator initiated or can be in response to a PA or RFA • R01 research plan proposed by applicants must be related to the stated program interests of one or more of the NIH institutes and centers such as the NIDCR • See parent FOA at /grants/guide/pa-files/PA-07-070.html
Exploratory/Developmental Research Grant Award (R21)	• Encourages new, exploratory, and developmental research projects by providing support for the early stages of project development. Sometimes used for pilot and feasibility studies • Limited to up to 2 years of funding • Combined budget for direct costs for the 2-year project period usually may not exceed $275,000 • No preliminary data are generally required • See parent FOA at /grants/guide/pa-files/PA-06-181.html
Small Grant Program (R03)	• Provides limited funding for a short period of time to support a variety of types of projects, including pilot or feasibility studies, collection of preliminary data, secondary analysis of existing data, small, self-contained research projects, development of new research technology, and so on • Limited to 2 years of funding

(Continued)

Table 5.2 Common NIH funding mechanisms (see also http://grants.nih.gov/grants/
funding/funding_program.htm#RSeries). (*Continued*)

	• Direct costs generally up to $50,000 per year
	• Not renewable
	• See parent FOA at /grants/guide/pa-files/PA-06-180.html
Research Project Cooperative Agreement (U01)	• Supports discrete, specified, circumscribed projects to be performed by investigator(s) in an area representing their specific interests and competencies
	• Used when substantial programmatic involvement is anticipated between the awarding institute and center
	• One of many types of cooperative agreements
	• No specific dollar limit unless specified in FOA
Small Business Research Funding Opportunities (R41, R42, R43, R44)	• Intended to stimulate technological innovation in the private sector and partnership of ideas and technologies between innovative small business concerns and research institutions
	• Depending on the specific award, phase I awards normally may not exceed $100,000 total for a period normally not to exceed 6–12 months. Phase II awards normally may not exceed $750,000 total for a period normally not to exceed 2 years
	• See NIH website for more information and parent FOA (http://grants1.nih.gov/grants/funding/sbir.htm)

a RFA and "set-aside" a specific amount in its budget for funding applications submitted in response to the RFA. A RFA specifies the amount of money that has been "set-aside" for the research and the approximate number of grants that are expected to be funded. Like a PAR, all grant applications received in response to a RFA are peer reviewed by a SRG convened by the issuing NIH institute or center. In contrast to a PA or a PAR, applications may only be submitted once in response to a RFA. However, NIH institutes can reissue a RFA to solicit additional applications if more are needed, if applications submitted in response to a RFA are not responsive to the RFA, or if the applications are judged by peer review to have insufficient scientific merit to warrant funding. Even though a RFA specifies "set-aside" funding, the issuing NIH institute is under no obligation to fund a specific number of grants or actually commit funding to grant applications received in response to a RFA.

Request for Proposals (RFP) for contracts   When the NIH or one of its institutes wishes to target a specific research need, it may issue a RFP for contracts. A contract obligates the successful applicant to provide a product or service defined in detail by the terms and conditions of the award. Thus, a RFP has information that allows applicants to prepare proposals for the specified contract research that includes descriptions and specifications of deliverables, expected performance schedule, and any other issues that could affect fulfilling the contract.

RFPs are published in the NIH Guide for Grants and Contracts and have a single application receipt date (NIH Guide for Grants and Contracts, 2008). Unlike grants, for which the research topic and plan are proposed by the applicant investigator, applicants bid on the research that is specified in the RFP. Proposals submitted in response to a RFP are reviewed by a special peer review group convened by the issuing NIH institute and are subject to close oversight by the NIH after the contract is awarded.

5.2.3   Industrial support for oral health research

The fundamental difference between government and industry-supported research is that funding for research by governmental agencies is generally obtained through an investigator-driven grant application process, whereas funding by industry is an integral component of product development and is generally "company driven." In many respects, therefore, industry-supported research is similar to a government research contract except that industry does not issue a public RFP.

Industry typically conducts and funds clinical research based on a product development timetable, rather than on the basis of a structured grant application process. Accordingly, for a clinical trial, industry would seek to identify study sites that have appropriate expertise and a solid track record of conducting clinical trials for specific product indications. Sites for a clinical trial are usually selected on the basis of expertise, publication history in the area of investigation, previous experience in working with industry, and, very importantly, having an established working relationship with the funding company. Prior to placing clinical studies at a new site, companies often conduct short "validation" studies to determine if the site is capable of sound execution and dealing with the logistical demands of a specific study.

While the process of selecting and funding clinical study sites is usually company driven, academic investigators with appropriate experience may contact companies to make them aware of potential new sites for clinical research. The importance of personal relationships in this process cannot be overestimated. Academic investigators seeking a relationship with industry should arrange to meet key corporate research and development directors to personally convey their qualifications. This is often done at meetings such as those held by the American and International Associations of Dental Research. Companies also rely on consultants to help identify additional study sites, especially when branching out into new products or when making new product claims for existing products.

Since industry is focused on product development with rigid timetables, it has some basic requirements for academic clinical study sites (Barnett, 1995, 2002). The study site should have an established infrastructure for conducting the clinical research, including a dedicated clinical trial facility, adequate support staff, and, very importantly, a demonstrated ability to meet timelines for recruiting the required number of qualifying subjects. Because product development timetables do not conform to academic schedules, principal investigators and support staff at academic sites must be flexible so studies can be initiated and completed within an acceptable time frame. The institution must also be in compliance with FDA regulations relating to good clinical practice as set forth in Title 21 Parts 11, 50, 54, 56, and 312 of the Code of Federal Regulations (CFR 21 Part 312 Investigational New Drug Application, 2008; United States Code of Federal Regulations Part 21, 2008) (see also Chapters 3 and 4 on institutional and federal regulations of clinical research).

Industry may provide a protocol to the academic investigator or it may collaborate with the academic investigator to create a new protocol. In either case, the investigator needs to propose a realistic study budget for consideration by the company. This can only be done after the protocol has been agreed upon. The budget should reflect costs of conducting the study and a reasonable indirect cost rate. Since most companies have considerable experience in funding research, investigators should not present an artificially low budget in the belief that this will help them "get" the study, nor should they propose a greatly inflated budget in the belief that companies have deep financial pockets. The investigator also should be aware that if the contractual budget is insufficient to cover study costs, his or her institution will be obligated to fund the deficit so the study can be completed as specified in the contract.

It is important that investigators who collaborate with industry avoid any misconceptions about the nature of the relationship. A common investigator misconception is that companies expect that tested products *must* be shown to be effective. This is definitely not the case. Reputable companies conduct studies to test hypotheses and support research that is based on rigorous scientific standards and guidelines. The investigator is obligated to conduct industry research in accordance with these standards so that the outcome is accurate, reproducible, and not the result of poor execution. Industry wants to obtain the most accurate product assessment, not necessarily the most favorable one.

5.2.4 Negotiating industrial agreements

Industry support of academic research involves a formal contractual agreement that specifies the obligations of each party and defines their relationship. The contract is generally negotiated by the company's legal department and the academic institution's office of sponsored research. It covers a wide range of study issues including study protocol and budget, payment terms, liability, number of subjects required to complete the research, study completion date, final study report requirements, confidentiality, publication and/or presentation of results, intellectual property rights, and dispute resolution.

Depending on the individual situation, academic investigators may or may not actively participate in the actual contract negotiations between their institution and a sponsoring company. However, it is imperative that they have input into the agreement and carefully review all its conditions prior to acceptance. This is especially important for subject recruitment and study completion timelines. If investigators are unrealistically optimistic in estimating the time required for subject recruitment, they will be unable to complete the study on schedule. Moreover, the company will lose confidence in the investigator and will be unlikely to support future research at the institution.

In order for a research contract to be agreed upon by both parties, it is necessary to have a study protocol and budget. It is critical that the principal investigator and company representatives agree on the study protocol and resolve any issues prior to ratifying the contract and initiating the study. Once the study begins, principal investigators are required to strictly adhere to the study protocol and cannot unilaterally change anything during the course of the study. If a protocol change is necessary, prespecified contractual provisions for changing the protocol must be followed. Regulatory agencies, such as the FDA, have strict requirements for conducting clinical trials, and failure to adhere to established protocols, including stipulations for revision, can invalidate trial results. The final protocol, negotiated study budget, and a payment schedule are included in the contract signed by the company and a legal representative of the principal investigator's institution. Investigators at academic institutions should never independently enter into contractual agreements with any organization or individual to support research unless they have specific and designated legal authority to act on behalf of their institution.

Contractual issues dealing with publication and/or presentation of study results are often controversial because the respective needs and values of academia and industry may appear to be in conflict. However, if each party understands the rationale of the other, issues of publication and presentation of results can usually be resolved satisfactorily. On the one hand, it is necessary for companies to recognize the importance of publications in faculty promotion and the academic tradition of open and free communication. Any blanket prohibition of publication is unlikely to be acceptable to an academic institution. On the other hand, there are circumstances under which it is reasonable for an industry sponsor to require a delay in publication or presentation of study results. Premature disclosure of results could jeopardize the patentability of a discovery and industry sponsors commonly request prior review of publications or presentations in order to prevent disclosure of information that could adversely affect intellectual property rights. Companies may also wish to have the right to provide nonbinding suggestions to the author.

There may be limited circumstances under which it is legitimate for a company to deny the right to publish study results. These include studies to validate a study site and exploratory studies conducted in the early stages of product testing. Unlike pivotal phase III clinical trials, these studies are not conducted to support product approval or claims and have little scientific or clinical value other than providing a company with proprietary information. It is important that investigators, their institutions, and industry sponsors agree on publication limitations *prior to* the start of the study *so that publication is not dependent upon study results.*

Investigators must be aware of contractual agreements of confidentiality that are made to prevent the dissemination of confidential information. In addition to this binding contract of confidentiality, investigators should always use discretion in disclosing anything but the most basic information about corporate research until the results are formally released to the public. This may seem contrary to the general spirit in academia of open communication and sharing, but it is another instance in which the needs and values of academia should be balanced with those of industry. The extremely competitive nature of product development and marketing must be recognized by academic investigators if they are to participate in industry-sponsored research. Indeed, dedicated clinical research facilities should operate in a way that visitors are unable to discern either the sponsorship or products being tested.

5.3   Grant-writing basics and developing research proposals

Funding agencies typically require specific procedures and formats for grant applications. In planning an application, it is important to ascertain the procedures and forms required by the specific funding agency. Since the NIH is the major public funder of oral health research in the world, tips for developing a successful NIH application will be outlined in this section. Prospective NIH grant applicants should access the NIH Office of Extramural Research (OER) websites (NIH Office of Extramural Research, 2008a, 2008c) for current information about applying for grants. It is also advisable to access specific NIH institute websites (e.g., NIDCR (National Institute of Dental and Craniofacial Research Homepage, 2008)) and contact NIH program officials for information and advice regarding applying for research support. Valuable grant-writing tutorials are available through various NIH institutes such as the National Institute of Allergy and Infectious Diseases (NIAID) (NIH National Institute of Allergy and Infectious Diseases, 2008a). Portions of the following section were developed using these resources.

5.3.1   Planning

5.3.1.1   What is the question?

Defining a significant, easily understood, and answerable research question is the most important, and often most difficult, part of any research proposal. Too often, applicants propose research that is based solely on available resources such as study populations or available expertise. While these are critical for any clinical study, unless the specific question to be answered is clearly defined, it is impossible to plan and design a sound research proposal. Defining the research question allows the hypothesis to be developed and the study designed appropriately. The research question should be clearly articulated in writing, preferably in one simple sentence, and must have clear significance for the funding agency. In the case of the NIH, answering the question must benefit clinical practice or the public health. In the case of industry, the question must be significant in terms of the specific product development goals of the company.

5.3.1.2   Time management

Investigators must be realistic about the time required to complete an application for research funding. It is very time consuming to get organized, refine ideas, collect preliminary data, write the application, and obtain institutional approval for the budget and Institutional Review Board (IRB) approval. To be successful, one must develop an internal timeline for each phase of application development and realistically assess if there is sufficient time available. In developing timelines, one must allow for unforeseen events that can, and usually do, occur. It is also important to know that successful applicants generally spend many evening and weekend hours preparing grant proposals. If insufficient time is available to develop a well-reasoned and well-written application, it will have little likelihood of funding and the time spent on preparing the application will have been wasted.

5.3.1.3   Planning within your institution

Researchers must plan funding applications in collaboration with their institution because research funding, whether from government or industry, is awarded to an institution or university and not to an individual such as the principal investigator (PI) or project director. The role of the PI is to prepare the application for funding and to conduct and direct the research project on behalf of his or her institution. The PI is responsible and accountable to the grantee institution and the sponsor for all aspects of the research. This includes obtaining necessary institutional approvals, financial management, treatment and evaluation of patients, assuring data integrity, adherence to research protocol, data analysis, and reporting results. If multiple PIs are designated by the applicant organization, they share authority and responsibility for leading and directing all aspects of the research project; each is responsible and accountable to the applicant organization and the sponsor for the proper conduct of the research.

Because there is such a close working relationship between the PI and the applicant organization, it is important that the PI begin working with their institutional office of sponsored research or grant support office while planning an application. The PI informs the institution about the budget and the type of grant or contract that is being considered while the institution's grant support office typically provides assistance in the application process, information about institutional deadlines, and advice on budget development. By meeting with their institutional grant support office, investigators can also plan their timeline so they can meet institution and sponsor deadlines for submission. It is especially important that new investigators become familiar with their institution's key contacts, internal procedures, and requirements for grant submissions, and develop working relationships with experienced people such as individuals in their grants support office, another investigator, or a departmental administrator who can help them prepare grant applications.

5.3.2   Key components of an application for research funding

Organizations that fund research have varying procedures for submitting funding applications. Many funding agencies follow the NIH format that requires a title, abstract, budget, background, specific aims, research design and methods, enrollment plans, and human subject assurances. Page limitations and type font are also specified by most funding agencies. Clear, concise writing is appreciated by reviewers. NIH applications are limited to a maximum number of pages that will be reduced from 25 to 12 pages beginning in January 2010 (Implementation Timeline for Enhancing Peer Review, 2008).

Anyone who is new to grant writing should seek a mentor who can provide guidance and assistance in preparing the application. This mentorship is fundamental to success and it is very important to have experienced grant writers read and critique applications prior to submission. Preferably, mentors will have served as peer reviewers and will share their previous successful (and unsuccessful!) grant applications and peer reviews of their applications.

5.3.2.1   Title

The title of a grant application should clearly and simply describe the topic of the research proposal. The title is important because it is the first thing read by reviewers and it gives a critical first impression. If the title does not clearly describe the proposed research or is difficult to understand, the chances of obtaining favorable peer review can be jeopardized from the outset. For example, a title such as "Changes in Periodontal Disease over Time" is simpler, more descriptive and easier to understand than a wordy and overly complex title such as "Prospective Longitudinal Temporal Variations in Periodontal Disease Parameters."

In general, it is better to have a shorter rather than a longer title. Funding agencies often specify limitations on title length that cannot be exceeded. Acronyms should never be used in titles and should only be used sparingly in the abstract or body of funding applications.

5.3.2.2 Abstract

The abstract is a critically important part of any proposal for research funding because, along with the title, it gives an important first impression to peer reviewers. A well-written abstract is vital to an application's success because it is usually read quickly by busy peer reviewers to get an overview of the proposed research. It must clearly state the rationale, long-term objective, specific aims, methods, and significance of the research. The abstract must also concisely describe why the proposed research is innovative and important. First-person tense should be avoided and past accomplishments of the investigator should not be included in the abstract.

If the abstract is difficult to understand, uses scientific jargon and acronyms, does not convey the importance of the proposed research, or does not clearly describe research aims and methods, it will have a negative effect on peer reviewers. If funded, the abstract of NIH applications become public information and it should be understandable to lay people and should not include proprietary or confidential information.

The abstract should be written before writing the application and then rewritten and finalized after the application is complete. Writing the abstract prior to beginning the application forces one to focus on the main points of the research and clearly articulate them in writing. As the application is developed, the emphasis or, indeed, the entire purpose or design of the proposed research may evolve into something entirely different than initially conceived. For these reasons, the final abstract should be the last thing that is written after the application has been completed. In writing the final abstract, one must make sure that the goals, objectives, specific aims, design, and significance of the research accurately reflect the proposed research. All too often, because of the need to meet application deadlines, abstracts are poorly written and do not accurately summarize the proposed research. This is a fatal flaw in any application. Most successful grant applicants have the final abstract critically reviewed by several colleagues who have peer review experience and who do not have a vested interest in the application.

5.3.2.3 Specific aims

The specific aims of a research proposal are the objectives to be accomplished by the proposed research. The specific aims must be clearly and concisely stated because successful research cannot be based on vague or unclear objectives. The specific aims should not be overly ambitious or confused with long-term research goals. They are concise statements of what is to be specifically accomplished by the research and can be thought of as "yardsticks" that will be used to measure success of the proposed research.

The specific aims section of a proposal usually begins with a sentence or two that states the long-term goal and specific hypothesis of the research project. This is followed by 3–4 specific aims that make it possible to answer the research question posed by the hypothesis. The specific aims should be listed and numbered in order of planned achievement. They should be written and organized so they can be easily understood by the target audience of peer reviewers. If the specific aims are stated in convoluted sentences or in a complex manner, the application will fail because the research expectations are unclear.

5.3.2.4   Background and significance

The purpose of this section is to summarize the available scientific knowledge related to the topic of the grant application and make a strong case to the funding organization for the importance of the proposed research. For NIH applications, the significance of the research must be to increase scientific knowledge and improve the public health, and must be related to the core mission of the institute to which the application is directed. It should be explicitly stated how achieving the specific aims will advance scientific knowledge or clinical practice. This section should be about 2–3 pages in length and should demonstrate familiarity with the field by critically reviewing the relevant scientific literature in a way that establishes a need for the proposed research. The applicant should be aware that if important work is omitted, reviewers will assume that the applicant is unaware of it or chose to ignore it, either of which will reduce enthusiasm for the research proposal.

The significance of the proposed research should emanate from the background that establishes the need for the proposed study or identifies gaps in existing knowledge. The background forms the basis for the importance of the study and frequently informs the design of the research plan. For example, if a phase III clinical trial is being proposed, pertinent animal research, human observational studies, and early clinical trials should be reviewed in the background section. It would be essential to review this literature so that a compelling argument for conducting a large, multicenter phase III trial could be made. Unless a clear and compelling reason for the research can be made based on existing science, there is little chance that an application will receive favorable peer review.

5.3.3   Preliminary studies/progress report

Although not an explicit requirement, peer reviewers generally expect R01 NIH applications to include preliminary data, preferably in published form. These data demonstrate that the proposed research is feasible and that the investigator has the ability to actually carry out the research plan. A critical interpretation of preliminary data also gives reviewers confidence that the applicant has carefully considered various design and methodological alternatives. It is always best to use one's own data and published work for preliminary studies, but it is also possible to use other published data as preliminary data. This is especially true for large epidemiologic projects or phase III clinical trials when data from studies published by other investigators can be particularly informative in designing research. Although preliminary data are not required for NIH R03 and R21 grant applications, it is usually helpful to include at least some data in these applications to assure reviewers that the proposed work is feasible and that the applicant is capable of actually doing the proposed research.

If the application is a renewal of an existing grant, a progress report must be included that gives the inclusive dates of the research project, a summary of progress toward the specific aims stated in the previously funded grant, and a list of publications based on the grant. It is important to bear in mind that future success is often based on previous performance. If a particular line of research or a specific investigator has not been productive in the past, future prospects for funding will be poor.

5.3.4   Research design and methods

The research design and methods section makes up most of the narrative portion of a grant application. Since reviewers tend to focus on this section, it must describe the research design and methods in sufficient detail so that they can evaluate the proposal. However, care must be taken not to include excessive methodological details or include anything that is not planned for the research project. Extreme detail is unnecessary, increases the chances of making mistakes, and gives reviewers more to criticize. Achieving the right balance in detail is important. Those who are new to grantsmanship should seek the advice of experienced grant writers concerning the level of detail needed for this section.

The research design, protocol, methods, procedures, data management, and analyses used to accomplish the specific aims of the project must be described. It is usually best to describe the overall design of the proposed research followed by a description of the methods that will be used to achieve each specific aim. To make it easy for reviewers, each specific aim should be listed and followed by a description of the proposed methods to achieve the aim. It is critical to describe how data will be collected, analyzed, and interpreted. If new technology is proposed, it is important to describe advantages over existing technology.

For clinical research, it is especially important to include a flow diagram and timetable of the proposed study because it makes it easy for reviewers to understand the design and methods. It also forces one to clearly conceptualize and plan research. The flow diagram should include the number of subjects to be enrolled, schedule of enrollment, baseline and follow-up assessments, measures to be recorded, and any interventions that might be planned. If a clinical trial is proposed, a CONSORT (Moher et al., 2003) type diagram should be included.

A detailed section must be included that describes data collection, data management, and statistical analysis. Sample data collection forms should be included in an appendix to demonstrate how data collection and management are planned. Applications are strengthened by validation of data forms in actual use.

It must be borne in mind that all applications for clinical research will have their data analysis plan peer reviewed. In order to receive a favorable review, a clear and rational statistical plan for data analysis must be included. Sample size estimates, sampling and research design, data definitions, and analytic models must be described. It is essential that the data analysis plan be reviewed, and preferably written, by a well-qualified biostatistician. Many peer reviewers feel that it is imperative that a biostatistician and a data manager be included as one of the key personnel in clinical research applications.

Many successful grantees feel that it is helpful to include a discussion of the potential difficulties and limitations of the proposed research. However, one must be careful to present any limitations or difficulties in a positive way that demonstrates how these issues will be addressed in the proposed study. If difficulties are acknowledged without a clear plan for dealing with them, peer reviewers will often use these issues to criticize the application.

5.3.5   Budget

Ideally, the research budget should be developed after the research plan and methods are completed. In reality, however, the budget is often developed simultaneously with the research plan because it is often subject to funding agency limitations. Prior to preparing a budget for an application, it is important to access current information on the funding agency's website and consult with funding agency staff. Because the PI's institutional grants management office or office of sponsored projects must approve the budget before it can be submitted on behalf of the institution, it is best to begin working with this office early in the process of preparing an application. Grants management personnel are very familiar with funding agency requirements and can provide current budgetary information such as personnel fringe benefit rates and facilities and administrative (F&A) costs that the institution has negotiated with the funding agency. The F&A costs are often referred to as "indirect costs" and can vary widely among institutions. All applications from institutions outside of the United States are limited to an 8% F&A cost rate.

With the exception of RFA and PA that may require detailed budgets and applications from foreign institutions, the NIH requires modular budgets in $25,000 increments for grants having annual direct costs of $250,000 or less in all years. Direct costs for NIH grants include:

- Salaries and fringe benefits of PI and supporting staff
- Equipment and supplies
- Travel expenses
- Fees and supporting costs for consultant services
- Contract services (also called subaward)
- Costs for consortium participants
- Inpatient and outpatient costs for human subjects
- Alterations and renovations to facilities
- Publications and other miscellaneous expenses

NIH modular budgets do not receive annual increases for inflation; all anticipated funding must be built into the original budget request. Usually, the same number of $25,000 modules is included each year, except for special needs such as equipment. A narrative statement is required to justify yearly variations in the number of modules. NIH budgets must also include justifications for personnel and consortium costs. All personnel, the number of months devoted to the project, and their roles must be specified in sufficient detail to justify their effort. Before preparing the personnel budget, current information regarding salaries and fringe benefits should be obtained from the PI's institution.

For NIH grant applications, detailed budgets are required if the annual direct budget exceeds $250,000 in any year of the proposed grant, if the application is from a foreign institution, or if it is a SBIR or STTR grant application. Instructions for preparing detailed budgets may be found at the NIH Office of Extramural Research Website (NIH Office of Extramural Research Modular Grant Applications, 2009). Prior approval for acceptance of grants seeking $500,000 or more (direct costs) is required from a NIH institute or center.

5.3.6   Other issues in grant preparation

For NIH grants, all investigators involved in human subjects' research must be certified as having completed training in human subject protection. All funders of human subjects' research require written assurance that the planned research has the approval of an independent ethics committee, commonly referred to as an IRB. Some agencies require that this approval be documented at the time of application submission, while others, such as the NIH, require IRB approval prior to actually making an award, but not when the application is submitted.

NIH applications require information on inclusion of children and vulnerable populations, enrollment projections by ethnicity and gender, plans for data sharing, and assurances regarding use of fetal tissue and embryonic stem cells. It is imperative that applicants check for updates regarding specific issues with program staff or on the appropriate NIH website prior to submitting their applications.

5.3.6.1   Peer review of NIH applications

The scientific merit of NIH applications is assessed through a rigorous process of peer review by independent experts who are drawn mainly from a wide range of academic institutions. These peer reviewers receive only modest payment for their services and share their time and expertise for the public good. Review criteria are transparent and published in NIH FOAs. Applications submitted under NIH Parent Funding Announcements and NIH PA are usually reviewed by a standing study section convened by the NIH CSR (NIH Center for Scientific Review (CSR) Homepage, 2008), and applications submitted in response to RFAs and PARs are reviewed by a SRG convened by the NIH institute that issued the RFA.

After discussion using specific and transparent review criteria, each peer reviewer assigns a scientific priority score to grant applications. These scores are then averaged for a final priority score that reflects the scientific merit of the application. If the application is reviewed by a standing CSR study section, it will also receive a percentile score that reflects how the application fared in comparison to other applications that were submitted. Not all applications are scored because applications receive a "streamlined review" if all peer reviewers agree that they are in the bottom one-half of applications being reviewed. Streamlined applications are not discussed and do not receive a priority score. However, all applicants receive a confidential critique of their application, known as a "Summary Statement," which contains a narrative critique of their application by the assigned reviewers.

While funding initiatives such as a RFA may list additional review criteria, investigator-initiated NIH research grant applications are reviewed using specific criteria as given below. These criteria are periodically modified and investigators should always check the NIH website for peer current review criteria prior to preparing an application:

1. **Significance:** Does this study address an important problem? If the aims are achieved, how will scientific knowledge or clinical practice be advanced? What will be the effect of these studies on the concepts, methods, technologies, treatments, services, or preventions that drive this field?

2. **Approach:** Are the conceptual or clinical framework, design, methods, and analyses adequately developed, well integrated, well reasoned, and appropriate to the aims of the project? Do the PI or PIs acknowledge potential problem areas and consider alternative tactics? For multiple PI applications, is the leadership plan consistent with and justified by the project's aims and each PI's expertise?

3. **Innovation:** Is the project original and innovative? For example, does it challenge existing paradigms or clinical practice or address an innovative hypothesis or critical barrier to progress in the field? Does the project develop or use novel concepts, approaches, methods, tools, or technologies?

4. **Investigators:** Are the PI or PIs and other key personnel appropriately trained and well suited to carry out this work? Is the work proposed appropriate to the experience level of the PI or PIs and other researchers? Do the PI or PIs and investigative team bring complementary and integrated expertise to the project (if applicable)?

5. **Environment:** Does the scientific environment or environments contribute to the probability of success? Do the studies benefit from unique features of the scientific environment or environments or subject populations? Do the studies use useful collaborative arrangements? Is there evidence of institutional support?

Reviewers also assess the involvement of human subjects and protections from risks related to participation in research, assess the adequacy of plans for including subjects from both genders, representative racial and ethnic groups, and children, and evaluate plans for recruiting and retaining subjects. The NIH website should always be reviewed for current information on these issues before submitting an application. Following peer review, applications receive secondary review by each NIH institute's National Advisory Research Council that may make recommendations for funding. Final funding decisions are made, however, by the individual NIH institutes, not by the Council.

Common problems cited by peer reviewers in NIH applications include the following (NIH National Institute of Allergy and Infectious Diseases, 2008b):

- Problem not important enough.

- Study not likely to produce useful information.

- Studies based on a shaky hypothesis or data.

- Alternative hypotheses not considered.

- Methods unsuited to the objective.

- Problem more complex than investigator appears to realize.

- Not significant to health-related research.

- Too little detail in the research plan to convince reviewers the investigator knows what he or she is doing, that is, no recognition of potential problems and pitfalls.

- Issue is scientifically premature.

- Overambitious research plan with an unrealistically large amount of work.

- Direction or sense of priority not clearly defined, that is, experiments do not follow from one another and lack a clear starting or finishing point.

- Lack of focus in hypotheses, aims, or research plan.

- Lack of original or new ideas.

- Investigator too inexperienced with the proposed techniques.

- Proposed project on a fishing expedition lacking solid scientific basis, that is, no basic scientific question being addressed.

- Proposal driven by technology, that is, a method in search of a problem.

- Rationale for experiments not provided, that is, why they are important or how they are relevant to the hypothesis.

- Experiments too dependent on success of an initial proposed experiment. Lack of alternative methods in case the primary approach does not work out.

- Proposed model system not appropriate to address the proposed questions.

- Relevant controls not included.

- Proposal lacking enough preliminary data or preliminary data do not support project's feasibility.

- Insufficient consideration of statistical needs.

- Not clear which data were obtained by the investigator and which were reported by others.

Whether from new or experienced researchers, most first submissions of NIH grant applications are not funded. Successful applicants must be able to deal with rejection and respond to specific peer review comments in an amended application. Simply stated, those who give up and are not persistent in seeking NIH funding will not be successful. *Successful applicants accept criticism and use it to their advantage. They do not give up!*

NIH policy allows one amended application to be submitted in response to scientific peer review. Applicants who fail to receive funding after two submissions may resubmit only if the application can be considered to be a new application by virtue of being substantially different in content and scope (DHHS NIH—New NIH Policy on Resubmission (Amended) Applications, 2008).

5.3.7   Industry review

Most often, industry supports clinical research at academic institutions based on an established protocol. This does not preclude an investigator from applying for support for research that may lead to a new product claim, help to elucidate a mechanism of action, or answer some other question of interest to a company. In such a case, a company might base its review on the study relevance to the company, investigator experience, regulatory implications for a new claim, and study cost. When proposing research to industry, particular attention should be paid to presenting a budget that truly reflects cost. When conducting studies at academic institutions, companies recognize that indirect cost rates can vary considerably among potential sites and often result in marked disparities in budget proposals from different institutions for the same protocol. All things being equal, this may place some institutions at a competitive disadvantage in obtaining industry support for clinical or translational research.

5.4   Oversight of funded clinical research

See also Chapter 3 on institutional guidelines for clinical research.

5.4.1   Industry

Monitoring of clinical trials is an essential component of good clinical practice as set forth in Title 21 subpart 312.56 of the Code of Federal Regulations (CFR) (CFR 21 Part 312 Investigational New Drug Application, 2008). Under this regulation, the sponsor (i.e., the company conducting the clinical trial) is required to monitor the progress of the clinical investigation to assure that it is being conducted in accordance with the study protocol and in compliance with all relevant good clinical practice provisions. Although CFR subpart 312.56 refers specifically to studies conducted by the sponsor under an investigational new drug (IND) application, it is customarily applied to *any* clinical trial conducted on behalf of a sponsor.

It is important that investigators understand oversight requirements so that the role of the study monitor is not misconstrued during site visits. The FDA has published guidance for sponsors concerning their obligations and the responsibilities of clinical trial monitors (DHHS FDA Guidance for Industry—Monitoring Clinical Trials, 1988). The fundamental role of the study monitor is to assure the integrity of the clinical trial, and to formally document the findings of site visits. The monitor serves as the primary interface between the sponsor and the clinical site and has responsibility for such items as assuring that the protocol is being followed, subject records are complete and up-to-date, IRB requirements are fulfilled, and that activities agreed to by the investigator have not been delegated to previously unspecified staff. The monitor has a key role in assuring that data submitted to the FDA, another regulatory body, and/or used for claim support are accurate and complete. It is, therefore, essential that the investigator understands and accepts his or her obligations when conducting a clinical trial and the need to work in concert with the study monitor to meet all FDA requirements.

5.4.2   Government grants management and oversight

See NIH National Institute of Allergy and Infectious Diseases, 2008c.

When a grant is awarded by the NIH, the institution receives a Notice of Grant Award that allows the PI to begin using government funds to conduct research proposed in the grant application. Grantees have considerable flexibility in making changes in their approved project or budget without NIH approval. With some exceptions, grantees can extend a project period without additional funds (no cost extension). Unless budgetary changes constitute a change in scope, grantees can also transfer work to a third party through consortium agreements and contracts and rebudget funds for expenses such as patient care or equipment. Specific NIH approval is required for spending money more than 90 days before the award date, changing the grantee organization, adding a foreign component to a domestic award, or making any change in the research project that constitutes a change in scope (such as changing the specific aims).

Once a NIH research project is underway, the PI and the grantee institution are required to submit a number of reports, including quarterly reports, financial status reports, invention reports, annual progress reports, continuation applications, and meet audit requirements. Annual certification of IRB approval must be submitted with each yearly continuation application. It is important to note that, although the PI has a major role in preparing the reports, they are actually submitted by the institution's grant support or business office. This is another reason why PI must have a close working relationship with the grants management office at their institution.

Unless there are allegations of research misconduct or financial mismanagement, the NIH does not usually conduct site visits for grants. However, the NIH frequently conducts site visits and interacts with investigators who have been awarded cooperative agreements and contracts. The purpose of these site visits is to assist the grantee institution and the investigators in carrying out the research specified in the contract or cooperative agreement. It also provides the NIH with an opportunity to assess whether the research is being conducted as planned in a timely manner. If adequate progress is not being made, the NIH has the authority to terminate contracts or cooperative agreements.

Clinical trials are a very special type of clinical research that require a data and safety monitoring plan approved by the granting institute of NIH and the applicant's IRB. This plan describes oversight and monitoring to ensure the safety of participants and the validity and integrity of the data. The level of monitoring must be consistent with the risks and the size and complexity of the clinical trial. Prior to the accrual of human subjects, a detailed data and safety monitoring plan must be submitted to the applicant's IRB and to the funding entity for approval. Adverse events must be reported to the IRB, the NIH funding Institute or Center, and other appropriate offices or agencies. This NIH policy requirement is in addition to any monitoring required by 45 CFR Part 46 (DHHS Title 45 Part 46 Protection of Human Subjects, 2008). NIH policy specifically requires the establishment of a Data and Safety Monitoring Board (DSMB) for multisite clinical trials involving interventions that entail potential risk to the participants, and generally for all NIH defined phase III clinical trials. The DSMB is appointed by the funding institute (such as the NIDCR) and primarily reports to it. The DSMB meets at least annually, and has regular communication with the investigator and the program official of the funding institute on issues related to patient safety and data integrity.

5.5   Conclusion

Adequate funding for clinical research is essential; without funding, research cannot be conducted. Support is available for clinical research, but investigators must take an active role in pursuing funding whether from government or industry. It is critical that clinical and translational researchers be aware of application procedures, requirements, review, and oversight of funded research projects. They must also seek the counsel of successful, experienced, and funded researchers, and their institution's office of sponsored research or grants management office. First and foremost, however, they need to understand that to be successful in obtaining public funding for research, they must submit carefully prepared grant applications, use peer review to their advantage, and be persistent.

References

Agency for Healthcare Research and Quality (AHRQ) Homepage. 2008. Available online at http://www.ahrq.gov/. Accessed November 2008.

American Dental Association Foundation. 2008. Available online at http://www.ada.org/ada/adaf/grants. Accessed November 2008.

Barnett ML. 1995. Ethical issues in sponsored clinical research. *Journal of Dental Research* 74: 1129–1132.

Barnett ML. 2002. University-industry relationships in dentistry: past, present, future. *Journal of Dental Education* 66:1163–1168.

CFR 21 Part 312 Investigational New Drug Application. 2008. Available online at http://www.accessdata.fda.gov/scripts/cdrh/cfdocs/cfcfr/CFRSearch.cfm?CFRPart=312. Accessed November 2008.

DHHS FDA Guidance for Industry—Monitoring Clinical Trials. 1988. Available online at http://www.fda.gov/RegulatoryInformation/Guidances/ucm126400.htm. Accessed November 2008.

DHHS NIH—New NIH Policy on Resubmission (Amended) Applications. 2008. Available online at http://grants.nih.gov/grants/guide/notice-files/NOT-OD-09-003.html. Accessed November 2008.

DHHS Title 45 Part 46 Protection of Human Subjects. 2008. Available online at http://www.access.gpo.gov/nara/cfr/waisidx_00/45cfr46_00.html. Accessed November 2008.

Grants.gov Homepage. 2008. Available online at http://www.grants.gov/applicants/search_opportunities.jsp. Accessed November 2008.

Implementation Timeline for Enhancing Peer Review. 2008. Available online at http://grants.nih.gov/grants/guide/notice-files/NOT-OD-08-118.html. Accessed November 2008.

Moher D, Schulz KF, Altman DG. 2003. The CONSORT statement: revised recommendations for improving the quality of reports of parallel-group randomised trials. *Clinical Oral Investigations* 7:2–7.

National Institute of Dental and Craniofacial Research Homepage. 2008. Available online at http://www.nidcr.nih.gov/. Accessed November 2008.

NIH Center for Scientific Review (CSR) Homepage. 2008. Available online at http://cms.csr.nih.gov/AboutCSR/Welcome+to+CSR. Accessed November 2008.

NIH Guide for Grants and Contracts. Available online at http://grants.nih.gov/grants/guide/index.html. Accessed November 2008.

NIH National Institute of Allergy and Infectious Diseases. 2008a. *All About Grant Tutorials*. Available online at http://www.niaid.nih.gov/ncn/grants/default.htm. Accessed November 2008.

NIH National Institute of Allergy and Infectious Diseases. 2008b. *Common Problems Cited by Peer Reviewers*. Available online at http://www.niaid.nih.gov/ncn/grants/cycle/part04.htm#e3. Accessed November 2008.

NIH National Institute of Allergy and Infectious Diseases. 2008c. *Managing Your Grant*. Available online at http://www.niaid.nih.gov/ncn/grants/cycle/part11a.htm. Accessed November 2008.

NIH Office of Extramural Research. 2008a. *Electronic Submission of Grant Applications*. Available online at http://era.nih.gov/ElectronicReceipt/prepare_app.htm. Accessed November 2008.

NIH Office of Extramural Research. 2008b. *Glossary and Acronym List*. Available online at http://grants.nih.gov/grants/glossary.htm. Accessed November 2008.

NIH Office of Extramural Research. 2008c. *Planning Your Application*. Available online at http://grants.nih.gov/grants/planning_application.htm. Accessed November 2008.

NIH Office of Extramural Research PA. 2008. Available online at http://grants.nih.gov/grants/guide/parent_announcements.htm. Accessed November 2008.

NIH Office of Extramural Research Modular Grant Applications, 2009. Available online at http://grants.nih.gov/grants/funding/modular/modular.htm. Accessed October 2009.

NIH Office of Extramural Research Small Business Research Funding Opportunities. 2008. Available online at http://grants.nih.gov/grants/funding/sbirsttr_programs.htm. Accessed November 2008.

United States Code of Federal Regulations Part 21. 2008. *Food and Drugs Parts 1–99*. Available online at http://www.access.gpo.gov/nara/cfr/waisidx_01/21cfrv1_01.html. Accessed November 2008.

U.S. National Institutes of Health Homepage. 2008. Available online at http://www.nih.gov/index.html. Accessed November 2008.

6

Data management in oral health research

Bruce A. Dye, DDS, MPH, **and Jules T. Mitchel,** MBA, PhD

6.1   Introduction

Good data management practice (GDMP) promotes the collection of quality data and facilitates meaningful data analysis. Data management is more than just the collection and manipulation of data, but a system that affects most aspects of a study—from study design and planning to data analysis and project termination. An important objective of data management is to prevent data entry and logic errors from being introduced to the data collection database. Another objective is to maximize the availability of clean and analyzable data that can be converted to an analytical database. It is at this stage that a database becomes available to investigators, statisticians, epidemiologists, and other data users.

Although the definition of "data management" seems intuitive, the term varies by research and informatics applications. Oral health research, like other health research activities, is conducted in a plethora of study designs, such as clinical studies, trials, survey research, and so on. Practicing good data management requires recognizing that study designs and requirements are case specific. While data management standards are useful, elements of "best practices" identified in one study design setting may not be applicable to another research activity.

Clarifying terminology and reviewing elementary concepts are essential to understanding GDMP. Data are defined as observations and facts consisting of numbers, text, graphics, and other images that are recordable, and a database is an organized collection of related data (Hoffer et al., 2002). Database management consists of identifying structures for data storage, processes for data manipulation, and implementing mechanisms that ensure data safety (Silberschatz et al., 2002). Although the term data management is ubiquitous in research, defining data management is more nuanced. For example, in research using existing data, which is often referred to as secondary data analyses, data management usually refers to those practices that lead to the building of an analytical data set for the study, such as acquiring and merging data sets, reviewing and adjusting for missing data, creating derived variables, and so on. For purposes of this chapter, we are including a discussion on defining variables in research protocol to illustrate key issues regarding data management in oral health research.

An awareness of some data management issues typically arises when the study protocol is being prepared. The study protocol is a comprehensive document describing the operational characteristics of the study, including outlining the rules for the conduct of the study. A detailed protocol promotes uniformity of data collection and minimizes misclassification when multiple examiners or interviewers are involved in data collection. A detailed protocol also promotes data quality during data handling and transfer to a master collection database when there are multiple study sites or multiple periods of data collection.

6.2   Developing a data management plan

GDMP begins with the development of a data management plan (DMP), which should be initiated after the study protocol is written. The DMP should not only describe the basic elements of data collection and analysis, but should also address data use and warehousing. Moreover, the plan should establish guidelines for accessing sensitive data and data sharing, which are important considerations for any IRB review. Figure 6.1 displays key concepts in developing a data plan. The essential features of a DMP include identifying study variables and designing data collection forms, describing the system architecture, identifying how data are to be entered and edited, describing the process for accessing the data for analysis, outlining controls to protect confidential information and minimize disclosure, and archiving of the data. The database architecture is essentially the hardware (the computing and processing systems) and software (the data manipulation applications) that are necessary to make the database functional. The final consideration in the development of a DMP focuses on creating an analytical database and providing data files for analyses.

The DMP should also identify the key personnel responsible for data processing and oversight. Typically, the data management responsibility for a study resides with the data manager. In smaller studies, the principal investigator (PI) or another research team member may also serve as the data manager. An important function of the data manager is to oversee the production of administrative or interim reports that assess the study's ongoing performance regarding enrollment and recruitment goals, as well as monitoring adverse effects and overall safety. The data manager regulates access to the database, ensures that the collection database does not contain perturbed data, and oversees the production of analytical databases for the research team and other investigators. These gatekeeper duties are essential in maintaining the integrity of the collected data for posterity. Additional activities in which a data manager may participate are (1) defining the study variables, (2) identifying the permitted responses or value ranges, (3) assigning the codes for data entry, (4) developing the data collection forms (paper or electronic), (5) designing the edit/validation check specifications, and (6) maintaining the audit system for data edits.

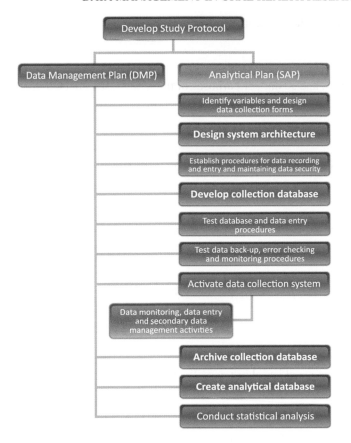

Figure 6.1 Diagram for key concepts in developing a data plan.

6.3   Defining variables

6.3.1   Creating a codebook

Coding the data is the process of taking observations or responses from study subjects and transforming this information into alphanumeric characters that can be entered into a computer. The size of a database is directly dependent upon the number of variables and permitted responses. Once the variables are identified, a codebook is created. The codebook is the data dictionary for the study and is considered an official record of the study. A codebook minimally contains the variable name and description, an abbreviated name, and the codes used for the permitted responses or values. In larger studies, the codebook may contain additional information describing variable source, hard edits, and so on. An example of a hard edit would be reporting the lower right first molar (#30) missing in the first sequence of a dental exam, and having the data collection system's software automatically code all subsequent observations for #30 as missing. Figure 6.2 displays examples of numerous types of variables created for the components of an oral health examination of the National Health and Nutritional Examination Survey (NHANES). For

Variable name	Abbreviated name	Permitted values	Code	Hard edit
Subject identifier—sequence number	SEQN	Range of values	–	–
Subject recumbent during exam	OHAPOS	Yes No Cannot assess	= 1 = 2 = 9	Missing if <5 years old
How would you describe the condition of your teeth? Would you say…	OHQ010	Excellent Very good Good Fair Poor Refused Do not know	= 1 = 2 = 3 = 4 = 5 = 7 = 9	Missing if <2 years old
Does your mouth feel dry when you eat a meal?	OHQ115	Yes No Refused Do not know	= 1 = 2 = 7 = 9	Missing if <18 years old
During the past 12 months, was there a time when you needed dental care but could not get it at that time?	OHQ770	Yes No Refused Do not know	= 1 = 2 = 7 = 9	If no, skip to end
What were the reasons that you could not get the dental care you needed?	OHQ780	Could not afford it Insurance did not cover it Dentist too far away Another dentist did not recommend it Unable to take time off from work Expected the problem to go away	= A = C = D = F = G = J	–
Upper right central incisor	OHX08TC	Primary tooth present Permanent tooth present Dental implant present Tooth not present Dental root fragment present Cannot assess	= 1 = 2 = 3 = 4 = 5 = 9	–
Subject is edentulous	OHXEDENT	Yes No Cannot assess	= 1 = 2 = 9	If yes or cannot assess, end exam
Presence of at least one tooth with decay	OHXDECAY	Yes No Cannot assess	= 1 = 2 = 9	–
Presence of at least one tooth with a dental restoration	OHXREST	Yes No Cannot assess	= 1 = 2 = 9	–
Caries experience category	OHDCE	Yes No	= 1 = 2	Missing if edentulous
Coronal caries: upper right central incisor	OHX08CTC	Sound primary tooth Missing due to dental disease Primary tooth with surface condition Missing due to other causes Missing due to dental disease but replaced Sound permanent tooth	= D = E = K = M = R = S	If "D, E, M, R, S, U X, Y" Skip OHX08CSC and code as missing

Figure 6.2 Selected oral health variables from the National Health and Nutrition Examination Survey (NHANES) Codebooks.

		Unerupted	= U	
		Missing due to other causes but replaced	= X	
		Tooth present, condition cannot be assessed	= Y	
		Permanent tooth with surface condition	= Z	
Coronal caries: surface calls for upper right central incisor	OHX08CSC	Lingual surface caries	= 0	–
		Facial surface caries	= 2	
		Mesial caries	= 3	
		Distal caries	= 4	
		Lingual surface restorations	= 5	
		Facial surface restorations	= 7	
		Mesial restoration	= 8	
		Distal restoration	= 9	
Caries experience: excluding third molars	OHDDMFT	0–28 teeth	= 0–28	Missing if edentulous
		Cannot calculate	= 99	
Upper right central incisor mid-facial pocket depth measurement	OHX08PCM	0–12 mm	= 0–12	Missing if <18 years old
		Cannot assess	= 99	
Upper right central incisor mid-facial recession measurement	OHX08CJM	–12–12 mm	= –12–12	Missing if <18 years old
		Cannot assess	= 99	
Upper right central incisor mid-facial loss of attachment	OHX08LAM	0–24 mm	= 0–24	Missing if OHX08PCM or OHX08CJM is missing or "99"
		Cannot calculate	= 99	
P. gingivalis (Pg) antibody titer level	DEPPG	Range of values	= 40–22885	–
Maximal incisal opening	OHXMAXIN	0–65 mm	= 0–65	If > 65, code 65
		Cannot assess	= 99	

Figure 6.2 (Continued)

instance, the administrative variable assessing if a subject received a recumbent dental exam, OHAPOS has the following three permitted responses: yes, no, and cannot assess. Each response is assigned a code value for data entry (yes = 1, no = 2, and cannot assess = 9).

6.3.2   Administrative/meta versus research data

Variables are typically classified as either administrative or research. Metadata or administrative data are information about the data and are often collected to monitor the performance of the data collection system and to assist in the management of the study (O'Carroll et al., 2003). The larger and more complex the study, the greater the amount of administrative data that will be collected. Administrative data include the personal contact information of study subjects as well as the time, date, and location of data collection. Quality control information such as a repeat examination, a duplicate test, or a second specimen collection that would be used to calculate reliability statistics is another example of administrative data. Another example of administrative data is the information collected during pharmaceutical studies and trials that is required to demonstrate regulatory compliance, such as adverse event monitoring data (Gallin and Ognibene, 2007).

The study subject's unique identifier is a key administrative variable. This unique identifier not only links various forms and tests results to the appropriate subject, but it also promotes data confidentiality by eliminating the need to inscribe forms, specimen containers, and other items with a subject's name. In large studies, the study subject may have a unique identifier for the data collection database, but a separate unique identifier for the analytical database. Data collection centers and laboratory facilities as well as examiners, interviewers, and other staff directly involved in data collection should have unique identification numbers. Having unique identifiers facilitates performance reporting and the ongoing review of the potential data errors. The early detection of errors allows for interventional measures, such as examiner retraining, which would assure the gathering of more accurate results during data collection.

Research data, on the other hand, are comprised of the outcome, explanatory, and exposure variables. These variables provide the information necessary to conduct data analyses relevant to the study's objectives. Although all members of the study team should have some input in identifying and selecting the research variables, it is the responsibility of the PI to remain cognizant of the data collection burden for study subjects and to prevent the data collection efforts from expanding exponentially beyond the scope of the study aims (McFadden, 2007). Likewise, failure to minimally collect important data during the active phase of the study will negatively impact future analyses. Consequently, under the management of the lead statistician, key members of the study team should prepare a draft Statistical Analytical Plan (SAP). This analysis plan will facilitate the identification of key variables required for analyzing the study aims and will minimize the possibility of collecting inadequate data during the study.

6.3.3   Questionnaire versus examination data

Typically, oral health research data are collected through two mechanisms: an examination or a questionnaire. Questionnaires may be constructed to use both close-ended and open-ended questions. A close-ended question is partnered with a set of permitted answers that the subject is asked to choose from. The variable asking a respondent to describe the condition of their teeth (OHQ010) is an example of a close-ended question and uses an ordinal scale to code the responses (Figure 6.2). An ordinal scale is a ranking of mutually exclusive categories into a measurement scale where there is a hierarchical relationship between the categories. For the variable OHQ010, the rank order ranges from excellent $(= 1)$ to poor $(= 5)$. Another example of a close-ended question is variable OHQ115, which asks the respondent if their mouth feels dry when eating a meal. The permitted responses for this variable are structured on a nominal scale, where yes $= 1$ and no $= 2$.

In contrast to close-ended questions, responses for open-ended questions are recorded using a subject's own words. The information collected is usually in literal or narrative form that is later transformed into alphanumerical code during data editing for the preparation of the analytical database. Because open-ended questions do not have responses that are standardized prior to data collection, there may be a level of uncertainty if a data user's categorization of the information does not capture the interpretation and message provided by the respondents. Occasionally, open-ended questions are asked in pilot studies or focus groups to ascertain a range of possible answers and to narrow those responses into a meaningful format that would permit the conversion of the open-ended question into a close-ended question.

The variable OHQ780 is an example of an open-ended question tested during a NHANES pilot study that was later developed into a close-ended question for the main study (Figure 6.2). The responses gathered during the pilot study were organized into major themes and then categorized into approximately a dozen permitted responses. In the example provided, if a study subject responded with a "yes" to the preceding question (OHQ770), they were asked the question that probed for reasons why they could not get the dental care that was needed (OHQ780). If they responded with a "no" to OHQ770, the interviewer skipped to the end of the questionnaire section.

6.3.4 Subject-level versus tooth-level data

Dental examination data are often collected either at the subject level or at the tooth level. Because the range of tooth-level information that can be collected is extensive, GDMP are required to optimize the efficiency of data collection and analysis. For example, to assess for the presence of primary or permanent teeth, constructing a tooth-level variable that can handle both tasks is better than having two variables assessing for each condition. The tooth count variable OHX08TC not only records the presence of either a primary or permanent upper right central incisor, but it also records if an implant or a root fragment is present (Figure 6.2). This arrangement permits for a more efficient collection of information.

The determination of whether to use subject-level or tooth-level variables for data collection is directly dependent upon the main aims of the study to be evaluated as well as any likely foreseeable secondary data analyses. To assess if the study subject was edentulous, one could use a subject-level variable such as OHXEDENT or one could create a derived variable using the "missing" information from all 32 tooth-level variables similar to OHX08TC. If edentulous status is primarily needed to determine eligibility for a particular assessment, such as a periodontal examination, then the edentulous subject-level variable would be sufficient.

One advantage of collecting data that is tooth based is that it permits aggregating information in more complex ways to describe the oral health status of the study subject. In essence, multiple tooth-level observations are made and later transformed into a derived subject-level variable. The classic oral health example is dental caries experience, which is based on the DMFT (number of decayed, missing (due to disease), and filled (permanent teeth) index introduced by Klein and colleagues 70 years ago) (Klein et al., 1938). The observed subject-level assessment for caries experience could simply be accomplished by ascertaining if the subject had at least one permanent tooth either missing, affected by untreated caries, or treated because of caries (filled). A slightly different approach to allow for the differentiation of either untreated caries or dental restorations at the subject level would be to collect data using variables for each. The variables OHXDECAY and OHXREST exemplify this approach (Figure 6.2). Aggregating information from both of these variables and accounting for any missing permanent teeth could be used to create the derived caries experience variable OHDCE for data analyses.

An alternate method for determining subject-level caries experience using a tooth-based approach is to collect data of the condition of each tooth. For instance, the variable OHX08CTC is used to assess for a variety of mutually exclusive characteristics for the upper right central incisor (Figure 6.2). Some of the permitted codes for observation include (1) a sound primary tooth (D), (2) missing tooth due to disease (E), (3) missing due to other causes (M), (4) not erupted (U), (5) sound permanent tooth (S), and (6) permanent tooth with surface condition (Z). Once the tooth-level condition is assessed, a second variable can be used to ascertain the surface condition of each tooth. Referring back to elementary dental anatomy, each anterior tooth is divided into four surface-level areas (lingual, facial, mesial, and distal) where the occlusal surface is added as the fifth area for posterior teeth. The OHX08CSC variable is used to assess the surface condition for the upper right central incisor. An example of permitted codes are (1) lingual surface caries present (0); (2) mesial surface caries present (3); (3) facial surface restoration present (7); and (4) distal surface restoration present (9). To carry the example forward, both variables OHX##CTC and OHX##CSC are designed to work together in sequence. If the examiner observes a class 3 carious lesion affecting the mesial surface on the upper right central incisor, the code called for OHX08CTC would be "Z" followed by a "3" for variable OHX08CSC. However, if the examiner did not observe any caries or restorations on tooth #8, only the code "S" for the variable OHX08CTC would be called and OHX08CSC would be left blank.

Using this paired variable scheme, data can be collected down to the surface level for each tooth with very good efficiency, using only 64 variables. With this approach, the researcher can calculate the subject-level DMFT score for each study subject, which then can be used to calculate means, and so on. The derived variable OHDDMFT has a range of 0–28 (Figure 6.2). Instead of using categorical variables as previously described to determine subject-level caries experience (OHDCE), the derived continuous variable representing the calculated DMFT score can be used. Utilizing this method to collect surface-level information also allows for the analysis of caries experience in finer detail by calculating a DMFS (surface) score. Finally, this method also permits the construction of a number of dental caries-based indices such as DT (number of decayed teeth), FS (number of filled surfaces), DS/DFS (proportion of decayed surfaces to total decayed and filled surfaces), and so on.

Another area of study in dentistry that often requires the collection of tooth-level information involves the evaluation of periodontal status. Unlike assessing caries experience with the DMFT index, there is no uniformly accepted standard for assessing periodontal disease. Although a number of methods have been proposed and implemented, many have faded from epidemiologic use as our understanding of periodontal disease evolves (Dye and Selwitz, 2005; Dye and Thornton-Evans, 2007). Measuring periodontal status will depend greatly on the study aims and analytical plan. A more comprehensive systematic approach to assess periodontal status is to make pocket depth (free gingival margin to sulcus base) and recession (free gingival margin to cemento-enamel junction) measurements at a number of periodontal sites that can then be used to calculate clinical attachment loss. When using this approach, the reference (gold) standard is to make measurements at six sites per tooth (mesio-facial, mid-facial, disto-facial, mesio-lingual, mid-lingual, and disto-lingual). Although a number of different site combinations could be used to produce a partial mouth design, the need for a full-mouth exam versus a partial mouth exam again will depend greatly on the study aims and analytical plan.

An important data management consideration for using site-based periodontal measurements is to determine how and when the clinical loss of attachment variable should be calculated. One approach would be to use paired data collection variables for pocket depth and recession, as similarly described for subject-level caries experience (tooth and surface condition variables). Instead of calculating attachment loss following the completion of data collection, an algorithm can be used to automatically calculate loss of attachment from each variable pair directly at the point of data collection if direct data entry is being performed.

For example, the variable OHX08PCM represents the mid-facial pocket depth measurement for the upper right central incisor (Figure 6.2). The permitted values are whole numbers in the range of 0–12 mm. Variable OHX08CJM represents the recession measurement for the same central incisor and the permitted values are -12–12 mm. Both pocket depth and recession variables measure periodontal characteristics using a numerical scale. An algorithm embedded into the data collection program will automatically calcu late attachment loss following data entry for OHX08CJM. In this example, the variable OHX08LAM is derived from the difference between the recession measure and the pocket depth measure (OHX08CJM$-$OHX08PCM $=$ OHX08LAM). This difference is then automatically transformed to an absolute value, thus, giving OHX08LAM a permitted range of values of 0–24 mm in whole numbers. Using embedded functions during direct data entry when numerous repetitive computations are required to produce derived variables is good data management. This practice facilitates data editing and provides the data manager with additional opportunities to perform error checking. Later, the PI or other analysts can aggregate any number of these periodontal variables to create a subject-level periodontal status definition pertinent to their data analysis.

Although pocket depth or attachment loss data are often statistically expressed in linear terms, for example, "mean" loss of attachment, the periodontal measurement variables are typically collected as discrete variables. For instance, the NHANES periodontal assessment protocol requires examiners to round down to the nearest whole number (Dye et al., 2007, 2008). Discrete data are collected in terms of whole numbers and there are a finite number of possible observations within the permitted range of values measured. Another example of an oral health discrete variable is caries experience based on the DMFT index (OHDDMFT). Continuous variables permit the collection of unrestricted observations along a linear scale. An oral health example of a continuous variable is DEPPG (Figure 6.2), which represents measurement data assessing the serum antibody level of *Porphromonas gingivalis* (Pg). Although the data collection variable for Pg permitted any titer value ≥ 0, the variable prepared for the analytical database restricted the range of permitted titer values from 40 to 22,885.

6.3.5   Formatting observed values

Formatting a variable's range of values can be done at different periods of data management. For instance, the variable OHXMAXIN (Figure 6.2), which measures the maximum incisal opening, had a permitted range of values ≥ 0 mm during data collection. However, when a value was called by the examiner that exceeded 65 mm, that observation was automatically converted by the data entry program to 65 mm, thus, effectively formatting the range of values from 0 to 65 mm for the variable. Likewise, while preparing data for the creation of an analytical database, a study subject's age may be "top coded" because limited numbers of older volunteers participated in the study. For instance, subjects whose age is greater than 85 years may be recoded to 85 years for age. Top coding is often done to improve statistical performance of the variable, manage outliers, or promote subject confidentiality by minimizing information disclosure.

6.4   Preparing the database for data entry

6.4.1   Data collection forms

Data entry is basically the manner in which responses and observations are recorded. This process begins with information being recorded on paper forms (hard-copy) or in electronic forms (direct data entry or electronic data capture (EDC)). Recording data on

Modified Gingival Index
OH_F7

Random half-mouth selected:

Upper right.....................1

Upper left.......................2

Lower left......................3

Lower right....................4

Upper quadrant:

	D	F	M	L		D	F	M	L		D	F	M	L		D	F	M	L
2M					1M					2B					1B				

	D	F	M	L		D	F	M	L		D	F	M	L
C					LI					CI				

Lower quadrant:

	D	F	M	L		D	F	M	L		D	F	M	L		D	F	M	L
2M					1M					2B					1B				

	D	F	M	L		D	F	M	L		D	F	M	L
C					LI					CI				

Figure 6.3 Basic layout for a data collection form using the Modified Gingival Index.

paper involves using forms designed to facilitate the recording of the information during data collection as well as entering the data into a computer database program. The layout of the paper form is critical to minimize data entry error by the clinical study site and maximize data entry efficiency for the data entry operators. If many forms are required for data collection, it is critical that all forms reflect a consistent design, especially in the use of headers, recording blocks for important identifiers, and numbering systems. Dates should be recorded uniformly and decimal points should be preprinted to clearly illustrate how many significant digits should be recorded. Figure 6.3 shows a basic hard-copy form layout for collecting data using the Modified Gingival Index. For larger studies, data managers coordinate the distribution and submission of paper forms for entering information into the collection database.

Recording source data on paper has benefits as well as limitations. When the study population size is small, study budget resources are limited, or the study environment cannot fully support the direct data entry infrastructure, the use of hard-copy forms for data collection does have an advantage compared to electronic data capture. However, illegible or ambiguous recordings can promote data entry error, paper forms can be lost or damaged prior to data entry, and additional resources are required to enter the source data into an electronic form by way of a computer data entry program.

6.4.2   Simple versus complex databases

When setting up a database for data entry, study managers need to determine if the basic structure of the collection database will be either a simple database or a complex database. A simple database may be a flat file, which basically stores information in one long text file, or a single table, which stores information in a spreadsheet format. Complex relational databases store information in multiple tables and permits greater flexibility and speed in manipulating data, especially in large studies. The database structure and data entry screens help to assure data quality. While simple databases are easy to set up, an EDC relational database management system can support a number of advanced study management needs, including an audit trail of changes. With clear data entry screens, data can be entered in a user-friendly manner. Simple range checks can be set up to alert the data entry clerk of any obvious error or missed data entry fields. This is needed in order to maintain data quality by assuring that data entered for a study subject are clearly associated with that subject and all changes to the data are clearly identified. There is much less control over the data entry process when using flat files and basic spreadsheets, which could lead to a greater likelihood of data entry errors and to longer data cleanup.

6.4.3   IT support

Another element of database architecture that PI and data managers will need to consider when setting up the database for data collection is the level of programming and informatics support that will be available and the operational platform of the computer systems. It is important to know if data handling will be performed using a single personal computer or a network of PCs, or other larger networked systems. The type of computing services planned and the size of the database estimated, which is directly related to the numbers of study subjects and variables, will directly impact the choice of software for data management. Data collection for small studies may be administered using data management resources available in statistical analysis software. For larger studies, data management needs may require more complex database software or more custom features that are developed specifically for data collection. Various components of data management may also be administered by other data support entities such as coordinating centers or contractors. Some larger academic and medical centers have clinical studies/data support centers that perform many of the day-to-day data management functions. This consolidates a number of data management staff over a number of studies and is intended to provide full-time professional data management at a reduced cost to clinical studies. Coordinating centers and contractors are more likely to be used in larger clinical studies and trials where data collection is more periodic and extensive, and requires the use of more complex databases.

6.4.4   Testing and validating the database

All databases must be validated for functionality as described in the database plan prior to their use in a study. Moreover, subsequent testing should occur to assure that the database is performing as designed. Pilot testing of the database(s) used for data collection is critical and standard operating procedures must be created to support this function. If a database is widely used in the public domain such as Microsoft SQL Server or Oracle Clinical, there is usually no need to fully validate the database. However, the data manager must ensure that the standard operating procedures outlined in the study's database plan clearly state if or when full validation is required.

GDMP also includes full end-to-end systems testing of data collection, data migration, and data aggregation functionality. When first using a database, it is always a good idea to fully test it with "mock" data. Mock data is basically a small data file that contains fictional, but plausible, responses for all of the variables to be used for data collection. This test is very useful for validating and testing skip patterns, variable range checks, and other variable attributes. Another good, basic test to conduct is to reproduce, at least in part, a study previously done with a different database to see if one gets the same outputs. For example, enter all the data for the first ten subjects of an actual study, export the data to a statistical software package (e.g., SAS) and do SAS Compare of the two studies. As long as there are no data entry errors and the data agree, then the database is properly performing as intended.

Database test plans should be formally established and performed across all databases used during the study. For instance, test scripts should be run from the initial point of data collection to the creation of the analytical database. This "end-to-end" testing is very important when multiple databases will be used during data collection. This process assures that all data elements are carried through data collection and handling, and the variables are properly named and that the basic functions work. Testing procedures with appropriate review by programming, data management, and statistical staff will assure quality and will minimize future problems at the data user end.

6.5   Using the database for data collection

6.5.1   Manual data entry

The main aim of data entry is to precisely and efficiently record information into the database (Hulley et al., 2001). This is accomplished by using appropriately designed paper and/or electronic forms, by recording data when the information is gathered, and by employing competently trained staff. Standardized procedures for data entry should be described in the DMP or study protocol. These procedures should clearly identify study staff responsible for data handling and the level of training that each staff member will receive. During data collection, errors transcribed on paper forms should be marked out with a single line with the correct information recorded near the erroneous entry. Additionally, paper forms should be periodically reviewed to identify errors or potentially unintelligible recordings prior to database data entry. All changes made to data collection forms following data collection must be inscribed with the date and name of the person making the change. Finally, the task of transferring data from paper forms into a database should be done in a timely and consistent manner to minimize data entry backlogs.

Traditionally, double-key data entry has been used to assure data quality for clinical studies that use paper forms. Double-key data entry is very efficient for verifying precision of numerical data and for data where there are predefined answers such as yes/no, or male/female. Single-key data entry is adequate for free text fields and for fields where the

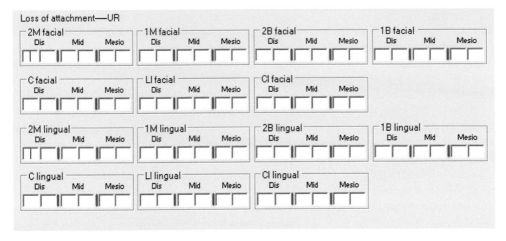

Figure 6.4 An EDC form example used for upper right quadrant full-mouth periodontal probing in a NHANES pilot study.

person entered symbols into the paper form, such as an arrow indicating "increased." The reason is that there are often so many errors in transcribing text fields that it is more efficient to enter the data once and complete a full quality control review of the variable field by someone knowledgeable in dental/biomedical terminology. Because free text data are also rarely analyzed, there is little likelihood that even if minor errors are recorded, these errors will impact on either the clinical or safety outcomes of the study. Nevertheless, the fewer the open-ended text entries there are, the better because coded data are less ambiguous and are more likely to be open to interpretation.

Technology now provides numerous opportunities for direct data entry on studies. Data recorders can enter information directly into the collection database at the time observations are made and responses are given. This eliminates the need for double-keyed entry and related tasks associated with collecting data on paper forms. With an electronic data entry system, not only can study information be entered from paper source documents, but data can also be directly entered into electronic forms and then immediately converted to the appropriate code. Because electronic forms can be created to resemble paper forms, a hard-copy readable form can be produced when needed for a study audit. Figure 6.4 shows a copy of an electronic form used to collect recession and pocket depth measures on a NHANES pilot study. Additionally, some direct data entry systems can be used by study subjects to enter their own responses into the collection database using portable computing or data entry devices. User-friendly forms, images, and even audio prompting can be used to facilitate accurate data collection. Computer-assisted data entry programs are particularly useful for collecting sensitive information and protecting respondents' confidentiality.

6.5.2   Electronic data capture

Electronic data capture is radically changing clinical research, data management, statistical analyses, medical writing, and even regulatory submissions and reviews (Mitchel, 2001, 2003a, 2003b, 2004a, 2004b, 2007). EDC solutions offer a convenient, cost-effective approach for streamlining areas such as management of subject enrollment, data entry, query management, communications, regulatory review, and project management. By reducing data entry errors through the use of electronic edit and logic checks at the time of data entry, there is improved data quality as well as a reduction in the time to prepare data for analyses. A critical difference between hard-copy data entry and EDC is that electronic data collection is quality assured and entered at the "front end" of the data collection system instead of at the "back end."

One of the main attributes of EDC is improved data quality. The main reasons for improved data quality are that (1) the people who know the data the best enter the data, and (2) the electronic edit and logic checks pick up missing, out of range, and potentially illogical data. EDC also promotes minimal transcription and spelling errors during free text data entry. Out of range, missing, and illogical data are addressed in the comment field at the time of data submission to the hosting server. There is, therefore, an online explanation for data exceptions that can then either be accepted as "OK AS IS" or queried by the monitor. Missing and out of range data can actually be addressed at the point of data collection. This assists data managers and other staff in preparing a "clean" data set for analysis by reducing the need for data retrieval or having to go back and revalidate or obtain missing inaccurate data. An example of a web-based EDC form is shown in Figure 6.5.

One significant advantage that EDC provides over using paper forms for collecting data is that data collection and management can occur via the internet. Online data collection facilitates rapid database updating when multiple data collection sites are used and promote ongoing data review by the data manager for potential errors. Online data entry reduces the need for multiple site visits to monitor data collection and entry, and provides near "real-time" project updates and status reports for the study managers. For larger studies,

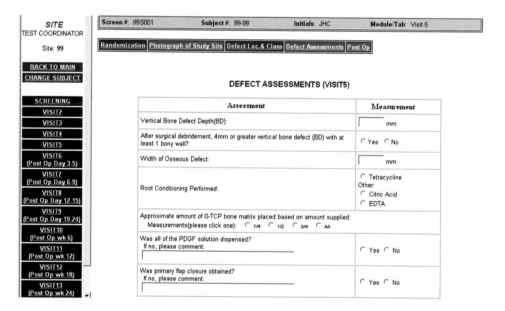

Figure 6.5 Web-based electronic form example used in a periodontal bone defect clinical trial.

online EDC provides rapid access to study subject enrollment data and summary reports that are accessible anytime, anywhere, and by anyone with proper authorization.

The potential for online treatment allocation (randomization) is one of the most powerful tools in EDC. Statisticians usually generate the randomization code in SAS®. While EDC systems can generate and/or control the treatment allocation assignments, if errors in randomization do occur, there could be instant notification to the appropriate study staff. Online randomization tools have practical application in studies where there is a central randomization schema and/or stratification to treatment. When subject allocation is performed online, there is instant knowledge that a subject has been allocated and there is no need to call or be routinely informed as to the subject's enrollment status.

Another important asset of EDC systems is rapid access to safety data. A web-based system can display nearly instantaneous updated health records and flag issues that might preclude a study subject to a particular examination or treatment allocation. This allows relevant medical monitoring to easily and effectively review for safety issues. For instance, during an interview, a series of questions could be asked to identify a subject who would require antibiotic prophylaxis prior to receiving an invasive dental examination, such as a periodontal probing. Depending upon the responses provided during the interview, the EDC system would not assign the subject to a periodontal examination. Another feature of web systems is that they can allow for event alerts via e-mail, phone, fax, or other media at the time of occurrence. One example is in patient dosing. When a drug is to be given per unit body weight, the system can automatically compare the actual dose with the calculated dose and send notice of any dosing errors.

6.5.3   Promoting data quality

Another activity related to data entry is the promotion of data quality. Although double-keyed data entry is designed to assure data quality, it is time consuming. When data are inscribed onto paper, there is no feedback at the time of data collection to identify possible transcription or logic errors. As a result, extensive secondary data management must be performed at the back end of data collection after the data elements are transcribed onto the paper. Initial quality assurance occurs when the data manager, the clinical research associate (CRA), or other study staff reviews the source documents for accuracy and precision. Following this task, the hard-copy documents and forms are ready for data entry. In large or multisite studies, these source documents are sent to a data management center, which logs in these items and enters the data twice into two parallel databases. Each "double entry" is then compared, usually using a data-compare program. If the two entries correspond to each other, the data are accepted. If the two entries do not match, the data manager or data entry clerk will need to determine which data elements are correct in order to correct the data entry error. If a data entry field is not legible, or the data are illogical or obviously incorrect, a query must be sent back to the examination team or clinical site to clarify or correct the data entry field.

In EDC systems, a large part of secondary data management, especially those tasks associated with double-key data are resolved at the time of data entry. Upon submission of the data through an interactive or web interface, the system automatically checks for inconsistent, illogical, or missing data, and will return an error message and provide a prompt for permitted values. The examiner, interviewer, or any other staff member authorized to collect data can then either change the data entry to match a permitted value or explain why their entry is the "correct" observation. If a potential error is discovered during data monitoring or during secondary data management activities, a query can be delivered electronically on the form level to the relevant data collection team member. This staff person can then respond to the query electronically where a "back-end" edit can be performed and all changes to the database are managed through an automatic audit trail that records the change, the time and date of the change, and if necessary, the reason for the change. The critical difference between an EDC system in comparison with a paper data collection system is that with EDC, all study data are initially quality assured when entered at the "front end" of the system instead of at the "back end."

Another key element of data quality assurance that directly impacts the development of a DMP is the type of subject-related repeat data that will be collected to perform inter- or intrarater reliability statistics. The collection of intrarater data is important to evaluate the potential for data variability that might occur within a single examiner or laboratory method. For instance, having a nonbiased subsample of study subjects return for a second dental examination to be conducted by the same examiner, or repeating the test using a sample from the same biological specimen source.

When a study utilizes multiple examiners, assuring clinical data reliability is critical to establishing internal validity within the study. There are two main methods for collecting interrater reliability data. Ideally, the better process is to require each examiner to independently repeat the dental examination on a randomly selected subsample of study subjects within a very narrow period of time. However, most studies that usually employ multiple examiners do so because either the primary data collection period is long or occurs over multiple study sites. To accommodate these studies, a reference or "gold-standard" examiner can be used to collect interrater reliability data. With this alternate approach, comparisons across examiners are made to the reference examiner. Regardless of the type of reliability data to be collected, when using a single database for data collection, multiple records will be established for each study subject. In other words, the database tabular format changes to where each data variable no longer resides in its own column, but in its own row. To avoid establishing multiple records in a single collection database, a "QA" parallel database or separate tables in relational database can be used.

6.5.4   Editing collected data

Once the data have been entered into the collection database, the data are exposed to a series of data editing and monitoring processes that are considered secondary data management activities. The main objective of secondary data management is to transform the collection database into a "clean" database that is primed for the preparation of analytical databases. As previously discussed, back-end data editing occurs when a recorded observation in the collection database is changed. All back-end edits must be properly documented. This includes recording the date, the name of the requestor, the affected variable, and a detailed explanation why the data were changed.

Data editing can be accomplished using three methods. The first is a manual process, where an expert reviewer examines the original data for biological nonplausibility, extreme outliers, or a combination of factors that might indicate potential data error. The reviewer may request to change an observation and this would be done manually as a back-end edit. This process relies on expert opinion. A more objective data editing process that can be used to produce clean data relies on automation. Automatic data editing uses small programs to scan incoming data to evaluate for nonconforming data. This process relies on range limits and logic checks. In EDC systems, automatic data editing is routinely conducted at the point of original data collection. The last data editing process is restricted to missing data and involves imputation. Imputation uses statistical procedures to estimate how a subject may have responded to a question if they would have chosen to answer that question. Imputation begins by evaluating responses to a key set of questions among a sample of study subjects who have complete information. An algorithm can be developed that will derive the best probable data for imputation based on the available information of those individuals with missing data. Imputation remains controversial and the PI must consider both the positive and negative aspects of producing a database with imputed data. When done improperly, imputation can introduce more error instead of reducing data error.

6.5.5 Data control mechanisms to minimize disclosure

A DMP should include guidance for managing confidential information and for minimizing the potential disclosure of a study subjects' identity. The key for managing confidential information is not to collect data or reports that have the subjects' name or any other key identifiers associated with it. However, when important individual identifiers, such as a name, social security number, or contact information, need to be obtained, they should be stored separately from the data collection database. Access to this information must be tightly controlled and limited only to key study personnel. When a subject is enrolled in a study, a unique study identifier should be assigned to the study subject. This unique number serves as a bridging variable, allowing a subject's information stored in various database tables or data files to be accurately matched. The unique study number is recorded in the data file containing the subject's confidential information and is the main identifier recorded on subsequent data collection forms. Some studies may include second tier identifiers to confirm that the appropriate individual is being interviewed, examined, or contributing a specimen. For example, only date of birth and/or gender information is recorded on the data collection form, but not the subject's initials. Study monitors should not see a subject's name during normal monitoring procedures.

When health records or other related documents are being abstracted as part of a study, it is imperative that confidential information is properly controlled and redacted from the data entry process. For instance, when incorporating photographs or radiographs that have patient names or their health record numbers recorded on the films, it is important to completely overwrite these identifiers so they are obliterated, while at the same time record the unique study number on the film to accurately assign each record to the study subjects. During abstraction, source documents should never leave the clinical site. Ideally, the data should be recorded on data entry forms instead of directly copying health records and submitting them for off-site data entry.

If information from health records is routinely abstracted during a study and those records are maintained electronically, using an EDC system could be advantageous if the information from an electronic health record (EHR) can be "linked" to a study's data collection system. When this happens, all information about a study subject will be sourced and updated electronically. This can facilitate evaluating an individual for inclusion/exclusion criteria as well as potential contraindications to subsequent assignments to treatment arms. The integration of the EDC and the EHR could benefit both study subjects and staff. A customized virtual personal health record that is available anywhere anytime will promote continuity of care if provided, reduce medical and prescribing error, and lead to better informed decisions. Furthermore, this eliminates the need for an intermediate data entry step and will allow the clinical site to maintain their source information about a study subject. Disclosure can be minimized by limiting access to the abstracted EHR to a limited number of key study personnel and by keeping the sourced information at the subjects' clinical site.

If biological specimens are being collected, the only individual identifier that should be recorded on the vial or container is the unique study number. If required for the test, the date of collection, date of birth, and gender could be recorded as well. Laboratories should return test results to the data manager or other staff responsible for data entry electronically with test results and other relevant information properly aligned with the unique study number to permit merging of the data into the main data collection database. Likewise, when radiographs or other images are sent to experts for reading, similar procedures should be followed.

The DMP should describe procedures for collecting and accessing sensitive data by the study staff. Sensitive data include information that could be associated with a societal stigma or illegal behavior. Examples of oral health assessments that may collect this type of information include evaluating methamphetamine use to investigate "Meth Mouth," using an oral rinse to sample human papilloma virus, or assessing for intraoral Kaposi's sarcoma as part of a HIV study. Because study subjects will be assured that this information will remain confidential, data management procedures must be fully documented to ensure that study staff understands the related data handling requirements and how the data will be made available for analyses. When the data are made available for analyses, especially to others outside the immediate study team, the data manager or PI should produce a shared data file that provides appropriate safeguards to prevent inadvertent subject disclosure. Some preventive measures include, but are not limited to, providing a data file containing no primary identifiers, restricting age to ranges instead of single-year ages, or not providing birth information.

6.5.6 Data archiving

One of the most important data management activities, but often overlooked, is data warehousing and archiving. It is vital to have a backup mechanism in place for all data systems. Unlike using paper forms for data collection, there is no inherent backup process for archiving data in electronic data systems. Consequently, data backup procedures must be developed and implemented for EDC systems. When using EDC, data entered directly into the database should be mirrored in real time to a server in another location to assure redundancy. In addition, all data must be backed up daily on tapes or equivalent media and then moved offsite at least weekly. These backup schedules should be modified depending on the needs of any individual program. Disaster recovery systems should also be in place so that data systems can be resurrected quickly in the event of a disaster. Servers should be in place in the designated disaster recovery center to facilitate the retrieval of study data. Minimally, the data plan should document standard operating procedures that support both data backup and recovery.

Not all databases require archiving. Through the course of data collection, handling, and analysis, many data files are produced. However, all data files associated with the collection of source data, primarily the collection database, must be archived. It is imperative that any secondary data management activities or analyses are not conducted on the original collection database. The original collection database should be duplicated and all other data management related functions should be performed on the duplicate database. Basically, all source data must be protected from the potential of permanent alteration. Once the original data collection base is finalized, the codebook for that database is archived as well. Likewise, when a database is prepared for analyses, the analytical database should be archived as well. This is particularly important if the database is small, is in a flat-file format, and has some statistical applications associated with the software that supports the data file. This preserves the original analytical data file and prevents the accidental permanent recoding of variables that always occurs during data analyses.

6.6   Using the data for analyses

6.6.1   Archiving analytical data files

As the analytical database is developed, the accompanying codebook will need to be updated and archived with the final analytical database as well. When the data manager creates the duplicate analytical database, the data set is almost ready for analyses. If the database is small, the PI and other study analysts will execute their analyses using all of the resident data. However, if the database contains a large number of variables and observations, the data manager may prepare smaller analytical data files "customized" for the study's analysts. If the analytical database is large or the software supporting the database does not contain statistical applications, the data file(s) will need to be converted to a file format supported by statistical programs, such as SAS©, STATA©, and so on. Given that data analyses investigating the main aims of a study should be driven by the study's SAP, the creation of analytical data file(s) should align with those prescripted analytical aims.

During data analysis, the analytical data file(s) may be repeatedly altered as variables are recoded and new ones are derived. For example, attachment loss variables are converted from a continuous variable to a categorical variable or the response of "don't know" to the question inquiring if a subject's mouth feels dry when eating is combined with "no." For this reason, either the data manager or the analyst will need to archive the source analytical data file(s). Following the completion of data analysis, the final working analytical data file should be archived by the researcher(s) as part of a manuscript, report, or other publications' permanent record.

References

Dye BA, Barker LK, Selwitz RH, Lewis BG, Wu T, Fryar CD, Ostchega Y, Beltran ED, Ley E. 2007. Overview and quality assurance for the National Health and Nutrition Examination Survey (NHANES) oral health component, 1999–2002. *Community Dentistry Oral Epidemiology* 35: 140–151.

Dye BA, Nowjack-Raymer R, Barker LK, Nunn JH, Steele JG, Tan S, Lewis BG, Beltran ED. 2008. Overview and quality assurance for the oral health component of the National Health and Nutrition Examination Survey (NHANES), 2003–2004. *Journal of Public Health Dentistry*, in press (available online-early press).

Dye BA, Selwitz RH. 2005. The relationship between selected measures of periodontal status and demographic and behavioral risk factors. *Journal of Clinical Periodontology* 32:798–808.

Dye BA, Thornton-Evans G. 2007. A brief history of national surveillance efforts for periodontal disease in the US. *Journal of Periodontology* 78:1373–1379.

Gallin JI, Ognibene FP. 2007. *Principles and Practice of Clinical Research*, 2nd edn. Burlington, MA: Academic Press, Elsevier, p. 74.

Hoffer JA, Prescott MB, McFadden FR. 2002. *Modern Database Management*, 6th edn. Upper Saddle River, NJ: Pearson Education, Inc., Prentice Hall, p. 4–5.

Hulley SB, Cummings SR, Browner WS, Grady D, Hearst N, Newman TB. 2001. *Designing Clinical Research*, 2nd edn. Philadelphia, PA: Lippincott Williams and Wilkins, p. 252.

Klein H, Palmer CE, Knutson JW. 1938. Studies on dental caries: I. Dental status and dental needs or elementary school children. *Public Health Reports* 53:751–765.

McFadden E. 2007. *Management of Data in Clinical Trials*, 2nd edn. Hoboken, NJ: John Wiley & Sons, p. 34.

Mitchel J, Ernst C, Cappi S, Beasley W, Lau A, Kim YJ, You J. 2004a. Implementing internet-based clinical trials. *DIA Forum* 40:22–23.

Mitchel J, Ernst C, Cappi S, Beasley W, Lau A, Kim YJ, You J. 2004b. Meeting the challenges of internet-based clinical trials. *Applied Clinical Trials* 13:44–53.

Mitchel J, Moncrieffe A, Kim YJ, Choi JH, Grimes I, Tantsyura V, Nadler D, Harnevo L, Bahagon Y. 2007. The paperless trial—past, present and future. *European Pharmaceutical Contractor* Autumn 72–74.

Mitchel J, You J, Kim YJ, Lau A, Cheng L, Fein S, Nardi R. 2003a. Clinical trial data integrity. Using internet-based remote data entry to collect reliable data. *Applied Clinical Trials* 12 Supplement:6–8.

Mitchel J, You J, Kim YJ, Lau A, Levinson B, Lynch S, O'Connor P. 2003b. Internet-based clinical trials—practical considerations. *Pharmaceutical Development and Regulations* 1:29–39.

Mitchel J, You J, Lau A, Kim YJ. 2001. Paper versus web; a tale of three trials. *Applied Clinical Trials* 10:34–35.

O'Carroll PW, Yasnoff WA, Ward ME, Ripp LH, Martin EL. 2003. *Public Health Informatics and Information Systems*. New York: Springer-Verlag Inc, pp. 728–729.

Silberschatz A, Korth HF, Sudarshan S. 2002. *Database System Concepts*, 4th edn. New York: McGraw-Hill Higher Education, p. 1.

7

Hypothesis testing and avoiding false-positive conclusions

Philippe P. Hujoel, DDS, PhD

7.1   Introduction

Hormone replacement therapy was suggested to reduce cardiovascular disease risk (Rossouw et al., 2002). Several vitamins were suggested to prevent cancer (The Alpha-Tocopherol Beta Carotene Cancer Prevention Study Group, 1994; Goodman et al., 2004; Bjelakovic et al., 2007). Vaccination was suggested to lower HIV infection risk (Macilwain, 1998; Barouch, 2008). These positive associations were derived from animal experiments, ecological studies, observational studies, and even large randomized controlled trials (RCT) (see Chapter 12). All these associations were ultimately proven to be false-positives by means of pivotal RCT. Publicity around these false-positives findings had nefarious consequences. From a public health perspective, scientific publications and press reports on the false-positive findings influenced physicians and laymen alike and ultimately led to hundreds of thousands of premature deaths. From a research perspective, the false-positives findings led to a loss of millions of dollars in pivotal randomized trials that should not have been initiated, and often multiple decades of lost time in the search for cures. It may not be surprising that controlling the rate of false-positives has been considered an important issue in clinical trial design for decades (Pocock, 1983; Ioannidis, 2005).

False-positive findings might be plaguing dental research just as much as medical research. Positive findings in randomized controlled trials suggested that chlorhexidine would lower caries risk (Sandham et al., 1991), that periodontal therapy would prevent low birth weight (Lopez et al., 2002), or that anti-inflammatory would control periodontitis (Jeffcoat et al., 1995). These findings came into question when larger, better controlled randomized trials were conducted (Forgie et al., 2000; Michalowicz et al., 2006). This chapter will review why the machinery of statistical hypothesis testing can lead to a preponderance of false-positive results and provide some approaches to reduce the incidence of false-positives.

7.2   How can hypothesis testing lead to an overabundance of false-positive leads?

A false-positive conclusion is defined here as a claim that an experimental intervention is superior to a control intervention, while in truth, the interventions have the same effectiveness, or more insidiously, that the control is superior to the experimental.

The publication biases toward positive findings—at the expense of negative findings—have been extensively reported on (Knight, 2003). There may be a continuing bias of journal editors and reviewers, commercial companies, and investigators against publishing negative results. Publishing exciting small research findings may generate future commercial and government funding, publicity and the attention of reporters, academic promotion, and increases in stock prices. In contrast, there are typically few incentives and several disincentives to publish negative results. The only time negative results appear of commercial interest is in equivalence trials where marketing advantages may exist.

There are many medical examples where pivotal trials go unpublished because of pressure by commercial interests or editor bias (Turner et al., 2008). The powerful biases against publishing negative results may be present in dentistry as much as in medicine. A negative finding in a large government-funded trial on oral hygiene and dental caries was rejected for publication in a premier dental journal (Silverstein et al., 1977). A negative finding on chlorhexidine rinsing and tooth loss (Hujoel et al., 2003) in another large government-funded trial was similarly rejected in another top-ranked dental journal. Yet, these same journals publish positive findings from small exploratory studies.

Given the all around unpalatable nature of negative results, it should not be surprising that many approaches have been devised to generate positive results. One approach to generate positive conclusions is to explore various patient subgroups, various end points, and various statistical techniques. For instance, analyses can explore the effects of treatment in patients with more severe dental disease, or dental patients with good oral hygiene, or other subgroups that lead to the desired results (Yusuf et al., 1991). Or, if the investigated treatments do not differ on the a priori defined end point, one can explore different end point definitions or switch to a different end point altogether. For instance, pretrial it may have been decided to consider a pocket reduction of >2 mm as a treatment success. This definition of success can be changed posttrial to a pocket depth reduction of >1 mm, a pocket depth reduction of >3 mm, or if neither leads to the desired result, to an evaluation of various cutoffs on probing attachment levels, radiographic bone levels, bleeding, or combinations of these. The possibilities to generate false-positives are almost infinite.

The saga of α-tocopherol (a form of vitamin E) demonstrates how even large-scale RCT can generate false-positive findings. One of the promising hypotheses of the twentieth century was that α-tocopherol could reduce lung cancer mortality. The results of the pivotal RCT on this hypothesis were disappointing; α-tocopherol increased overall mortality risk (Miller et al., 2005), increased the risks for serious adverse events such as heart failure (Lonn et al., 2005), and did not impact lung cancer mortality rates (The Alpha-Tocopherol Beta Carotene Cancer Prevention Study Group, 1994). Nonetheless, secondary data analyses on two of these randomized trials—data explorations without prespecified hypotheses—led to the observation that α-tocopherol was associated with a decreased risk for prostate cancer (The Alpha-Tocopherol Beta Carotene Cancer Prevention Study Group, 1994; Duffield-Lillico et al., 2003). These positive results were considered sufficiently promising to initiate "the largest individually randomized cancer prevention trial ever conducted," the SELECT trial (Gann, 2008).

The results of the SELECT trial (Lippman et al., 2009) may well be the ultimate confirmation of Yusuf's 1991 report: positive findings from post hoc generated hypotheses in RCT are unreliable; the equivalent of betting on the horse after the race is over (Yusuf et al., 1991). If anything, the results of the SELECT trial indicated that α-tocopherol increased rather than decreased prostate mortality risk (Lippman et al., 2009).

The excess of false-positive results in the literature is in part caused by fitting causal explanations to observed chance associations. There is a difference between testing a hypothesis against data that will be collected versus the manufacturing of a hypothesis tailored to the data that have been analyzed. Formulating a specific hypothesis *prior* to data collection is a quintessential feature of scientific experimentation. In medical and dental research, it provides investigators with the opportunity to predict how patients with predefined characteristics will respond to two or more interventions with respect to a prespecified clinical outcome. These predictions can then be compared to the observations collected during the clinical experiment, and lead to reliable inference. Fitting a causal explanation post hoc is a treacherous exercise, as a large number of hypotheses can be consistent with an observed association, only one of which is accurate.

Statistical techniques themselves can be bent to provide positive results. Different statistical techniques can be explored with respect to their impact on p values; parametric or nonparametric, one-sided versus two-sided tests, with and without adjustment for baseline covariates, site based or patient based, and if site-based analyses are selected, various correlation structures can be assessed. Such cherry-picking of statistical analyses can often switch marginally significant results to the magical $p < 0.05$ conclusion.

Actual flaws or deceptions—intended or not—in the design or data analysis (Pocock, 1983) can similarly lead to false-positive findings. Controls groups can be contrived, randomization can be tampered with (Nowak, 1994), and inappropriate statistical methods can be employed to try to squeeze significance out of a data set. Contrived control groups typically revolve around tampering with the effectiveness of the control group. For instance, instead of using an experienced surgeon for the control intervention, the control procedure could be performed by a lesser qualified person. Or, instead of using the standard dose of a painkiller, or an antibiotic, the dose could be halved, thereby increasing the likelihood that the experimental treatment will be effective. Several articles have reviewed the use of inappropriate statistical methods in dental research and noted the continued high prevalence of such practices (Lesaffre et al., 2007). Motives for using inappropriate statistical technique can be as simple as picking the method that provides statistical significance, regardless of appropriateness.

When the above approaches are mixed and matched, the possibilities to generate false-positive findings are endless. Reducing false-positive findings can be achieved in part by the a priori specification of nine elements: (1) the subject characteristics, (2) the experimental treatment, (3) the control treatment, (4) the primary outcome by which the effectiveness treatment will be judged, (5) the magnitude of the difference between treatments considered clinically significant (Δ), (6) the type I error rate (α), (7) the type II error rate (β), (8) the likelihood of finding a positive association (π), and (9) the analytic method. Any post hoc deviation from these nine elements increases the risk for false-positive conclusions.

7.3   Quantifying the false-positive rates; the theory

The type I error rate (α), the type II error rate (β), and the "a priori" likelihood that the null hypothesis is false (π) determine the false-positive error rates.

The *type I error rate* (α) is the probability of rejecting the null hypothesis, when it is true. Note that α is a probability that is conditioned on the information that the null hypothesis is true. Thus, for instance, a type I error rate of 5% indicates that, *if the null hypothesis is true*, the chance for rejecting the null hypothesis is less than 5%. The type I error rate is a *conditional* probability. One does not know when conducting an experiment whether the null hypothesis is true or false. The experiment is designed to modify our belief that the null hypothesis is true.

The *type II error rate* (β) is the probability of accepting the null hypothesis, when it is false. The type II error rate is also a *conditional* probability. The type II error rate is conditioned on the knowledge that the null hypothesis is false and that there exists a given difference between the experimental and the control group. For instance, a type II error rate of 20% indicates, that *if* the null hypothesis is false and if there exists a given difference between the investigated treatments, there is less than 20% chance to accept the null hypothesis. The power of an experiment is one minus the type II error rate ($1 - \beta$).

The "a priori" likelihood that the null hypothesis is false (π) is the third factor that determines the likelihood of false-positive and false-negative conclusions. In order to provide an intuitive sense on π, two extreme examples may provide a useful illustration. First, assume you are the all-supreme ruler of knowledge and that you know of a type of dental or medical disease for which *no* effective treatment exists. For instance, maybe there is a type of leukemia that leads to bleeding gingival tissues for which no type of locally administered periodontal treatment is effective. All treatments, when compared to the control treatment, are ineffective against this type of leukemia-induced periodontal disease. Under this scenario, π equals 0. We can do a million randomized trials, all trials should lead to the same conclusion; the experimental treatment does not work. In such a situation, all positive conclusions reached in clinical trials will be false-positives. Regardless of whether the type I error rate is 1% or 5%, and whether the type II error rate is 80% or 99%, the rate of false-positive conclusions will be 100%.

A second extreme example is where *all* experimental treatments, when compared to the control treatment, are effective. The local mechanical treatments, the drug treatments, the combination of local and drugs treatments are all effective at dealing with a particular dental disease, when compared to no treatment. Under this circumstance, π equals 1. All treatments, when compared to the control, will be truly effective. Under this situation, there will be no false-positive conclusions and all negative conclusions are false-negatives. All treatments identified as effective will truly be effective. Regardless of whether the type I error rate is 1% or 5%, or whether the type II error rate is 80% or 99%, the false-positive error rate will be 0%.

In real life, π falls somewhere between these two extremes. The history of clinical trial results in the different chronic disease areas provides some estimate of the likelihood that the experimental treatment is effective. In general, statisticians with experience in randomized controlled trials for chronic human diseases (e.g., cancer, AIDS, rheumatoid arthritis) generally consider π to be small. For cancer trials, the a priori probability that a novel treatment is better than a standard treatment (π) has been reported to be in the range of 0.1–20% (Staquet et al., 1979; Fleming, 1982; Simon, 1982).

In dental research, it would be useful to have some discussion on the range of plausible π values for the family of dental interventions. The history of randomized controlled trial results on a particular treatment can provide an estimate of π. A first small trial may be suggestive that the experimental treatment works. Our estimate of π may go up ($\pi > 0$). We do more clinical trials, and if all clinical trial results remain positive, our estimate of π may keep increasing. Translating our degree of belief in an actual value of π is subjective, but required to estimate the likelihood of obtaining false-positive conclusions.

This estimate of π can affect whether the conduct of randomized controlled trials is considered ethically feasible. For a nonfatal disease where effective treatment(s) exists, a clinician may be uncomfortable to randomize patients unless there is a 50-50 chance that the new experimental treatment is as effective as the standard. In this situation, an assumption of $\pi = 0.5$ may be desired to convince an ethical review board that a randomized trial is appropriate.

On the other hand, for a fatal disease, a clinician may be comfortable to randomize patients to a novel experimental treatment even when he believes the experimental treatment has a less than 1% chance of being effective. The more desperate the clinical situation becomes, the larger the willingness of both patient and clinician to try anything (even for treatments where π is close to 0).

The false-positive and false-negative error rates depend on the type I error rate (α), the type II error rate (β), and the a priori likelihood that experimental treatment is better than control treatment (π). A 2×2 table illustrates these relationships for n experimental treatments (Table 7.1). Among the n experimental treatments, $\pi \times n$ treatments will be truly effective and $n \times (1 - \pi)$ treatments will be truly noneffective. For the $\pi \times n$ truly effective treatments, a certain proportion will be incorrectly classified as noneffective. This proportion is determined by the power of the experiment. If the power of the experiment is 80% (type II error rate of 20%), 80% of the $\pi \times n$ treatments will be correctly classified as being effective, and 20% of the $\pi \times n$ treatments will be incorrectly classified as noneffective.

Analogously, there will be $n \times (1 - \pi)$ experimental treatments that are truly noneffective. The proportion of these that will be correctly classified depends on α (the type I error rate). Of the $n \times (1 - \pi)$ noneffective treatments, $n \times (1 - \pi) \times 0.05$ will be incorrectly classified as effective if the type I error rate is 5%, and $n \times (1 - \pi) \times 0.95$ will be correctly classified as noneffective (Table 7.1).

A common problem is to misinterpret a p value less than 0.05 as a reflection that the chance of a false-positive conclusion is less than 5%. This is not the case. Under most circumstances, the likelihood for false-positive conclusions is higher than the

Table 7.1   The relationship between α (say 0.05), β, and π, and the false-positive and false-negative error rates.

| p value | True relationship between experimental and control treatment | | |
	Effective	Noneffective	
≤0.05	$\pi\, n(1-\beta)^a$	$n\,\alpha\,(1-\pi)^b$	$\pi\, n(1-\beta) + n\,\alpha\,(1-\pi)$
>0.05	$\pi\, n\, \beta^c$	$n\,(1-\pi)^a(1-\alpha)^a$	$\pi\, n\, \beta + n\,(1-\pi)\,(1-\alpha)$
	$\pi\, n$	$n\,(1-\pi)$	n

Based on the type I error rate (α), the type II error rate (β), and the a priori likelihood that experimental treatment is better than the control treatment (π), the false-positive probability equals $\frac{(1-\pi)\alpha}{(1-\pi)\alpha+\pi(1-\beta)}$ (1) and the false-negative probability equals $\frac{\pi\beta}{(1-\pi)(1-\alpha)+(\pi\beta)}$ (2) (Staquet et al., 1979; Ioannidis, 2005).
[a]Correct conclusion on the effectiveness/noneffectiveness of the treatment.
[b]False-positive conclusion.
[c]False-negative conclusion.

type I error rate of 5%. The lower the probability that treatment differences exist (i.e., the smaller π), the more challenging it is to find effective treatment for the chronic disease under investigation, and the higher the likelihood for false-positive conclusions. Before proceeding with suggestions on how to decrease the false-positive rates in dental research, an example of the false-positive rate for a typical small periodontal trial may be useful.

7.3.1   Quantifying false-positive rates; a periodontal example

In most periodontal trials, the classical significance level (α) of 0.05 is selected as the type I error rate. The typical exploratory randomized periodontal trial in the not-so-distant past had 15 subjects (DeRouen et al., 1995; Hujoel, 1995), have variability estimates that can be abstracted from the published periodontal literature (Table 7.2), and considered 0.2 mm pocket depth difference clinically significant (Williams et al., 2001). For the plaque index, a 15% difference (mean plaque index = 1.0) was considered clinically significant. For bleeding on probing, a 15% difference (30% reduction in bleeding on probing) was considered clinically significant. For simplicity's sake, a parallel arm design is assumed (Table 7.2).

Based on α and β, one can calculate the false-positive error rate for a small periodontal trial (formula 1). For π = 0.1%, a larger than 99% false-positive error rate is present. When π is raised from 0.1% to 1%, 2–3% of the significant treatment effects reported reflect truly effective treatments, and 97% of the reported significant results are false-positives. When π is 10%, the false-positive rate varies between 62% and 83%.

These false-positive error rates are valid if there is one a priori defined hypothesis. The number of *reported* hypotheses tested in randomized periodontal trials is typically 15 (Hujoel, 1995). The number of unreported statistical tests is probably higher. Such multiple testing impacts false-positive error rates. For 15 independent tests, the probability of making at least one type I error is not 5% but 54%, the type II experimentwise error rate is not 20% but close to 0%. As the number of statistical tests increases without controlling for the experimentwise error rate, the type I error rate (α) approaches 1, and the power approaches

Table 7.2 Typical power (1 − β) of exploratory trials for studies with a sample size of 15 subjects (30 patients total) lasting 6 months or more.

End points	SD	Δ	Power (1−β) (%)	False-positive error rate		
				Π = 0.1% (%)	Π = 1% (%)	Π = 10% (%)
Mean pocket depth 5–6 mm	0.6	0.2 mm	15	>99	97	75
Mean pocket depth ≥7 mm	1.0	0.2 mm	9	>99	98	83
Mean probing attachment level 5–6 mm	0.7	0.2 mm	12	>99	98	79
Mean probing attachment level ≥7mm	1.1	0.2 mm	8	>99	98	85
Mean recession 5–6 mm	0.7	0.2 mm	12	>99	98	79
Mean recession ≥7mm	0.8	0.5 mm	11	>99	98	80
Sillness and Loe Plaque Index	0.62	15%	11	>99	98	80
Bleeding on probing	0.29	15%	28	>99	98	62

Δ = clinically significant difference.

1. In the limiting case of $\alpha = 1$ and $\beta = 0$, the false-positive rate equals $1 - \pi$, the a priori probability of no difference between experimental and control treatments. Thus, if the probability that the novel treatment is more effective than the standard is 5%, then 95% of all claims of significance will be false-positive claims.

7.4   Minimizing false-positive conclusions; π, registries, surrogates, randomization

The goal in clinical trials is to minimize the risk of false-positive conclusions. In order to achieve this goal, there should be one a priori defined hypothesis. The situation where there is more than one a priori hypothesis raises the complexity substantially and will not be discussed here. The following steps can reduce the likelihood of false-positive conclusions in the published literature.

7.4.1   Reporting π and its impact on α and β

Specifying the likelihood that a dental treatment is effective (π) is useful in terms of determining α and β and also in directing research funding. This process is currently an area where every effort is done "to prove" that π is high, and any effort at refutation may be considered counterproductive in the sense that it reduces the chances of funding for a clinical trial. Ranges of priors could be determined for the likelihood that anti-infective approaches reduce caries risk ($\pi < 1\%$?), that antibiotics reduce tooth loss in patients with periodontitis ($\pi < 5\%$?), or that regenerative periodontal treatments reduce tooth loss.

In the beginning, controversy may exist on values of π, but as evidence becomes available, controversy may decrease. For instance, why give a $\pi < 1\%$ for anti-infective caries treatments? Despite labeling caries as an infectious disease for decades and a multitude of clinical trials on anti-infective approaches, none have provided unequivocal evidence of effectiveness (Zero, 2004). If the estimate of π keeps decreasing with each additional randomized controlled trial, it has two consequences. First, upcoming pivotal trials on anti-infective approaches for dental caries need to specify a very small α and β to decrease the large risk for false-positives (given that $\pi < 1\%$). Second, as π keeps decreasing, research funding may increasingly focus on non-anti-infective approaches such as sealants and fluorides where the likelihood for identifying effective treatments (i.e., π) is larger. Similarly, that rationale for suggesting that antibiotics are unlikely to decrease tooth loss in periodontitis patients is based on the evidence that in cohort studies antibiotics appear to increase tooth loss (Cunha-Cruz et al., 2008), and that systematic reviews of the short-term clinical trials are inconsistent and report at best small changes in surrogate end points (Herrera et al., 2002; Haffajee et al., 2003). Or, finally, take the example of regenerative periodontal products. If a truly effective treatment for periodontal regeneration existed, there would *not* be such a therapeutic diversity and the half-life of the regenerative products that reached the market place would be longer. For regenerative periodontal trials, π may be less than 1% suggesting that α and β should be specified as small as possible to avoid the false-positive findings.

7.4.2 Prevalent diseases with low morbidity/mortality require trials with small α and β

The prevalence and the morbidity and mortality of the disease determine the level of concern for false-positive findings and side effects. For a rare and fatal disease such as Creutzfeldt–Jakob disease for which no effective treatment exists, there is minimal concern regarding side effects of promising treatments. Both common and serious side effects and a high chance for false-positives are acceptable given that the alternative to treatment is certain death. On the other hand, for a widely prevalent benign disease such as the common cold, there is almost no tolerance for side effects, even if they are extremely rare. Even a side effect as rare as Reye's syndrome with an incidence of less than 1.1 per million can become unacceptable, even when treatment is effective.

Since dental conditions such as gingivitis are—in terms of clinical significance—closer to a common cold, than Creutzfeldt–Jakob disease, there should be more certainty regarding the safety and effectiveness of the treatments. Dental treatments such as toothpastes or fillings are used almost worldwide, sometimes resulting in almost life-long exposures. As a result, ineffective products (e.g., products on the market as a result of false-positive findings) and rare side effects can have a substantial adverse impact in terms of wasted health care resources and common adverse events.

In dental research, the selection of α and β should be guided by the anticipated prevalence of the population exposure to the investigated treatment (or market penetration) and the seriousness of the condition under investigation. A clinical trial on a novel toothpaste should specify a much smaller α and β (e.g., $\alpha = 0.001$ and $\beta = 0.05$) than a clinical trial on a novel treatment for pemphigoid (e.g., $\alpha = 0.05$ and $\beta = 0.20$).

7.4.3 Proper randomization and intent-to-treat

Randomization is a delicate process that can easily be tampered with, and allegedly was in medical trials where clinicians have been reported trying to circumvent the process of randomization (Nowak, 1994). The process of randomization may leave much to be desired in periodontal trials where only 7% of the studies provide evidence on allocation concealment (Montenegro et al., 2002).

An important corollary to randomization is the intent-to-treat principle. The most perfect randomization scheme is useless if the analysis is based on a set different than the randomized set. For dental trials, which rely extensively on surrogate end points, every randomized patient and site should be accounted for in the analyses. It is used to be common that once a patient became edentulous, or when a patient lost a tooth, the patient or tooth would be dropped from the analysis. There was the mistaken belief that the split-mouth design would protect against such biases (Hujoel and DeRouen, 1992). Both a proper randomization and an intent-to-treat analysis are critical as deviations prohibit reliable information on treatment effectiveness and may increase the likelihood of false-positive conclusions.

7.4.4 Trial registration and negative results; is there a solution?

A 1997 review came to the conclusion that nonsteroidal anti-inflammatory medications (NSAIDS) have been "unequivocally" shown to have "primary therapeutic efficacy for periodontitis in humans (Salvi et al., 1997)." A casual PUBMED search may further identify small exploratory trials suggesting that such treatments are "a useful adjunct in the treatment of rapidly progressive periodontitis" (Reddy et al., 1993). Some clinicians may have been tempted to extrapolate such reports and prescribed rofecoxib based on the positive findings of *in vitro* evidence (Tipton et al., 2003). Yet, what was not published in the literature was that at least two large multicenter pivotal trials were conducted whose results were to the best of our knowledge not published. As a result, the published evidence consists of the small exploratory trials and the enthusiastic expert reviews; the unpublished evidence consists of the large multicenter studies with negative findings whose results disappeared into a black hole.

Such selective publication bias endangers a fair assessment of harms and benefits. Periodontal patients prescribed NSAIDS can expect a fourfold increased risk of serious gastrointestinal complications (Hernandez-Diaz and Rodriguez, 2000). For every 57 periodontal patients prescribed rofecoxib for up to 3 years, one patient can be expected to have a fatal or nonfatal myocardial infarction or stroke or a death from an unknown cause (Baron et al., 2008) as a direct result of taking rofecoxib. Such risks may be acceptable to some clinicians if indeed anti-inflammatory medications are effective against periodontitis. However, the nonpublication of pivotal trial results raises substantial doubt on the question of effectiveness.

The ongoing efforts at clinical trial registration and repositories for clinical trial results go a long away at solving such problems. However, even in medicine, it is realized that the current systems is still far from perfect ("No more scavenger hunts," 2008) and that the black hole for negative results is ever present. In dental research, where trials are conducted across the globe in locations ranging from China to Middle America to Eastern European countries, the potential for black holes appear at least as large as in medicine. Unless government organization such as the Food and Drug Administration, professional organizations such as the American Dental Association, and leading dental journals insists on pretrial registration of a protocol, and on the mandatory reporting of negative results, false-positives will continue to crowd out negative findings, and a warped reality will remain present in the published literature. Until solutions for this challenging problem are found, what is not published may remain more informative than what is published.

7.4.5   Size of the treatment effect and surrogates; how it relates to hypothesis testing?

Both the type of end point and the size of the treatment effect impacts on when to use statistical hypothesis testing and on what to specify for α and β (Newman et al., 2006). Four situations are differentiated and listed in order of decreasing clinical importance.

7.4.5.1   Clinical importance level 1

Bone marrow transplantation for leukemia, or tooth extraction for resolving the pain of acute pulpitis, is an example where treatment has a large impact on a clinically relevant outcome. Rigorous clinical trial design, hypothesis formulation, or issues such as α and β are largely irrelevant for establishing effectiveness. However, the less morbidity and mortality involved with the disease under investigation, the more important safety issues become.

The use of amalgam in dentistry offers one example where safety, and not effectiveness, was the primary reason to conduct randomized controlled trials (DeRouen et al., 2002).

7.4.5.2   Clinical importance level 2

Reliable detection of small treatment effects on true end points requires the conduct of randomized controlled trials, formal hypothesis formulation, and specification of α and β. Such an approach minimizes the risk for false-positive conclusions. Trials designed on true end points are typically large in sample size allowing for the reliable detection of side effects, a key issue for dental products with large market penetration.

Findings on surrogate end points are of a lesser clinical importance than findings on true end points. As a result, there is a more stringent need to have evidence on the absence of long-term adverse patient outcomes. Results on surrogate end points are classified depending on the size of the effect.

7.4.5.3   Clinical importance level 3

A 10+ mm reduction in probing depth or a 90% reduction in incidence of caries lesions that extend into the dentin are examples of large effects on surrogates. No hypothesis formulation, RCT, or specification of α and β are required to reliably detect or document such effects. The unforeseen long-term consequences on morbidity or mortality are of concern and cohort studies or case-control studies are needed to ensure that the large surrogate effects translate into a large patient benefits. For instance, while bone marrow transplants resulted in large amount of periodontal regeneration, longer follow-up indicated that up to 50% of such teeth were lost due to root resorption.

7.4.5.4   Clinical importance level 4

The conduct and analysis of the randomized controlled trials designed to detect small effects on surrogate end points should be most rigorous and specify small α and β as even tiny biases can increase the risk in false-positive conclusions. Use of sophisticated measurement techniques may allow for the design of studies where subtle treatment effects can be detected with small sample sizes. Such studies, however, cannot reliably detect side effects. Specifying small α and β will not only allow to reduce the rate of false-positive, but also to detect side effects more reliably.

7.5   Conclusion

Hypothesis testing and randomization are two key elements that provide a probabilistic basis for calculating false-positive and false-negative error rates. Reliable inference on the safety and the effectiveness of treatments is possible if the hypothesis is specified prior to the data collection, if the outcome is a true end point, if the likelihood for identifying effective treatments is large, and if all clinical trial results are reported, not just the positive ones. Potential solutions to reduce the rate of false-positive conclusions include providing a range for π prior to the initiation of the trial, a requirement to register clinical trials and their primary hypothesis prior to the conduct of the study, an ability to access *all* registered clinical trial results, specifying small α and β, and usage of true rather than surrogate end points. The ongoing changes in the drug and device approval process in the medical arena may ultimately lead to the implementation of some of these issues in dental research and thereby lead to a reduction in false-positive results.

References

Baron JA, Sandler RS, Bresalier RS, Lanas A, Morton DG, Riddell R, Iverson ER, Demets DL. 2008. Cardiovascular events associated with rofecoxib: final analysis of the APPROVe trial. *The Lancet* 372(9651):1756–1764.

Barouch DH. 2008. Challenges in the development of an HIV-1 vaccine. *Nature* 455(7213):613–619.

Bjelakovic G, Nikolova D, Gluud LL, Simonetti RG, Gluud C. 2007. Mortality in randomized trials of antioxidant supplements for primary and secondary prevention: systematic review and meta-analysis. *The Journal of the American Medical Association* 297(8):842–857.

Cunha-Cruz J, Hujoel PP, Maupome G, Saver B. 2008. Systemic antibiotics and tooth loss in periodontal disease. *Journal of Dental Research* 87(9):871–876.

Duffield-Lillico AJ, Dalkin BL, Reid ME, Turnbull BW, Slate EH, Jacobs ET, Marshall JR, Clark LC. 2003. Selenium supplementation, baseline plasma selenium status and incidence of prostate cancer: an analysis of the complete treatment period of the Nutritional Prevention of Cancer Trial. *BJU International* 91(7):608–612.

DeRouen TA, Hujoel PP, Mancl LA. 1995. Statistical issues in periodontal research. *Journal of Dental Research* 74(11):1731–1737.

DeRouen TA, Leroux BG, Martin MD, Townes BD, Woods JS, Leitao J, Castro-Caldas A, Braveman N. 2002. Issues in design and analysis of a randomized clinical trial to assess the safety of dental amalgam restorations in children. *Controlled Clinical Trials* 23(3):301–320.

Fleming TR. 1982. Historical controls, data banks, and randomized trials in clinical research: a review. *Cancer Treatment Reports* 66(5):1101–1105.

Forgie AH, Paterson M, Pine CM, Pitts NB, Nugent ZJ. 2000. A randomised controlled trial of the caries-preventive efficacy of a chlorhexidine-containing varnish in high-caries-risk adolescents. *Caries Research* 34(5):432–439.

Gann PH. 2008. Randomized trials of antioxidant supplementation for cancer prevention: first bias, now chance—next, cause. *The Journal of the American Medical Association* 301:102–103.

Goodman GE, Thornquist MD, Balmes J, Cullen MR, Meyskens FL Jr., Omenn GS, Valanis B, Williams JH Jr. 2004. The beta-carotene and retinol efficacy trial: incidence of lung cancer and cardiovascular disease mortality during 6-year follow-up after stopping beta-carotene and retinol supplements. *Journal of National Cancer Institute* 96(23):1743–1750.

Haffajee AD, Socransky SS, Gunsolley JC. 2003. Systemic anti-infective periodontal therapy. A systematic review. *Annals of Periodontology* 8(1):115–181.

Hernandez-Diaz S, Rodriguez LA. 2000. Association between nonsteroidal anti-inflammatory drugs and upper gastrointestinal tract bleeding/perforation: an overview of epidemiologic studies published in the 1990s. *Archives of Internal Medicine* 160(14):2093–2099.

Herrera D, Sanz M, Jepsen S, Needleman I, Roldan S. 2002. A systematic review on the effect of systemic antimicrobials as an adjunct to scaling and root planing in periodontitis patients. *Journal of Clinical Periodontology* 29(Suppl. 3):136–159; discussion 160–162.

Hujoel PP. 1995. Definitive vs. exploratory periodontal trials: a survey of published studies. *Journal of Dental Research* 74(8):1453–1458.

Hujoel PP, DeRouen TA. 1992. Validity issues in split-mouth trials. *Journal of Clinical Periodontology* 19(9 Pt 1):625–627.

Hujoel P, Kiyak A, Persson R, Persson G, Noonan C, Macentee MI, Wyatt C. 2003. Do dental chemotherapeutics provide real benefits? The need for large, simple trials. *Journal of Dental Research* Abstract 618.

Ioannidis JP. 2005. Why most published research findings are false. *PLoS Medicine* 2(8):e124.

Jeffcoat MK, Reddy MS, Haigh S, Buchanan W, Doyle MJ, Meredith MP, Nelson SL, Goodale MB, Wehmeyer KR. 1995. A comparison of topical ketorolac, systemic flurbiprofen, and placebo for the inhibition of bone loss in adult periodontitis. *Journal of Periodontology* 66(5):329–338.

Knight J. 2003. Negative results: null and void. *Nature* 422(6932):554–555.

Lesaffre E, Garcia Zattera MJ, Redmond C, Huber H, Needleman I. 2007. Reported methodological quality of split-mouth studies. *Journal of Clinical Periodontology* 34(9):756–761.

Lippman SM, Klein EA, Goodman PJ, Lucia MS, Thompson IM, Ford LG, Parnes HL, Minasian LM, Gaziano JM, Hartline JA, Parsons JK, Bearden JD 3rd, Crawford ED, Goodman GE, Claudio J, Winquist E, Cook ED, Karp DD, Walther P, Lieber MM, Kristal AR, Darke AK, Arnold KB, Ganz PA, Santella RM, Albanes D, Taylor PR, Probstfield JL, Jagpal TJ, Crowley JJ, Meyskens FL Jr., Baker LH, Coltman CA Jr. 2009. Effect of selenium and vitamin E on risk of prostate cancer and other cancers: the selenium and vitamin E cancer prevention trial (SELECT). *The Journal of the American Medical Association* 301(1): 39–51.

Lonn E, Bosch J, Yusuf S, Sheridan P, Pogue J, Arnold JM, Ross C, Arnold A, Sleight P, Probstfield J, Dagenais GR. 2005. Effects of long-term vitamin E supplementation on cardiovascular events and cancer: a randomized controlled trial. *The Journal of the American Medical Association* 293(11):1338–1347.

Lopez NJ, Smith PC, Gutierrez J. 2002. Periodontal therapy may reduce the risk of preterm low birth weight in women with periodontal disease: a randomized controlled trial. *Journal of Periodontology* 73(8):911–924.

Macilwain C. 1998. Clinton 'is failing to honour pledge on AIDS vaccine'. *Nature* 393(6682):199.

Michalowicz BS, Hodges JS, DiAngelis AJ, Lupo VR, Novak MJ, Ferguson JE, Buchanan W, Bofill J, Papapanou PN, Mitchell DA, Matseoane S, Tschida PA. 2006. Treatment of periodontal disease and the risk of preterm birth. *New England Journal of Medicine* 355(18):1885–1894.

Miller ER, 3rd, Pastor-Barriuso R, Dalal D, Riemersma RA, Appel LJ, Guallar E. 2005. Meta-analysis: high-dosage vitamin E supplementation may increase all-cause mortality. *Annals of Internal Medicine* 142(1):37–46.

Montenegro R, Needleman I, Moles D, Tonetti M. 2002. Quality of RCTs in periodontology—a systematic review. *Journal of Dental Research* 81(12):866–870.

Newman MG, Takei HH, Klokkevold PR, Carranza FA. 2006. *Carranza's Clinical Periodontology*, 10th edn. Philadelphia: W.B. Saunders Co.

No more scavenger hunts. 2008. No more scavenger hunts. *Nature* 452(7183):1.

Nowak R. 1994. Problems in clinical trials go far beyond misconduct. *Science* 264(5165):1538–1541.

Pocock SJ. 1983. *Clinical Trials: A Practical Approach*. Chichester [West Sussex]; New York: Wiley.

Reddy MS, Palcanis KG, Barnett ML, Haigh S, Charles CH, Jeffcoat MK. 1993. Efficacy of meclofenamate sodium (Meclomen) in the treatment of rapidly progressive periodontitis. *Journal of Clinical Periodontology* 20(9):635–640.

Rossouw JE, Anderson GL, Prentice RL, LaCroix AZ, Kooperberg C, Stefanick ML, Jackson RD, Beresford SA, Howard BV, Johnson KC, Kotchen JM, Ockene J. 2002. Risks and benefits of estrogen plus progestin in healthy postmenopausal women: principal results from the women's health initiative randomized controlled trial. *The Journal of the American Medical Association* 288(3):321–333.

Salvi GE, Williams RC, Offenbacher S. 1997. Nonsteroidal anti-inflammatory drugs as adjuncts in the management of periodontal diseases and peri-implantitis. *Current Opinion in Periodontology* 4:51–58.

Sandham HJ, Brown J, Chan KH, Phillips HI, Burgess RC, Stokl AJ. 1991. Clinical trial in adults of an antimicrobial varnish for reducing mutans streptococci. *Journal of Dental Research* 70(11):1401–1408.

Silverstein SG, S, Heilbron D, Nelms D, Wycoff S. 1977. Effect of supervised deplaquing on dental caries, gingivitis, and plaque (abstract). *Journal of Dental Research* 56(Special Issue A):A85.

Simon R. 1982. An evaluation of clinical trial designs that randomize composite units rather than individual patients. *Experientia Supplementum* 41:318–326.

Staquet MJ, Rozencweig M, Von Hoff DD, Muggia FM. 1979. The delta and epsilon errors in the assessment of cancer clinical trials. *Cancer Treatment Reports* 63(11–12):1917–1921.

The Alpha-Tocopherol, Beta Carotene Cancer Prevention Study Group. 1994. The effect of vitamin E and beta carotene on the incidence of lung cancer and other cancers in male smokers. The alpha-tocopherol, beta carotene cancer prevention study group. *New England Journal of Medicine* 330(15):1029–1035.

Tipton DA, Flynn JC, Stein SH, Dabbous M. 2003. Cyclooxygenase-2 inhibitors decrease interleukin-1beta-stimulated prostaglandin E2 and IL-6 production by human gingival fibroblasts. *Journal of Periodontology* 74(12):1754–1763.

Turner EH, Matthews AM, Linardatos E, Tell RA, Rosenthal R. 2008. Selective publication of antidepressant trials and its influence on apparent efficacy. *New England Journal of Medicine* 358(3):252–260.

Williams RC, Paquette DW, Offenbacher S, Adams DF, Armitage GC, Bray K, Caton J, Cochran DL, Drisko CH, Fiorellini JP, Giannobile WV, Grossi S, Guerrero DM, Johnson GK, Lamster IB, Magnusson I, Oringer RJ, Persson GR, Van Dyke TE, Wolff LF, Santucci EA, Rodda BE, Lessem J. 2001. Treatment of periodontitis by local administration of minocycline microspheres: a controlled trial. *Journal of Periodontology* 72(11):1535–1544.

Yusuf S, Wittes J, Probstfield J, Tyroler HA. 1991. Analysis and interpretation of treatment effects in subgroups of patients in randomized clinical trials. *The Journal of the American Medical Association* 266(1):93–98.

Zero DT. 2004. Sugars—the arch criminal? *Caries Research* 38(3):277–285.

8

Outcomes in oral health research

Amid I. Ismail, BDS, MPH, MBA, DrPH

8.1   Introduction

Research is a systematic method for asking and answering questions. It is a method of enquiry that follows protocols to control and eliminate biases and increases the probability of making the least biased decisions. The foundation of clinical research is based on asking focused and clinically relevant questions; postulating hypotheses and alternative hypotheses (see Chapter 7); defining outcome measures; and testing or evaluating interventions. The use of a systematic approach to define, measure, and analyze the outcomes of interest is crucial for the success of any research endeavor (Platt, 1964, Chapter 18).

Unfortunately, there is limited evidence and research on methods of assessing outcomes in dental research. By and large, researchers have focused on consistency of methods to assess "outcomes" and comparability among studies. There is limited development and discussion on what are the appropriate outcomes in dental research as well as on research to develop new methods that are more suited for contemporary research questions.

A major challenge in clinical research is the understanding of the term "outcome." Outcomes are the consequences or results of interventions (Bader and Ismail, 1999). While this definition may appear simple, a deeper understanding of the "consequences of interventions" is required to appreciate the full depth of the process for determining how to assess outcomes. Some health conditions assessed in clinical research progress slowly (caries clinical trials, e.g., require at a minimum 2 years). In such cases, either process or surrogate outcomes (change in behaviors, dietary intake, infection with cariogenic bacteria; salivary flow) may be measured provided that these can be influenced in shorter time frames than the final health outcomes. (A surrogate outcome is a measure that is related to and can be used as a substitute for the "true" outcome.) Another challenge is that some outcomes, such as the quality of life, can be difficult to measure using simple indicators because they assess multidimensional domains. Quality of oral health status is measured using questions that assess different dimensions such as oral symptoms, functions, social, and behavioral affects that impact positively or negatively on the quality of life (Locker and Slade, 1993; Locker et al., 2004). Such scales require complex validation and evaluation of their internal consistency (Allen et al., 1999; Foster Page et al., 2005) and validity.

In many areas of clinical research, identifying outcomes is a crucial process for understanding the disease process and its management. For example, in caries research, the primary outcome in clinical trials have been the increment (increase) in the number of decayed, missing, and filled teeth or tooth surfaces (DMFT or DMFS). This is an end-stage outcome (equivalent to death). An alternative outcome could be the reduction in the initiation and progression of early caries. Such an outcome may not only reduce the length of time required to show an effect in caries clinical trials but may also lead to developing interventions that promote remineralization or arrestment. Using standard or traditional assessment methods in order to ensure comparability does not help in the evaluation of efficacy of new interventions. In periodontal research, the presence of loss of attachment or pathological pockets may not be as important as assessing the probability of progression of loss of periodontal attachment (disease activity).

The measurement of oral health outcomes is of considerable importance to the success of any research project. A fatal error in research design is the failure to define the appropriate outcomes and how best to measure them validly and reliably. Also, defining what outcomes to measure has implications on all aspects of the design of a clinical research project. Sample size and power calculations depend on the expected changes and degree of variance of the outcome measures.

This chapter provides an introduction to the field of outcome assessment to enable the readers to understand the relevant questions and issues that should be addressed when clinical research projects are developed. This chapter does not cover in depth the topic area and research on methods to assess oral health outcomes and it does not present any statistical background for how outcomes are validated, assessed, or analyzed. Readers are advised to consult with textbooks that deal with these topics (Nezu and Nezu, 2008; McDowell and Newell, 1996).

8.2   Classification of outcomes

Bader and Ismail (1999) presented a framework for evaluation of dental outcomes using four dimensions: biological, clinical, psychosocial, and economic costs (Table 8.1).

The biological dimension includes outcomes associated with the pathological, physiological, microbiological, immunologic, genetic, or sensory effects of health or disease. These outcome domains have been widely used in dental research because they can show an impact after short exposure to an intervention. For example, in recent clinical trials on periodontal diseases, biological outcomes used were the extracellular matrix metalloproteinase inducer (EMMPRIN) in gingival crevicular fluid (GCF) (Emingel et al., 2008) and serum markers of acute-phase inflammatory and vascular responses (Ide et al., 2003). In dental caries, the reduction in cariogenic bacterial levels, such as streptococcus mutans, has been used as a microbiological outcome (Derks et al., 2008). The problem with using surrogate outcomes is that while an agent, such as antimicrobial varnish or

Table 8.1   Classification of outcomes of oral health care.

Dimension	Examples
Biological	
Physiological	Salivary flow and consistency, demineralization, inflammation
Microbiological	Oral microflora composition, presence of specific pathogens
Sensory	Presence of pain, parathesia
Clinical status	
Survival	Longevity/loss of tooth, pulp, tooth surface, restoration
Mechanical	Smoothness of margins, conformation of contours
Diagnostic	Presence of pathology, caries, periodontal diseases
Functional	Ability to chew, speak, swallow
Psychosocial	
Satisfaction	Satisfaction with treatment, dentist, oral health
Perceptions	Esthetics, oral health self-rating
Preferences	Values for health states and health events
Oral health-related quality of life	Ratings of how oral health affects life
Economic costs	
Direct	Out-of-pocket payments, third party payments
Indirect	Lost wages, transportation, child care expenses

Courtesy: Bader and Ismail (1999).

salivary flow, may be impacted by an intervention, the effect on the final clinical outcomes may not occur. There is definitely need for validation of all surrogate outcome vis-à-vis the final clinical outcome. Validation should be replicated under different clinical conditions.

Clinical outcomes are most widely reported in dental clinical trials. These outcomes can be classified into survival outcomes (longevity of restoration or loss of tooth or restoration); mechanical outcomes (smoothness of margins, conformation of contours, mobility of teeth); diagnostic outcomes (presence of pathology, caries, periodontal disease, open bites, crossbites, malocclusion); and functional outcomes (chewing of foods; speaking, swallowing after cancer treatment).

A significant interest has emerged during the last decade in evaluating psychosocial outcomes. Oral health and dental care influence the quality of life and assessment of this outcome is necessary to understand the full impact of dental interventions on patients' well-being. Hence, it is now customary in clinical trials to assess quality of life and answer the question of whether the intervention improves the quality of oral health-related quality of life. Psychosocial outcomes include satisfaction with treatment, providers, or outcomes of interventions. Perception outcomes are related to how people feel about esthetics and their oral health status. Preference for outcome states is another important, but not yet fully developed research area. Preference refers to the choices that individuals make between two or more outcomes under conditions of uncertainty (probability of success is known but it varies). There are different methods to assess preferences including health time equivalents, willingness to pay (WTP), and quality-adjusted life (tooth) years, among others (Birch and Ismail, 2002; Birch et al., 2004; Ismail et al., 2004). Utility assessment measures the expected effect of undertaking an intervention on an individual's assessment of his or her well-being. The trade-offs between two interventions depends on whether the well-being associated with a treatment more than offset the reduction in well-being associated with the additional cost and discomfort, and inconvenience associated with an alternative treatment. This is an important dimension of assessing outcomes in clinical research because, while a new treatment may be more effective than the standard of care, the associated loss of well-being may be higher, and hence, patients will continue to prefer the standard of care, even though it is less effective. Hence, by focusing only on physical outcomes, the full impact of newly discovered interventions on oral health will not be known.

Psychosocial outcome assesses the impact of an intervention on individuals' lives and daily living. One of the widely used tools in dentistry to measure quality of oral health is the Oral Health Impact Profile (OHIP) (Slade and Spencer, 1994). Like all quality of life measures, OHIP does not assess the trade-off in individuals' well-being between two interventions, and hence, it cannot provide information on direct comparability between two interventions (Birch and Ismail, 2002).

Economic outcomes are objective measures of the costs (Bahrami et al., 2004), effectiveness relative to cost (Simon et al., 2008), and return on investment associated with any intervention (Finkelstein and Trogdon, 2008). Cost-effectiveness analysis focuses on the cost of achieving one unit improvement in a clinical outcome or health status. The best interventions are the ones that achieve the improvement in outcomes with the lowest cost. Return on investment is a business outcome that can be assessed in health programs. It measures the profits (health benefits in dollars) generated with a health intervention compared with the direct and indirect costs of the intervention. For example, Finkelstein and Trogdon (2008) measured the return on investment to reduce childhood obesity by assessing the cost of the programs versus savings of later or delayed costs of treating obesity. In making these economic analyses, it is imperative to consider not only direct costs but also indirect costs such as cost of transportation, lost wages, and child care expenses (Bader and Ismail, 1999). Another factor that is often missed is the opportunity cost, which is the cost of foregoing another intervention or another activity.

8.3   Measurements of outcomes

The decision on which outcome(s) to assess in a clinical study depends on the research question. After the question for a clinical research project is defined, the next step is to state a hypothesis. The hypothesis should define the outcome measure(s) that will answer the question. For example, in a randomized controlled trial reported by Truelove et al. in 2006, the objective was to compare different types of occlusal splints with self-care on temporomandibular disorders (TMD-related pain and self-reported TMD symptoms). The researchers defined the outcomes in the hypotheses as "short-term improvement in self-reported pain and in clinical measures such as range of motion, [and] palpation pain." These are specific and measurable outcomes.

Outcomes may either be quantitative or qualitative. Quantitative outcomes are those that can be expressed with numbers. For example, the number of carious tooth surfaces, depth of pockets, and pain intensity are some of the quantitative measures used in dental clinical studies. Qualitative outcomes are verbal or categorical representations of nonquantifiable characteristics such as gender, race, and satisfaction. Some outcomes such as pain can be measured using qualifiers (Truelove et al., 2006) or quantitatively (Yamamoto et al., 2006). The choice of scale is important in answering the question. If the question calls for evaluating the effectiveness of fluoride varnish on the incidence of children with new caries lesions, then the outcome variable is different from the question that asks if the severity of new carious lesions will be reduced by the fluoride treatment. The first scale is a count (number of children with new lesions divided by the total number of children), whereas the second scale is quantitative (the number of tooth surfaces with new carious lesions). The reason why scales are important is because they influence the choice of appropriate statistical methods.

Qualitative outcomes can be classified into nominal measures such as gender (male vs. female) or presence or absence of pain. These outcomes should not be averaged; rather, frequencies or probabilities should be computed. Nominal outcomes can be modeled in linear equations (such as logistic regression) to identify the risk factors associated with high probability of developing disease or being in a disease state.

Outcome measures that provide information or order the data or observations are referred to as ordinal. These outcomes present sequential ascending or descending order of a disease state or risk factor. For example, education can be measured by the level of highest attainment (less than elementary, elementary school completed, less than high school, high school completed, some college, and college degree completed). Ordinal data should not be averaged as well and can be analyzed using frequency counts or median or mode.

Quantitative outcome measures are classified into internal or ratio scales. An interval scale has rankings, just like an ordinal scale, but the distance between adjacent points on the scale are equal. For example, the difference between a temperature of 10 degree on the Fahrenheit scale and 20 degrees is equivalent to the difference between 30 and 40 degree. However, 20 degrees is not as twice as hot as 10 degrees because there is no meaningful zero point. A zero Fahrenheit does not mean that there is no temperature. When an interval measure has a real zero (e.g., zero age), an individual who is 20 years old is twice as old as someone who is 10 years old. Ratio scales have all the characteristics of nominal, ordinal, and interval scales. Both ratio and internal scaled variables can be averaged.

In understanding scales and how they relate to statistical analysis, it is imperative to appreciate that there are many compromises. For example, in dental research, gingival bleeding may be measured at each tooth surface using a nominal scale (present, absence). Each tooth may have one or more of these measures based on the number of sites assessed in a study. Analysts may sum up the scores and create an average number of bleeding site. Currently available statistical techniques, such as General Estimating Equation, can analyze data from each tooth site and account for the clustering of disease within a single mouth (Hanley et al., 2003); however, these techniques are not widely used in dental research. In other cases, outcome measures that are generally ordinal are analyzed as if they are interval scales. For example, in evaluating satisfaction with dental care, or pain, the scales are ordinal but are analyzed as interval scales.

In assessing outcomes that are affected by more than one construct, such as quality of life, or outcomes where there is no one question or indicator to classify the presence or absence of a condition, such as depression, researchers have developed methods to validate multidimensional scales. For example, depression is measured using a 20-item questionnaire that has been validated and can generate a single score that classify the symptoms of depression (Radloff, 1977; Hann et al., 1999). The Center for Epidemiologic Studies Depression (CES-D) scale can generate a score between 0 and 60 and measures symptoms in four somatic symptoms: appetite, bothered, effort, and sleep (Radloff, 1977).

The CES-D scale has item consistency measured using the Cronbach's alpha (α) coefficient (>0.85) (Hann et al., 1999) indicating that the 20 questions cluster as a group and can be used to validly measure the symptoms of depression. A score of more than 16 indicates that there are symptoms of depression but that does not mean that a patient has depression.

Outcome measures or scales for psychosocial or behavioral outcomes should not be accepted at face value. Researchers should critically evaluate each measure applicability and utility for their research project. Standard categorization of outcome measures, such as the CES-D, for example, should be tailored to differences among population groups. For South Koreans, for example, the suggested cutoff point is 24–25 instead of 16 that is recommended for the CES-D (Cho et al., 1998). Also, it is imperative to evaluate whether validation of an outcome measure was conducted with a similar patient or population groups to those targeted in a research project. Validation of an outcome measure among whites may not be applicable to other groups. Similarly, cross-country or cross-cultural validation is recommended before selecting outcome measures in any clinical study. This caution applies to clinical criteria as well.

8.3.1   Validity

A valid outcome measure truly assesses the disease, condition, or health state that it purports to measure. Imagine observing an archer in the Olympics. She is "valid" when her arrows hit the center of the target (the bull's eye) (Figure 8.1a).

She is also reliable. Reliability is how clustered are the arrows of the Olympian around the target area (Figure 8.1b). Reliability is the inverse of the degree of inconsistency, or variation, of the Olympian. If she hits the bull's eyes, what is the percentage or probability that she will hit the same target area? An outcome measure may be reliable but not necessarily hitting the target (Figure 8.1c). In this case, the measure is invalid. To achieve validity, the outcome measure must be reliable.

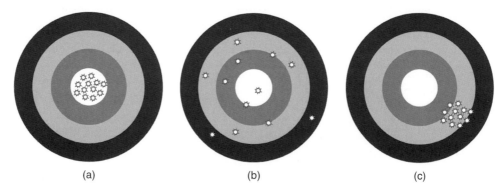

(a)   (b)   (c)

Figure 8.1 Reliability and validity. (a) An example of a highly valid and reliable outcome measure. (b) An example of a highly unreliable outcome measure. The measure cannot be considered valid because of its high unreliability. (c) An example of highly invalid but highly reliable outcome measure.

The previous example is oversimplistic because most of what we measure in clinical research cannot be equated with the "bull's eye." Often we do not know what the "true" status is or we measure a multidimensional condition (such as pain) where there is no one "true" state. In some cases, it is not feasible to assess validity for ethical or practical reasons. Hence, validation is usually carried out using multiple approaches.

Clinical researchers should always ask the question of whether the outcome measure (e.g., criteria for assessing caries) has content validity. Stated differently, do the criteria measure the caries process as it is currently understood based on the scientific evidence? In evaluating 29 criteria systems for caries assessment, the majority of these were found to have low content validity (Ismail, 2004). Criteria used for detection of caries that have been developed during the last 10 years have higher content validity (Ismail, 2004) than older criteria systems.

Content evaluation is usually conducted by experts in the field or area of research. It is a subjective process and does not involve statistical evaluations. In evaluating questionnaires, experts check for comprehensiveness of the items and whether they measure all factors associated with the condition being considered (Radloff, 1977, has the questions used in the Center for Epidemiological Studies Depression questionnaire).

Statistical evaluation of validity can be divided into either criterion or construct evaluation. Criterion validity requires comparing the instruments with a "gold standard." A simple approach to criterion validity is based on correlating the new instrument or criteria or outcome measure with the findings obtained by using a "gold standard." This process is also referred to as correlational validity. This validation approach can also be divided into "concurrent" or "predictive" validity depending on whether the new instrument, criteria, or questionnaire purports to assess current or future status.

Unfortunately, in evaluating new outcome measures, a "gold standard" may not always be available, or if available, it may be prone to random errors; in other words, it is "fuzzy" (Phelps and Hutson, 1995). A fuzzy gold standard could generate over- or underestimation of the true correlation between a new outcome measure and the standard. The direction depends on the correlation between the errors of each measure (Phelps and Hutson, 1995). Correction methods have been proposed for either case (Phelps and Hutson, 1995).

The design of correlational validation studies depends on the time frame. In concurrent validation studies, the new instrument or questionnaire is compared with the results of the "gold standard." In predictive validation, the new test is applied in a prospective study in which the measurements obtained at the start of the study are compared with subsequent outcomes. However, such design may present an ethical paradox in that once a patient is found to be at risk of developing disease; intervention must be provided and that will change the course of disease overtime. To resolve this problem, predictive validation studies should be of short duration and patient welfare should be protected.

A common correlational validation method of diagnostic tests (or outcomes) depends on estimating the sensitivity and specificity of tests to differentiae between people who are sick from those who are well. Sensitivity is defined as the proportion individuals who are diseased and are correctly identified by the test, and specificity is the proportion of individuals who are healthy and are correctly classified by the new test. Estimating sensitivity and specificity requires classifying individuals into two categories: healthy or diseased. If a test provides a continuum of data, such as blood pressure, a prior decision should be made on what cutoff point designate an individual to be healthy or diseased. That is usually arbitrary and can be problematic. A solution to this problem involves changing the cutoff points and estimating sensitivity and specificity for each point. A graph depicting the two parameters (sensitivity against 1-specificity) at different cutoff points is referred to as the receiver operating curve (ROC). The area under the curve (AUC) provides a measure of how good the new test is in detecting disease. If the AUC is 50%, then the new test is as good as flipping a coin. An AUC of 70–90% is usually considered acceptable and a test with an AUC of 90% or higher is considered highly accurate.

The best design for a sensitivity and specificity validation is to apply the new and standard test on individuals who are randomly selected from a population that has a wide array of severity of the diseased state and represents the target users of the tests. This design may not always be feasible because of the cost of applying the standard test or ethical concern. An alternative design is to select patients (cases) using the new test and then confirm the diagnosis using the standard test. A random sample of patients classified as healthy also receives the standard test. This design may suffer from selection bias and may lead to inflation of the sensitivity coefficient.

Conditions such as pain, quality of life, depression, stress, anxiety, satisfaction, and others do not have gold standards. They can be compared with standard tests if both tests measure the same dimensions. Construct validation of these outcomes begins with conceptual mapping of the condition or phenomenon. The mapping of constructs or domains also includes identifying the potential theoretical relationships among the components. The correlations among the constructs are studied to evaluate whether the theoretical basis is accurate for the outcome or risk factor being evaluated.

Factor analysis is often used to select constructs or factors that represent significant domains to be included in a new scale. Factor analysis uses responses to identify groupings of indicators with high correlations that are also different from other subgroups or factors. There are requirements for conducting appropriate factor analyses (Comrey, 1978; Boyle, 1985). The questions or items to be analyzed should be measured at the interval scale and the responses should be normally distributed. There should be a large enough sample size (more respondents than variables). Most factor analyses of categorical responses violate the first two requirements. Studies with large sample size may yield indicators that are close to normally distributed. For binary data, latent trait analysis or item response theory can be used for data reduction (reducing data to be collected by identifying factors or questions to be measured that provide the same power to detect differences, data exploration, and theory confirmation (a check on whether the hypothesized questions are important factors) (Uebersax, 1993, Uebersax and Grove, 1993). The standardized tests such as the Graduate Record Examination (GRE) are developed using latent trait analysis.

8.3.2   Cautions

Validation of outcome measure is a complex and time-consuming endeavor. Designing new questionnaires should never be viewed as a simple task of writing questions. This is scientifically naïve and dangerous. Waste of respondents' time by collecting data using a poorly constructed questionnaire can result when the instrument is not well developed and validated. There are always biases that could result when a validated instrument is applied in a different setting or with different population group than those who share the same characteristics as those engaged in developing the instrument. Prevalence of the condition measured may be different between the original study and the new one and that results in bias. Hence, validation of outcomes measures or assessments of risk factors should always be carried out in different settings.

Prior to selection of an outcome measure for a study, it is imperative that hypotheses and goal of assessment are defined. Systematic approaches to construct validation have been proposed (Kantz et al., 1992; McHorney et al., 1993).

8.3.3   Reliability and internal consistency

In a previous discussion of validity and reliability, the dispersion around a target (Figure 8.1) was used to describe the degree of unreliability. The less the inconsistency or variation in measuring the desired outcome or risk factor, the higher is the reliability or consistency. There are different reasons why an outcome measure is rated as unreliable. The measure itself or the individual who is assessing it may suffer from systematic errors or is consistently biased. These errors are due to a flaw in the measure itself or the examiner or interviewer. For example, an examiner in a caries study may suffer from color blindness and hence cannot differentiate between "white" and "brown" caries lesions. The examiner is biased (he will not measure the "true" state of caries all the time).

The reliability error that can be reduced and assessed is caused by random error. An examiner may be tired, a patient may be difficult to examine, or the tooth status may be unique or different from average teeth examined before. The examiners' random error is not related to the severity of disease (error is not greater in patients with high diseases compared with other patients). Random errors also balance out if large enough observations are made. There is always safety in numbers, even when reliability is assessed!

In dental research, reliability is usually assessed by examining about 10% of the subjects. However, this goal may not always be possible because sometimes it may be difficult to recall children or adults for reliability assessment.

The common model for assessing reliability of criteria and examiners is the test–retest model (Bland and Altman, 1986). The examiner repeats the examination after a reasonable period (a day to a week) (intra-examiner) or two examiners sequentially examine the same patients (inter-examiner reliability). A statistically better approach would be to estimate a sample size for a hypothesized level of examination reliability and the width of the confidence interval, which is influenced by the sample size for a given type I error ($\alpha = 0.05$) (Flack et al., 1988). For evaluation of questionnaires, the focus is usually on the consistency of the interviewers in following protocols. This type of evaluation requires monitoring the fidelity of the interview process using either audio or videotaping.

There is often some misunderstanding of the difference between agreement and association. Agreement refers to the degree with which two measures of the same conditions differ. For each individual examined in a study, the scores (e.g., pocket depth) can be graphically plotted for first and second examinations (assuming that there are two examinations). The difference between the scores is a measure of the degree of agreement. It is expected that 95% of the difference in scores will lie within two standard deviations of the mean. The standard deviation of the difference can be computed by squaring the differences, dividing by the total number of observations, and taking the square root (Bland and Altman, 1986).

An association between two clinical measures assessed by two examiners, or one examiner assessing the same condition twice, within reasonable time frame, refers to the linear relationships, rather agreement, between the two scores. For example, the Pearson correlation coefficient is a measure of association that may indicate high level of linear relationship between two scores when the two scores consistently have low agreement. To illustrate, in assessing pocket depth, one examiner consistently overestimate pocket depth and another consistently underestimate pocket depth, the relationship will be high (because of the consistency) but low in agreement (because of examiners' systematic error).

In assessing reliability, it is imperative to know (or decide) on the scale of the outcome measures. For binary nominal scale (yes vs. no), the best measure of agreement is the Cohen's Kappa (κ) coefficients (Cohen, 1960). The widely used κ coefficient measures the level of agreement that exceeds chance and it includes information from scoring of all categories of the scale. There are accepted general guidelines of what is considered a good or excellent κ (Landis and Koch, 1977). A κ lower than 0.4 is considered to be an indicator of poor agreement while a κ coefficient higher than 0.6 is rated as very good (substantial) agreement. For multinomial scales, the weighted κ is the recommended statistics (Fleiss, 1971). A weighted κ assigns values to each deviation from perfect agreement (the diagonal cells in an agreement table). Weights are computed using formula by major statistical analysis packages. The two commonly used are the Fleiss et al. (2004) or the Cicchetti and Allison (1971), which yield more conservative estimate of reliability than the Fleiss method.

κ coefficients are recommended for assessing reliability of all the scores in nominal or ordinal scales. κ coefficients, however, should not be used to assess the reliability of a single code in an ordinal scale. For example, κ as a statistic is not recommended for assessing the reliability of examiners on detecting early carious lesions in a system that measures the stages of dental caries, because when the scale is dichotomized, the degree of consistency is dependent on the full range of the scores (e.g., early carious lesions versus all other lesions). A crude approach to address this issue is to present the agreement on a single score to report proportions of agreement (of all incipient caries lesions detected by examiner A, how many were detected by examiner?). However, these simple proportions should be presented with the proportions showing the direction and degree of misclassification either within the same examiner or among examiners.

κ coefficients are often reported without any evaluation of whether there is marginal homogeneity in the distribution of the scores between the same examiners or in case of inter-examiner reliability two examiners. While this condition was challenged by Gwet (2002) who found that κ coefficients are more affected by the propensity for positive classifications (or identifying disease state(s)) rather than by marginal homogeneity (Gwet, 2002), it is imperative to remember that the prevalence of the condition should really be monitored when assessing examiner reliability (Ludbrook, 2004). This means that similar numbers of diseased and healthy teeth or subjects should be examined by all examiners. For ordinal scales, such as those that stage the disease as none, medium, and high, there should be relatively balanced distribution among all examinations. To achieve this goal, reliability assessment should be conducted using a selection of teeth or patients that represent the disease and healthy states rather than conducted using convenience samples.

For interval data, the best approach is to estimate the intraclass correlation coefficient (ICC), which is a measure of the explained variance of the interval scale that is attributable to the two time points (in a test–retest model of assessing reliability) (Shrout and Fleiss, 1979). It is the ratio of between groups (or two time periods for the same examiner) to total variance. If the examiner agrees 100% with her previous scores, then the ICC will be equivalent to 1.0, indicating perfect reliability. That is rarely achieved, and if reported in a study, the reader should feel extremely suspicious of the data. Formulas for computing the

ICC for a specific study are available (Walter et al., 1998; Bonett, 2002) and are based on power level (e.g., 0.8), magnitude of the predicted ICC, and type I error (0.05). The ICC is interpreted like a correlation coefficient. An ICC of 1.0 indicates that the raters (or two time periods) are fully homogenous or their scores are the same for each subject. More details on how to compute and interpret the ICC scores can be found in Shrout and Fleiss (1979).

8.3.4   Internal consistency

In evaluating the reliability of outcome measures with multiple domain or dimensions, such as the CES-D questionnaire, the recommended approach is to evaluate the internal consistency of the questionnaire. Test–retest reliability is not recommended because the subjects in a study may change their answers after the first administration. Computing all possible correlation among all pairs of questions, the internal consistency of the data can be assessed. Cronbach's α is a widely used measure of internal consistency (Cronbach, 1951). The α coefficient is a measure of reliability and it provides an estimate of how good are the variables (e.g., questions) in measuring a single latent concept (e.g., pain intensity or depression). Cronbach's α has similar foundation as factor analysis. It is equivalent to unidimensional factor analysis. In constructing a scale, a set of questions are analyzed to identify clusters of questions that are measuring the same "factors." Investigators label the different sets, if possible, and then compute the Cronbach's α to check for internal consistency of the newly developed scale. Before using a questionnaire to measure multidimensional indicators of an outcome (e.g., depression), it is advisable that the internal consistency be evaluated.

8.4   Dental and oral health outcomes in clinical research

This section presents examples of some contemporary outcome measures of dental caries, periodontal diseases, and temporomandibular disorders/facial pain. Full details on the measures and their validity and reliability are not discussed in this chapter. Readers should survey the literature on methods of outcomes assessed in current studies before launching a clinical research project. I also advise researchers to focus on the research question and hypothesis proposed in a study and select (or develop) outcome measures that can validly and reliably assess the impact of an intervention or provide information to answer the question or test an hypothesis.

8.4.1   Dental caries

Dental caries is a complex disease (Selwitz et al., 2007) with different manifestations (noncavitated, cavitated, filled, missing) involving any of the 20 primary or 32 permanent teeth or their tooth surface. The unit of analysis in clinical studies has been the total caries experience per individual that is summarized by the number of decayed (D or d), missing due to caries (M or m), and filled (F or f) teeth or tooth surfaces (DMFT or DMFS for permanent teeth and dmfs or dmft for primary teeth). Each component of the DMF score (D, M, or F) has potential measurement errors and is subject to random variation.

The assessment of presence or absence of dental caries on nonrestored or restored tooth surfaces follows defined criteria. Ismail (2004) evaluated 29 criteria systems commonly used in dental epidemiological or clinical studies and found that most of them, especially those widely used in the United States, lack current content validity. New criteria in clinical studies should assess different stages of the caries process from clinically noncavitated to cavitated lesions (Pitts and Stamm, 2004). Except for some recent criteria (Nyvad et al., 2003; Ekstrand et al., 2007), the existing definitions do not differentiate between actively progressing and nonactive carious lesions.

All of the current criteria for detection of caries measure one (cavitated) or more (noncavitated and cavitated) disease stages, if they are applied consistently and correctly by the examiners. The criteria, however, differ in the way the disease is measured (dry vs. wet teeth and use of explorers) (Ismail, 2004).

An attempt to develop contemporary definitions and requirements for detecting caries was launched in 2002 by the International Caries Detection and Assessment System (IC-DAS) (Ismail et al., 2007). ICDAS was designed to detect six stages of the carious process (Table 8.2), ranging from clinically visible early carious demineralization to extensive cavitation. Detection of caries using ICDAS is a two-stage process. The first decision is to classify each tooth surface as sound, sealed, restored, crowned, or missing. The second decision is the classification of the carious status on an ordinal scale (codes 0–6) (International Caries Detection and Assessment System, 2005). The κ coefficients for six examiners using ICDAS were between 0.59 and 0.82 (Ismail et al., 2007). ICDAS has been shown to be correlated with histological detection of caries in enamel and dentin (Ekstrand et al., 1997; Ricketts et al., 2002) and has discriminatory validity (Ismail et al., 2008).

The ICDAS status for each tooth surface can be used to compute the total number of decayed, missing due to caries, or filled teeth or tooth surfaces. The DMFS or DMFT (or dmft or dmfs for primary teeth) are outcome measures of the severity of dental caries but not prevalence (prevalence is the number of individuals with a disease state). For primary teeth, counting of missing teeth can be confounded by natural exfoliation, and hence sometimes only teeth extracted due to caries (e) before their exfoliation age are counted instead of missing teeth in a mouth. For adults, sometimes it is difficult to determine whether teeth were missing because of caries or due to other reasons. As far as counting of filled tooth surfaces or teeth, the real reason why a filling was placed cannot be determined at the time the clinical examiners in a research project conduct the evaluation. There is good evidence that dentists vary significantly in when they restore or not restore a tooth and misclassification is a problem (Bader and Shugars, 1997).

In clinical trials or longitudinal studies, the outcome measure is the increment in DMF scores (Δ DMFS). The increment should not be computed by subtracting the DMFS score at follow-up from the score at baseline because the transitions (reversals) between the different states of the D, M, and F, as well as between noncavitated and cavitated caries status may not always be logical. For example, a tooth surface may be scored filled at baseline and sound at follow-up, and a cavitated lesion could illogically move toward noncavitated status at follow-up. There is currently no standard method for handling these reversals; however, they must be included in the computation of the so-called "net" increment because if the examiners erred in classifying a filled tooth surface at baseline sound at follow-up, it is expected that they also erred sometimes in the opposite direction.

There are two approaches that can be recommended for handling reversals. The first approach uses a weight for each possible transition. The weight can range from -1 to $+1$.

Table 8.2   Diagnostic levels of dental caries measured using the International Caries Detection and Assessment System.

Code	Description
0	Sound tooth surfaces There should be no evidence of caries (either no or questionable change in enamel translucency after air drying for 5 seconds). Surfaces with developmental defects such as enamel hypoplasia, fluorosis, tooth wear (attrition, abrasion, and erosion), and extrinsic or intrinsic stains are recorded as sound
1	First visual change in enamel When seen wet, there is no evidence of any change in color attributable to carious activity, but after air drying for 5 seconds, a carious opacity is visible that is not consistent with the clinical appearance of sound enamel
2	Distinct visual change in enamel When viewed wet, there is a carious opacity or discoloration that is not consistent with the clinical appearance of sound enamel (*Note*: the lesion is still visible when dry). This lesion may be seen directly when viewed from the buccal or lingual direction. In addition, when viewed from the occlusal direction, this opacity or discoloration may be seen as a shadow confined to enamel, seen through the marginal ridge
3	Initial breakdown in enamel due to caries with no visible dentin Once dried for 5 seconds, there is distinct loss of enamel integrity, viewed from the buccal or lingual direction. These lesions may also have a discolored dentine shadow beneath the marginal ridge
4	Noncavitated surface with underlying dark shadow from dentin This lesion appears as a shadow of discolored dentin visible through an apparently intact marginal ridge, buccal, or lingual walls of enamel. The darkened area is an intrinsic shadow that may appear as gray, blue, or brown in color
5	Distinct cavity with visible dentin Cavitation in opaque or discolored enamel with exposed dentine in the examiner's judgment
6	Extensive distinct cavity with visible dentin Obvious loss of tooth structure, the extensive cavity may be deep or wide and dentine is clearly visible on both the walls and at the base. The marginal ridge may or may not be present. An extensive cavity involves at least half of a tooth surface and possibly reaching the pulp

Courtesy: Ismail et al. (2007).

The negative weights are assigned to illogical transitions. By multiplying the weights by the number of surfaces in each cell of a transition matrix, an adjusted increment is computed. This adjusted increment should be used to assess the outcomes of a clinical intervention.

Another approach is to use an adjustment formula to account for the illogical reversals using data from each tooth surface. Beck et al. (1995) developed a method to correct reversals in caries increment due to examiner misclassification. The method assumes that (1) the frequency of an examiner reversal (caries is present at baseline but the examiner misclassifies the status at follow-up) is positively related to baseline caries prevalence, and (2) there is a negative relationship between the frequency of a false positive classification (or examiner increment when the examiner misclassifies a tooth as carious at follow-up when tooth that was sound at baseline and follow-up) and the baseline caries prevalence. These assumptions may be difficult to verify because of the lack of data (e.g., examiner misclassification).

The following formula can be used for the adjustment:

$$\text{Adjusted caries increment (ADJCI)} = y_2 - y_2 \left(\frac{y_3}{y_3 + y_4} \right)$$

where

y_1 Sound → Sound,
y_2 Sound → Carious/filled/missing,
y_3 Carious/filled/missing → Sound,
y_4 Carious/filled/missing → Carious/filled/missing.

The formula should be adjusted if dental caries is measured at two stages (noncavitated and cavitated).

Outcomes in clinical studies on dental caries can vary depending on the objectives or hypotheses. In addition to the increment described before, outcomes may focus on the increment in each of the component of the DMF score, decayed only, on unrestored or restored teeth. Moreover, there is high interest in assessing outcomes indicating remineralization before the stage of cavitation. For such studies, the increment in noncavitated carious lesions can be used.

Epidemiological studies rarely use radiographs because of ethical reasons. However, radiographic changes in enamel and dentin have been used in clinical trial to add to the visual clinical data (Morgan et al., 2008), which usually underestimate the presence of caries (Poorterman et al., 1999). Like all detection tools, the use of radiographs requires diligence with training of technicians and examiners as well as assessment of their reliability. The use of standard scales for rating of caries progression in enamel or dentin is recommended (Ekstrand et al., 1997).

Criteria for assessment and summary measures of increment in root caries have not yet been well developed. ICDAS has proposed a system based on existing evidence and expertise (International Caries Detection and Assessment System, 2005). Markers of root caries activity have been used in a recent study by Ekstrand et al. (2008). Both ICDAS and Ekstrand et al. use the surface texture (hard, leathery, soft), cavitation, distance from the gingival margins, and color of the lesion (dark brown/black vs. light brown/yellowish) to differentiate between active and inactive root caries lesions.

8.4.2   Periodontal diseases

Like dental caries, outcome measures of periodontal disease attempt to summarize complex and multidimensional assessments of changes in status of the periondontium. The two conditions that are usually assessed in clinical trials are gingivitis and periodontitis. While there are different classifications of these conditions (Armitage, 2004), the clinical manifestations in terms of gingival inflammation or loss of periodontal attachment or alveolar bone height are assessed using the same methods. The case definition of periodontal severity and extent varies among clinical studies. The question is how many sites should be affected and at what severity level should disease be defined as present? Using different case definitions may impact on the statistical power of studies to detect significant associations between risk factors, such as preterm birth, and periodontal diseases (Manau et al., 2008). Researchers in this field should rely on current case definitions that are reported in referred journals. The research question and hypothesis should guide the selection of the appropriate case definition.

The measurement of gingivitis and periodontitis is dependent on the study. In a randomized controlled trial evaluating repeated antimicrobial therapy in the treatment of perioimplantitis, the two disease conditions were measured as follows (Renvert et al., 2008):

Bleeding on sampling (BOS) was recorded as 0 (no bleeding) or 1 (bleeding) after microbial sampling. At baseline, PD [pocket depth] was recorded (in millimeters) as the distance from the gingival margin to the base of the periodontal pocket, and readings were rounded up to the nearest millimeter. Four sites were measured on each implant: mesial, distal, facial, and oral. The full-mouth bleeding score (FMBS) was calculated based on scores of 0 (no bleeding) or 1 (bleeding) after probing for PD. Bleeding on probing (BOP) was recorded as 0 (no bleeding) or 1 (bleeding) after probing for PD. The full-mouth plaque score (FMPS) was determined by the presence or absence of plaque on four surfaces at each tooth and/or implant. The local plaque score (LPS) was recorded as 0 (no plaque) or 1 (plaque) at facial, oral, mesial, and distal sites on study implants. Standardized radiographs of study implants were taken using a long-cone technique.

This trial has used an all-or-none case definition for presence of bleeding on probing, and pocket depth was measured to the nearest millimeter. In selecting cutoff points, a review of the reliability of the examiners is important because it is not advisable to assess disease at a level that the examiner was not reliably assessing. However, cutoff points selected for any study can be challenged by others and there are no standards used to evaluate reliability data in dental research.

In another recent trial, the issue of calibration of the examiners to a specified level of reliability was described (Bogren et al., 2008):

Clinical examinations were performed prior to any intervention at baseline and included full-mouth recordings of plaque, BOP [bleeding on probing], PD [pocket depth], and the position of the gingival margin (GM). The assessments were made at four sites per tooth (buccal and lingual aspects of proximal sites) at all teeth except third molars. Plaque was scored as present if detected when a probe was run along the tooth surface at the GM. BOP was scored positive if a site bled immediately after probing or at completion of the probing of a jaw quadrant. PD and GM were measured twice at each visit to the nearest millimeter with a manual probe. GM was defined as the distance between the soft tissue margin and the cemento-enamel junction/border of a restoration. A negative value for GM was given when it was located apical to the reference point on the tooth.

Prior to the study, the examiners were trained to levels of accuracy and reproducibility for the various clinical parameters to be used. Calibration sessions were also scheduled during the study period. For inter- and intra-examiner reproducibility, the standard deviation for PD and GM measurements had to be <0.6 and <0.8 mm, with an agreement within 2 mm for ≥99% and ≥96% of sites examined, respectively.

These two studies have used bleeding on probing to evaluate the presence of gingival inflammation. This indicator was found to be the most reliable compared with other indices (Marks et al., 1993). Gingival bleeding is a valid measure of inflammation. The standard evaluation of loss of periodontal attachment relies on measuring the depth of pocket and the distance between the gingival margin and the base of the pocket or the distance between the cemento-enamel junction and gingival margin. Random error accounts for most of variance of these measurements (Grossi et al., 1996).

Outcome measures such as alveolar bone height and furcation involvement are not discussed in this chapter. See Chapter 9 on Examiner Training and Standardization for more detail.

8.4.3   Temporomandibular disorders/facial pain and dysfunction

The conditions known as temporomandibular disorders (TMD) represent multiple dimensions that cannot be captured by one outcome measure. In 1992, a multidisciplinary team of clinicians and behavioral scientists (LeResche and Von Korff, 1992) designed a two-dimensional system for assessing indicators of TMD that can be used to evaluate outcomes. The research diagnostic criteria/TMD (RDC/TMD) assess two axes of the disorders. The first axis, the clinical axis, focuses on assessing muscle pain with or without limited opening, disc displacements, and arthralgia, arthritis, and arthrosis. The second axis, pain-related disability and psychological status, focuses on assessment of pain intensity, pain-related disability, depression, and nonspecific physical symptoms. For each of the axes, the RDC/TMD provide measurement criteria and scales for classification of the condition.

The conditions included in axis II were evaluated for their concurrent validity with established measures of depression, somatization, and graded chronic pain (Dworkin et al., 2002b). The RDC/TMD was found to discriminate between two groups of patients receiving different levels of care after 1 year of therapy (Dworkin et al., 2002a). The RDC/TMD components were evaluated for their predictive validity of joint-related diagnoses (Schmitter et al., 2008). Several indicators were found to provide sufficient discrimination among patients with arthrosis or disc displacement with or without reduction. The indicators were maximum unassisted jaw opening, maximum assisted jaw opening, history of locked jaw, joint sound with and without compression, joint pain, facial pain, pain on palpation of the lateral pterygoid area, and overjet (some of these indicators were measured on both sides of the mouth). The reliability of the assessment of examiners' decisions was "satisfactory" (intraclass correlation coefficients of 0.4).

8.5   Outcomes and causal pathways

Outcomes, such as reduction in dental caries or incidence of periodontal diseases, are achieved through steps, or intermediate outcomes, that are linked to and are prerequisites to achieving the final outcome. For example, health literacy is an important intermediate outcome required for achieving health. Health literacy is an intermediate outcome to achieving better utilization of health care services (Paasche-Orlow and Wolf, 2007a, 2007b), understanding of disparities (Osborn et al., 2007), and in promoting early screening or detection (Aggarwal et al., 2007).

Developing and analyzing causal pathways assist in understanding the biological and nonbiological systems leading to specific outcomes. Causal pathways connect biological pathways with clinical outcomes. Interventions that are designed without due consideration of the biological mechanisms of disease will most likely not produce significant outcomes. For example, the failure to incorporate information on the dental biofilm (Ten Cate, 2006) in designing interventions, such as the delivery of chlorhexidine, may fail to reduce the burden of dental caries. Dental caries is caused by multiple bacterial species and many of them develop resistance to chlorhexidine (Deng et al., 2007). Causal pathway analysis is an important part of designing research projects that aim to reduce the burden of disease.

8.6   Final comments

The scientific method is founded on three principles: hypotheses generation, design of studies to reduce biases and errors, and measurement of outcomes. An important general theme in research is the "RE" in research, which stands for replication and retrying. This chapter provides a synopsis to the field of outcome assessment in dental research. It was not designed to provide a comprehensive thesis on the topic, but rather it is an introductory chapter. Outcomes should be defined based on the research question and potential clinical applications of the research project. Always ask how the results will be implemented in clinical care. In areas where clinical applications have not yet been envisioned, it is important to consider what will be the alternative hypotheses that should be tested if the current hypothesis of a project is rejected or accepted. Understanding and analysis of causal pathways should be a prerequisite learning requirement for all students of science.

References

Aggarwal A, Speckman JL, Paasche-Orlow MK, Roloff KS, Battaglia TA. 2007. The role of numeracy on cancer screening among urban women. *American Journal of Health Behavior* 31(Suppl. 1):S57–S68.

Allen PF, McMillan AS, Walshaw D, Locker D. 1999. A comparison of the validity of generic- and disease-specific measures in the assessment of oral health-related quality of life. *Community Dentistry and Oral Epidemiology* 27:344–352.

Armitage GC. 2004. Periodontal diagnoses and classification of periodontal diseases. *Periodontology* 34:9–21.

Bader JD, Ismail AI. 1999. A primer on outcomes in dentistry. *Journal of Public Health Dentistry* 59:131–135.

Bader JD, Shugars DA. 1997. What do we know about how dentists make caries-related treatment decisions? *Community Dentistry and Oral Epidemiology* 25:97–103.

Bahrami M, Deery C, Clarkson JE, Pitts NB, Johnston M, Ricketts I, MacLennan G, Nugent ZJ, Tilley C, Bonetti D, Ramsay C. 2004. Effectiveness of strategies to disseminate and implement clinical guidelines for the management of impacted and unerupted third molars in primary dental care, a cluster randomised controlled trial. *British Dental Journal* 197:691–696.

Beck, JD, Lawrence HP, Koch GG. 1995. A method for adjusting caries increments for reversals due to examiner misclassification. *Community Dentistry and Oral Epidemiology* 23:321–330.

Birch S, Ismail AI. 2002. Patient preferences and the measurement of utilities in the evaluation of dental technologies. *Journal of Dental Research* 81:446–450.

Birch S, Sohn W, Ismail AI, Lepkowski JM, Belli RF. 2004. Willingness to pay for dentin regeneration in a sample of dentate adults. *Community Dentistry and Oral Epidemiology* 32:210–216.

Bland JM, Altman DG. 1986. Statistical methods for assessing agreement between two methods of clinical measurement. *The Lancet* 1(8476):307–310.

Bogren A, Teles RP, Torresyap G, Haffajee AD, Socransky SS, Wennström JL. 2008. Locally delivered doxycycline during supportive periodontal therapy: a 3-year study. *Journal of Periodontology* 79:827–835.

Bonett DG. 2002. Sample size requirements for estimating intraclass correlations with desired precision. *Statistics in Medicine* 21:1331–1335.

Boyle GJ. 1985. Self-report measures of depression: some psychometric considerations. *British Journal of Clinical Psychology* 24:45–59.

Cicchetti DV, Allison, T. 1971. A new procedure for assessing reliability of scoring EEG sleep recordings. *American Journal of EEG Technology* 11:101–109.

Cho MJ, Nam JJ, Suh GH. 1998. Prevalence of symptoms of depression in a nationwide sample of Korean adults. *Psychiatry Research* 81(3):341–352.

Cohen J. 1960. A coefficient of agreement for nominal scales. *Educational and Psychological Measurement* 20:37–46.

Comrey AL. 1978. Common methodological problems in factor analytic studies. *Journal of Consulting and Clinical Psychology* 46:648–659.

Cronbach LJ. 1951. Coefficient alpha and the internal structure of tests. *Psychometrika* 16:297–334.

Deng DM, Ten Cate JM, Crielaard W. 2007. The adaptive response of Streptococcus mutans towards oral care products: involvement of the ClpP serine protease. *European Journal of Oral Science* 115:363–370.

Derks A, Frencken J, Bronkhorst E, Kuijpers-Jagtman AM, Katsaros C. 2008. Effect of chlorhexidine varnish application on mutans streptococci counts in orthodontic patients. *American Journal of Orthodontics and Dentofacial Orthopedics* 133:435–439.

Dworkin SF, Huggins KH, Wilson L, Mancl L, Turner J, Massoth D, LeResche L, Truelove E. 2002a. A randomized clinical trial using research diagnostic criteria for temporomandibular disorders-axis II to target clinic cases for a tailored self-care TMD treatment program. *Journal of Orofacial Pain* 16:48–63.

Dworkin SF, Sherman J, Mancl L, Ohrbach R, LeResche L, Truelove E. 2002b. Reliability, validity, and clinical utility of the research diagnostic criteria for temporomandibular disorders axis II scales: depression, non-specific physical symptoms, and graded chronic pain. *Journal of Orofacial Pain* 16:207–220.

Emingil G, Atilla G, Sorsa T, Tervahartiala T. 2008. The effect of adjunctive subantimicrobial dose doxycycline therapy on GCF EMMPRIN levels in chronic periodontitis. *Journal of Periodontology* 79:469–476.

Ekstrand K, Martingon S, Pedersen P-H. 2008. Development and evaluation of two root caries controlling programmers for home-based frail people older than 75 years. *Gerodontology* 25:6–75.

Ekstrand KR, Martignon S, Ricketts DJ, Qvist V. 2007. Detection and activity assessment of primary coronal caries lesions: a methodologic study. *Operative Dentistry* 32:225–235.

Ekstrand KR, Ricketts DN, Kidd EA. 1997. Reproducibility and accuracy of three methods for assessment of demineralization depth of the occlusal surface: an *in vitro* examination. *Caries Research* 31:224–231.

Finkelstein EA, Trogdon JG. 2008. Public health interventions for addressing childhood overweight: analysis of the business case. *American Journal of Public Health* 98:411–415.

Flack VF, Afifi AA, Lachenbruch PA. 1988. Sample size determination for two rater kappa statistics. *Psychometrika* 53:321–325.

Fleiss JL. 1971. Measuring nominal scale agreement among many raters. *Psychological Bulletin* 76:378–382.

Fleiss JL, Levin B, Cho Paik M. 2004. *Statistical Methods for Rates and Proportions*, 3rd edn. New York: Wiley.

Foster Page LA, Thomson WM, Jokovic A, Locker D. 2005. Validation of the child perceptions questionnaire (CPQ 11–14). *Journal of Dental Research* 84:649–652.

Grossi SG, Dunford RG, Ho A, Koch G, Machtei EE, Genco RJ. 1996. Sources of error for periodontal probing measurements. *Journal of Periodontal Research* 31(5):330–336.

Gwet K. 2002. Statistical methods for inter-rater reliability assessment. Inter-rater reliability: dependency on trait prevalence and marginal homogeneity. STATAXIS Consulting. No. 2. Available online at http://www.stataxis.com/files/articles/inter_rater_reliability_dependency.pdf. Accessed on July 14, 2008.

Hanley JA, Negassa A, Edwardes MD, Forrester JE. 2003. Statistical analysis of correlated data using generalized estimating equations: an orientation. *American Journal of Epidemiology* 157:364–375.

Hann D, Winter K, Jacobsen P. 1999. Measurement of depressive symptoms in cancer patients: evaluation of the Center for Epidemiological Studies Depression Scale (CES-D). *Journal of Psychosomatic Research* 46:437–443.

Ide M, McPartlin D, Coward PY, Crook M, Lumb P, Wilson RF. 2003. Effect of treatment of chronic periodontitis on levels of serum markers of acute-phase inflammatory and vascular responses. *Journal of Clinical Periodontology* 30:334–340.

International Caries Detection and Assessment System. 2005. Criteria Manual. Appendix I. In: Stookey G (ed.). *Proceedings of the Seventh Indiana Conference*. Indianapolis, IN, pp. 190–222.

Ismail AI. 2004. Visual and visuo-tactile detection of dental caries. *Journal of Dental Research* 83:C56–C66.

Ismail AI, Birch S, Sohn W, Lepkowski JM, Belli RF. 2004. Utilities of dentin regeneration among insured and uninsured adults. *Community Dentistry and Oral Epidemiology* 32:55–66.

Ismail AI, Sohn W, Tellez M, Amaya A, Sen A, Hasson H, Pitts NB. 2007. The International Caries Detection and Assessment System (ICDAS): an integrated system for measuring dental caries. *Community Dentistry and Oral Epidemiology* 35:170–178.

Ismail AI, Sohn W, Tellez M, Willem JM, Betz J, Lepkowski J. 2008. Risk indicators for dental caries using the International Caries Detection and Assessment System (ICDAS). *Community Dentistry and Oral Epidemiology* 36:55–68.

Kantz ME, Harris WJ, Levitsky K, Ware JE Jr., Davies AR. 1992. Methods for assessing condition-specific and generic functional status outcomes after total knee replacement. *Medical Care* 30(Suppl.):MS240–MS252.

Landis JR, Koch GG. 1977. The measurement of interrater agreement for categorical data. *Biometrics* 33:159–174.

LeResche L, Von Korff MR. 1992. Research diagnostic criteria. *Journal of Craniomandibular Disorders* 6:327–334.

Locker D, Jokovic A, Clarke M. 2004. Assessing the responsiveness of measures of oral health-related quality of life. *Community Dentistry and Oral Epidemiology* 32:10–18.

Locker D, Slade G. 1993. Oral health and the quality of life among older adults: the oral health impact profile. *Journal of Canadian Dental Association* 59:830–833.

Ludbrook J. 2004. Detecting systematic bias between two raters. *Clinical and Experimental Pharmacology and Physiology* 31:113–115.

Manau C, Echeverria A, Agueda A, Guerrero A, Echeverria JJ. 2008. Periodontal disease definition may determine the association between periodontitis and pregnancy outcomes. *Journal of Clinical Periodontology* 35:385–397.

Marks RG, Magnusson I, Taylor M, Clouser B, Maruniak J, Clark WB. 1993. Evaluation of reliability and reproducibility of dental indices. *Journal of Clinical Periodontology* 20:54–58.

McDowell I, Newell C. 1996. *Measuring Health. A Guide to Rating Scales and Questionnaires.* New York: Oxford University Press.

McHorney CA, Wae JE Jr., Raczek AE. 1993. The MOS 36-item short form health survey (SF 36). 1993. II. Psychometric and clinical tests of validity in measuring physical and mental health constructs. *Medical Care* 31:247–262.

Morgan MV, Adams GG, Bailey DL, Tsao CE, Fischman SL, Reynolds EC. 2008. The anticariogenic effect of sugar-free gum containing CPP-ACP nanocomplexes on approximal caries determined using digital bitewing radiography. *Caries Research* 42:171–184.

Nezu M, Nezu CM. 2008. *Evidence-Based Outcome Research.* New York: Oxford University Press.

Nyvad B, Machiulskiene V, Baelum V. 2003. Construct and predictive validity of clinical caries diagnostic criteria assessing lesion activity. *Journal of Dental Research* 82:117–122.

Osborn CY, Paasche-Orlow MK, Davis TC, Wolf MS. 2007. Health literacy an overlooked factor in understanding HIV health disparities. *American Journal of Preventive Medicine* 233:374–378.

Paasche-Orlow MK, Wolf MS. 2007a. Health literacy, health inequality and a just healthcare system. *American Journal of Bioethics* 7:5–10.

Paasche-Orlow MK, Wolf MS. 2007b. The causal pathways linking health literacy to health outcomes. *American Journal of Health Behavior* 31:S19–S26.

Phelps CE, Hutson A. 1995. Estimating diagnostic test accuracy using a "fuzzy gold standard". *Medical Decision Making* 15:44–57.

Pitts NB, Stamm JW. 2004. International consensus workshop on caries clinical trials (ICW-CCT)—final consensus statements: agreeing where evidence leads. *Journal of Dental Research* 83(Spec. Iss. C):C125–C128.

Platt JR. 1964. Strong inference. *Science* 146:347–353.

Poorterman JH, Aartman IH, Kalsbeek H. 1999. Underestimation of the prevalence of approximal caries and inadequate restorations in a clinical epidemiological study. *Community Dentistry and Oral Epidemiology* 27:331–337.

Radloff LS. 1977. The CES-D scale: a self-report depression scale for research in the general population'. *Applied Psychological Measurement* 1:385–401.

Renvert S, Lessem J, Dahlén G, Renvert H, Lindahl C. 2008. Mechanical and repeated antimicrobial therapy using a local drug delivery system in the treatment of peri-implantitis. *Journal of Periodontology* 79:836–844.

Ricketts DNJ, Ekstrand KR, Kidd EAM, Larsen T. 2002. Relating visual and radiographic ranked scoring systems for occlusal caries detection to histological and microbiological evidence. *Operative Dentistry* 27:231–237.

Schmitter M, Kress B, Leckel M, Henschel V, Ohlmann B, Rammelsberg P. 2008. Validity of temporomandibular disorder examination procedures for assessment of temporomandibular joint status. *American Journal of Orthodontics and Dentofacial Orthopedics* 133:796–803.

Selwitz RH, Ismail AI, Pitts NB. 2007. Dental caries. *The Lancet* 369:51–59.

Shrout PE, Fleiss JL. 1979. Intraclass correlations: uses in assessing rater reliability. *Psychological Bulletin* 86:420–428.

Simon J, Gray A, Clarke P, Wade A, Neil A, Farmer A. 2008. Diabetes Glycaemic Education and Monitoring Trial Group. Cost effectiveness of self monitoring of blood glucose in patients with non-insulin treated type 2 diabetes: economic evaluation of data from the DiGEM trial. *British Medical Journal* 336:1177–1180.

Slade G-D, Spencer AJ. 1994. Development and evaluation of the oral health impact profile. *Community Dental Health* 11:3–11.

Ten Cate JM. 2006. Biofilms, a new approach to the microbiology of dental plaque. *Odontology* 94:1–9.

Truelove E, Huggins KH, Mancl L, Dworkin SF. 2006. The efficacy of traditional, low-cost and nonsplint therapies for temporomandibular disorder: a randomized controlled trial. *Journal of the American Dental Association* 137(8):1099–1107; quiz 1169.

Uebersax JS. 1993. Statistical modeling of expert ratings on medical treatment appropriateness. *Journal of the American Statistical Association* 88:421–427.

Uebersax JS, Grove WM. 1993. A latent trait finite mixture model for the analysis of rating agreement. *Biometrics* 49:823–835.

Walter SD, Eliasziw M, Donner A. 1998. Sample size and optimal designs for reliability studies. *Statistics in Medicine* 17:101–110.

Yamamoto N, Itoi E, Minagawa H, Seki N, Abe H, Shimada Y, Okada K. 2006. Objective evaluation of shoulder pain by measuring skin impedance. *Orthopedics* 29:1121–1123.

9

Examiner training: standardization and calibration in periodontal studies

Niklaus P. Lang, DDS, MS, PhD**, Mary P. Cullinan,** BDS, MSc, FADI**, Douglas W. Holborow,** BDS, FDSRCS, **and Lisa J.A. Heitz-Mayfield,** BDS, MDSc, Odont Dr

9.1 Rationale

Clinical studies are usually carried out over a prolonged period of time. It is, therefore, of crucial importance that examiners be reproducible to a high degree and that there are no significant differences between the scorings of different examiners assessing the same parameters in larger studies when multiple examiners have to be used for logistic reasons. Moreover, it is imperative that examiners be accurate in their assessment of parameters, that is, they can distinguish between healthy and diseased conditions. To obtain such knowledge and skills, examiner training followed by standardization and calibration procedures are prerequisites for a proposed study of high quality. Furthermore, examiner training may, indeed, lead to increased reproducibility (Abbas et al., 1982). In 1994, the Task Force on Design and Analysis in Dental and Oral Research has proposed guidelines for acceptance of products by the American Dental Association (seal of approval) for professional, nonsurgical treatment of adult periodontitis (Imrey et al., 1994a, 1994b). These guidelines gained a lot of attention internationally and have influenced the conduct of clinical trials ever since.

Clearly, it was stated that quality control in conducting and documenting clinical studies cannot simply be replaced by investigator background or experience. Quality control exercises should be performed prior to and, depending on its duration, during a trial without involving actual study subjects.

It is the purpose of this chapter to emphasize quality control, to promote and outline standardization and calibration exercises, and to improve the reliability of data gathering in clinical trials.

9.2   Instruments

Since it is the first description in newer times (Black, 1913) and despite significant limitations, the periodontal probe has remained the main instrument for the clinical evaluation of periodontal tissues in health as well as in disease. Originally, periodontal probes were uncalibrated, but later, various incremental marks were added to the probes to accurately determine distances, gingivo-apically either for penetration (pocket, probing) depth or for measuring to what extent fibers of the periodontal ligament have been detached (loss of attachment). Incremental markings on the probe include a variety of systems. Millimeter markings (PCP-UNC: U of North Carolina 15) are usually difficult to read for the examiner, and hence, other increments have been applied (e.g., 2 mm: U of California). Also, variable incremental units characterize some periodontal probes, such as 3-6-8-11 mm (U of Michigan M1) or 3-6-9-12 mm markings. Some probes employ color coatings for easier readability.

The shape (round vs. flat) and the dimensions of probes may also vary. Today, slightly tapered metal cylinders with a point diameter of 0.4–0.5 mm are preferred in clinical research and dental practice. Regarding the markings, it has to be realized that increased readability may be at the expense of measurement accuracy.

It is evident that one type of measurement instrument has to be selected for a clinical study and applied by all examiners. As manufacturers work with some tolerance in accuracy, it cannot be expected that all instruments of the same type present accurate and identical markings and/or dimensions, even when from the same brand (Ramfjord, 1974). Hence, it is imperative to select study instruments and to verify the accuracy of dimensions and markings on the instruments prior to examiner training. Depending on the manufacturer, it can be anticipated that only approximately 70% of instruments yield identical markings and dimensions.

Manual probing generally allows the distinction of 1-mm increments for a single reading. The standard deviation for a single measurement has been reported to be in the range of 0.4–1.0 mm (Glavind and Löe, 1967; Abbas et al., 1982; Haffajee et al., 1983; Badersten et al., 1984; Osborn et al., 1990; 1992). Novel probe tip designs (flat and rounded) may have greater validity, good reproducibility, and may produce less patient discomfort (Vartoukian et al., 2004) than conventional probes hitherto used. Electronic probes, on the other hand, may improve the resolution up to 0.2–0.3 mm (Clark et al., 1992) and, hence, may be more suitable to detect smaller changes of probing depth (PD) or clinical attachment level over time (Jeffcoat and Reddy, 1991; Marks et al., 1991; Clark et al., 1992; Mombelli et al., 1997).

9.3   Components of assessment

The components of the assessment of periodontal conditions usually include the evaluation of clinical features such as (a) accumulation of biofilms, (b) signs of gingival inflammation, and (c) damage to the periodontal tissues. The management of these data is critical (patient based and site based) and is described below and in Chapter 6 on data management.

9.3.1   Accumulation of biofilms

Owing to the fact that microbial challenge is essential for the initiation of periodontal diseases (Löe et al., 1965; Seymour, 1991; Seymour et al., 1996; Page and Kornman, 1997), it is logical to assess the accumulation of soft and hard biofilm deposits on the teeth. Basically, two different methods for evaluating plaque deposits have been advocated. One method assesses the extension of plaque growth from the gingival margin in the occlusal or incisal direction (i.e., Quigley and Hein, 1962; Greene and Vermillion, 1964; Turesky et al., 1970), while the other method focuses on the assessment of the thickness of biofilm formation at the gingival margin (i.e., Silness and Löe, 1964). While the former techniques generally evaluate a tooth as a single unit, the latter uses the tooth site or surface as a unit of examination. In the range of moderate plaque amounts, these two methods correlate well. Indeed, between a Plaque Index (PlI; Silness and Löe, 1964) of 0.5–2.0, the correlation was almost linear (Lang et al., 1972). However, for early plaque formation and minor deposits, the PlI was the more sensitive method of assessment. On the other hand, with large amounts of plaque deposits exceeding PlI = 2.0, the indices assessing occlusal extension of plaque were more discriminating (Lang et al., 1972). As the biofilm starts to accumulate at the gingival margin (Lang et al., 1973; Mombelli et al., 1990), the assessment *at the gingival margin* appears to be the relevant evaluation in clinical oral health studies. Nevertheless, the occlusal extension indices still enjoy widespread popularity in studies designed for testing antiplaque effects of antimicrobial or cleansing products (Biesbrock and Bartizek, 2005; Mallatt et al., 2007). Study protocols need to state clearly the purposes of a given study and index systems designed appropriately. Standardization of examiners requires a clear understanding of the criteria and application of the appropriate index system chosen (Fischman, 1986).

9.3.2   Gingivial inflammation

Plaque-induced periodontal diseases represent opportunistic infections that exhibit signs of clinical inflammation (Seymour, 1991; Seymour et al., 1996). Consequently, a means of assessing and recording signs of clinical inflammation is essential for assessing the health or disease status of the periodontal tissues in oral health studies.

The four cardinal signs of inflammation were presented by Celsus (30 BC–AD 38) more than 2,000 years ago: (1) redness (*rubor*), (2) swelling (*tumor*), (3) heat (*calor*), and (4) pain (*dolor*). In addition, Galenus (AD 129–201) added the fifth sign of "loss of function" (*Functio laesa*) to the cardinal signs of inflammation.

When assessing periodontal tissues, it has to be realized that "heat," "pain," and "loss of function" are of limited value. Pain is only observed under very few and specific circumstances, while "loss of function" probably equates with the terminal phase of periodontal disease, that is, imminent tooth loss. On the other hand, "bleeding on probing" is due to increased vascularity in the tissues, while suppuration and the production of gingival fluid may be considered as additional specific signs of inflammation of the periodontal tissues.

The evaluation of periodontal tissues must certainly incorporate all the known signs of inflammation. If one or more of those these signs are present, the tissues are not healthy. Conversely, the definition of gingival health is dependent on the absence of *all* signs of inflammation.

While signs of inflammation such as *color* and *swelling* can sometimes be subtle and are, therefore, rather *subjective* criteria, *bleeding on probing* may be a more *objective* criterion provided that the technique of the gingival challenge prior to the bleeding assessment is standardized (Chaves et al., 1993). However, it is well established that these factors may vary substantially for the same examiner at different times as well as between examiners (Imrey et al., 1994a, 1994b).

As no assessment of gingival inflammation is fully objective, special training exercises should be performed to standardize examiners prior to their involvement in clinical oral health studies. Assessment of examiner training and examiner variability may be performed on a subject or site level. Appropriate statistical methods have to be chosen for the evaluation of the reliability of index systems of gingival inflammation (Kingman, 1986).

9.3.3   Damage to periodontal tissues

Plaque-induced periodontal diseases are usually placed into two categories of (a) gingivitis without and (b) gingivitis with concomitant loss of connective tissue attachment to the tooth, that is, periodontitis.

Sites with periodontitis always exhibit signs of inflammation, but in addition, a pathological dissolution of connective tissue (collagen) fiber attachment to the cemental surface has occurred resulting in a *loss of attachment* that is usually measured in a linear fashion and expressed in millimeters. Apical migration of the junctional epithelium is another feature leading to increased probing pocket depth, likewise measured in a linear fashion and expressed in millimeters. The inflammatory processes may also result in resorption of the coronal portions of the tooth-supporting alveolar bone. Increased probing pocket depth represents the expression of present periodontal disease and indicates possible future attachment loss (LA) (Cullinan et al., 2003), while loss of attachment also indicates the history of past disease.

The assessment of *probing depth* and *loss of attachment*, therefore, represent indispensable components of the evaluation of periodontal tissues in clinical oral health studies. As the key issue in this assessment is the identification of the cemento-enamel junction as a reference from which attachment loss is estimated, special emphasis has to be given to the accurate identification of this structure during examiner training.

Most methods of assessment of periodontal conditions used in clinical oral health studies apply categorical parameters. However, the assessment of probing depth and loss of attachment are continuous parameters. Consequently, in the evaluation of examiner variability, the nature of the parameters utilized will have to be considered and appropriate statistical methods have to be applied (Kingman, 1986; 1993; Kingman et al., 1991).

9.4   Bleeding on probing

Monitoring inflammation of the gingival tissues is best documented by the parameter of *bleeding on probing* (for review, see Lang et al., 1996).

The histologic characteristics of the gingival tissues associated with *bleeding on probing* have been presented (Greenstein et al., 1981). Sites that bled following probing with a light pressure being applied to the tissues (0.25 N) were associated with a significantly increased percentage of a cell-rich and collagen-reduced connective tissue, but no increase in vascularity or vessel lumen size that could justify the bleeding tendency. Obviously, *bleeding on probing* may be provoked by trauma to the tissues using a periodontal probe. Hence, the probing pressure to be applied to the tissues when evaluating *bleeding on probing* should not exceed the pressure that may create trauma rather than provoking tissues to bleed because of increased fragility of the blood vessels due to the presence of inflammation. In periodontally healthy young subjects (Lang et al., 1991) and in periodontally treated, but healthy middle-aged subjects (Karayiannis et al., 1992), it was demonstrated that *bleeding on probing* with pressures greater than 0.25 N would result in false-positive readings, that is, trauma to the tissues. An almost linear correlation existed with these two different subject cohorts between the percentage of sites with *bleeding on probing* and the probing pressure applied. By incrementally increasing the pressure by 0.25 N, an increase of approximately 13% *bleeding on probing* sites was noted (Lang et al., 1991).

As various factors, such as probe dimension, angulation of the probe, and applied pressure, may affect the assessment of gingival inflammation (Van der Weijden et al., 1994), it is imperative to standardize for *bleeding on probing* using well-defined forces, preferably not exceeding 0.25 N. Standardization exercises for applying a "light" force of that order of magnitude may include the practicing of probing pressures on a balance, both for verifying the avoidance of too high pressures and for determining reproducibility of the examiner to be trained (Marks et al., 1991).

9.5   Probing pressure and probe angulation

The definition of probing pressure is relevant not only for the evaluation of gingival health or inflammation in order to avoid false-positive readings, but also for the assessment of damage to the periodontal tissues (Mombelli, 2005). The development of periodontal pockets and the loss of connective tissue attachment are pathognomonic features of periodontal disease, and hence, the assessment of their magnitude is a key task for the clinical researcher as well as the practicing dentist.

Probing the periodontal tissues is a site-specific assessment and the estimation of the "histological" attachment level provides a gold standard for such assessments. However, the measurements can—in the best case scenario—only provide an approximation of the "true" histological attachment level. Rather, the penetration depth of the periodontal probe exposed to a defined probing pressure is assessed and related to the landmark of the cemento-enamel junction, the identification of which may be obscured by calcified deposits or restorations. Hence, various factors affect the measurements, and attempts to control these should be part of the standardization process of clinical examiners. Probe dimensions and incremental measurement units have been discussed above.

Factors further affecting the outcome of probing measurements are the applied pressure to the tissues and the angulation of the probe tip (Grossi et al., 1996). Special efforts have to be made to control these two variables. Finally, it has been demonstrated that the inflammatory state of the gingival tissues affected probing measurements the most (Listgarten et al., 1976; Armitage et al., 1977; Garnick et al., 1980; Magnusson and Listgarten, 1980; Fowler et al., 1982; Aguero et al., 1995). In untreated periodontitis, probe tips penetrated through the connective tissue attachment and stopped in the connective tissue exceeding the "histological" attachment level by approximately 0.5 mm (Armitage et al., 1977). In contrast, in pockets without signs of inflammation, probe penetration applying standardized forces of 0.2–0.25 N did not reach the apical termination of the junctional epithelium (Armitage et al., 1977; Fowler et al., 1982).

It is evident that probing measurements are usually reduced after periodontal therapy and clinical attachment gain claimed. Such attachment gain cannot be attributed to a gain in "histological" attachment, but rather to an increase in density of the tissues in the apical region of the periodontal pocket affecting penetration depth of the probe.

As the location of the probe penetration is highly variable in healthy versus diseased tissues, appropriate patients with similar levels of disease to the patient cohort to be examined in the clinical study should be chosen for calibration exercises.

Probing force obviously affects probe penetration and has to be standardized prior to performing clinical studies. The question arises as to which probing force should be chosen to reveal the changes being investigated, for example, effects of therapy rather than to identify the "histological" attachment level.

Without special training, probing forces applied by clinical researchers and clinicians vary considerably (Gabathuler and Hassel, 1971; Hassel et al., 1973; Freed et al., 1983).

Force-controlled probes may reduce possible errors due to varying probing forces both within and between examiners (Gibbs et al., 1988; Walsh and Saxby, 1989; Jeffcoat and Reddy, 1991; Bergenholtz et al., 2000). It is, therefore, imperative to validate probing forces of various examiners following practicing and standardization of exercises.

By recording probe penetration as a function of force (Mombelli and Graf, 1986; Mombelli et al., 1997), it can be appreciated that probing depths depend on the forces applied. Since depth–force curves follow the characteristics of saturation curves that flatten with increasing probing forces, small probing forces have a greater impact on reproducibility of probing depth measurements in the low-force range. Conversely, at high probing forces, reproducibility is generally higher than at low forces.

Since depth–force characteristics may vary before and after therapy, the measurable treatment outcome expressed as the difference in probing depth and clinical attachment levels depends on the probing force chosen. If therapy produces shrinkage of the tissues, the minimum force to be applied to detect the treatment outcome would have to be 0.25 N (Mombelli et al., 1992). In this situation, lower probing forces would be inappropriate. With higher forces, the treatment effect may be underestimated. Hence, examiners should be trained to apply 0.25 N for determining both probing depth and loss of attachment.

Angulation of the probe during assessment of probing depth and attachment loss severely affects the outcome. Again, standardization of the location of probing and the angulation of the probe to be applied are of critical importance. To identify the cemento-enamel junction, the probe has to be angulated (45° to the root surface), whereas to determine probe penetration (PD), the probe should be guided along the long axis of the tooth. This is most reproducible when measuring at the line angles adjacent to the contact area rather than aiming at the deepest penetration depth in the interproximal region. However, it has to be realized that some more advanced lesions in the interproximal area may be missed in favor of a higher reproducibility of measurements. The decision regarding the location of probing in the interproximal region and its angulation needs to be discussed in standardization exercises prior to the launch of a clinical study (Watts, 1989). To even further increase reproducibility, stents may be applied with engraved indentations for the probe (Marks et al., 1991). However, the true benefit of these costly devices in clinical trials is still subject to debate (Watts, 1987; Pihlstrom, 1992). They do not appear to affect reproducibility, but only reduced variability slightly (Watts, 1987). Moreover, they are only of value in studies of relatively short duration as tooth movement or tooth loss limits their usefulness in long-term studies.

9.6   Patterns of examiner bias

In order to determine the proficiency of gingivitis examiners and to validate various index systems for assessment of gingivitis, a clinical model was developed (Sturzenberger et al., 1985; Bollmer et al., 1986). In this model, two groups of subjects were subjected to appropriately timed-staggered dental prophylaxes to create a gingivitis treatment effect between the two groups. The first group received dental prophylaxes immediately after baseline, approximately 5–6 weeks before the second group. Four to 10 days after the second group had received dental prophylaxes, both groups were examined independently by multiple examiners. This delayed prohylaxis design created a difference in the healing responses between the two groups. Significantly less gingivitis was noted in the second group receiving a prophylaxis shortly before the follow-up examination as expressed by significantly fewer bleeding sites. This was demonstrated by all examiners who utilized *bleeding on probing* as a criterion in their assessment. These differences were, however, not revealed by examiners who assessed the gingival tissues strictly visually without the use of a probe to provoke bleeding. It appears, therefore, that for the assessment of gingivitis, the evaluation of the bleeding tendency following probing is a necessity.

In a more recent study (McClanahan et al., 2001), the style of assessment and the effect on statistical outcomes and the magnitude of treatment differences were analyzed using five different studies with the same clinical model and 12 experienced examiners for the GI (Löe and Silness, 1963). In these studies, the interval between the two examinations was 8 weeks and the interval of the prophylaxis of the second group before the follow-up examination was 5–7 days. All 12 examiners observed statistically significant differences between the prophylaxis treatment groups at the final visit for both mean number of bleeding sites and mean GI. This, in turn, means that all 12 experienced, but blinded, examiners were able to identify the known differences between the two groups, but with a huge range varying from 21.5% to 84.6% for mean number of bleeding sites and from 9.4% to 39.2% for mean GI. Based on the frequency that a given GI score (0, 1, 2, or 3) was attributed by a clinician, four distinct styles employed were identified and characterized for these experienced clinicians (Figure 9.1). These styles included three modalities in which the examiners preferred to use predominantly a pair of scores, such as the style 0–1, style 0–2, and style 1–2. The fourth style, however, utilized more of the index system, that is, 0–1–2. Scores of GI = 3 were not noted in these studies. Apparently, the examiners consistently applied the same examiner style that did not vary across time. Intra-examiner calibration is, therefore, influenced by the examiner style. The use of Kappa (κ) statistics to assess intra-examiner agreement of repeated measurements will tend to result in higher κ values when the index system is more broadly used than when reduced to only a pair of scores (McClanahan et al., 2001).

Hence, it is recommended to identify the style of an examiner if results of calibration exercises are to be interpreted in a meaningful way.

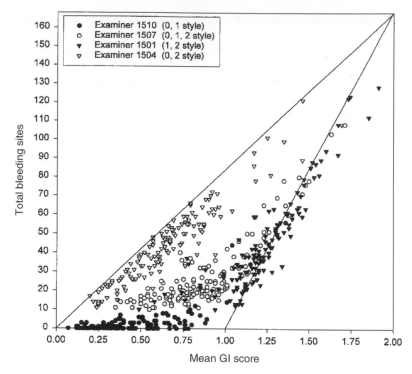

Figure 9.1 Based on data from a prospective clinical study, four distinct examiner styles could be identified by 12 examiners. As examples, Examiner 1510 displayed a style by which GI scores of 0 and 1 were predominantly (98%) called and GI = 2 was called only in 2%, representing the 0–1 examiner style. Examiner 1507 (and six further examiners) used the full spectrum of GI scores 0, 1, and 2. GI = 0 scores were given between 25% and 75% of the time representing the most frequently encountered 0–1–2 examiner style. Examiner 1501 (and one other examiner) preferred a style that favored the GI scores of 1 and 2 with <25% calls of GI = 0, representing the 1–2 examiner style. Examiner 1504 (and one other examiner) called predominantly GI scores of 0 and 2 with >75% calls of GI = 0, representing the 0–2 examiner style. Adapted from McClanahan et al., 2001.

9.7   Subjects for examiner training

For standardization as well as for assessment of intra- and inter-examiner agreement, it is preferable to select subjects who are not enrolled or going to be enrolled in a subsequent study (Imrey et al., 1994b). A spectrum of subjects ranging from health, gingivitis to periodontitis that is comparable to that found on the protocol of a given study should be selected. If examiner training prior to a therapeutic study in patients with periodontitis is to be performed, the subjects selected for calibration likewise should be in good general health, and exhibiting periodontal sites with simultaneous evidence of clinical attachment loss, periodontal inflammation, and probing depth of at least 5 mm (Imrey et al., 1994a). However, if examiner training is performed prior to a study with preventive agents and aimed at gingivitis patients, subjects with various stages ranging from health to generalized gingivitis should be chosen.

While standardization of new examiners to experienced examiners generally requires large patient cohorts, the assessment of intra-examiner agreement may be performed with small numbers of subjects chosen appropriately for the purpose of the subsequent study. Often, repeated assessments are made during the actual study with a limited number of patients (Kingman et al., 1991). While not ideal from a training and standardization point of view, this method of duplication during the study may provide adequate data to determine intra-examiner reproducibility of an experienced examiner.

The determination of an adequate number of subjects to be incorporated in a calibration exercise is based on specific margin of error (half-width of the 95% confidence interval (CI) of the percentage agreement within 1 mm). It may be necessary to conduct a pilot study to calculate point estimates and design effects for examiner reliability measures of interest. On the basis of these, the sample size required to achieve a desired margin of error (half-width of the 95% CI) in the examiner reliability estimates (Hill et al., 2006) can be determined.

9.8   Standardization versus calibration

Standardization of clinical examiners should be performed prior to a planned study in order to minimize the impact of examiner style (McClanahan et al., 2001). For multicenter studies where multiple examiners are employed, such standardization is of utmost importance and should include not only the evaluation of the various index systems or measurements used, but also a detailed understanding of the procedures to be performed during the planned study.

A number of difficulties arise in dealing with these issues. For example, due to the subjective nature of the Gingival Index, there is no established and objective standard to which examiners should be standardized. Consequently, an experienced, standardized, and reproducible examiner is arbitrarily identified and taken as a "gold standard." Usually, such examiners were able to detect known treatment differences in previous studies or because of their reproducibility as opposed to their accuracy in detecting clinical inflammation.

Following standardization, a common style of examination may often be achieved, even though it is unclear which is the most appropriate style for the planned study.

Calibration of an examiner follows standardization exercises. In this process, the reproducibility, rather than the accuracy of an examiner to detect signs of health and/or disease, is evaluated. Calibration without prior standardization may falsify the image of the true tissue conditions present. The examiner may reach high reproducibility with an index system without correctly appraising the relevant clinical changes.

In an extreme situation, the majority of sites may be given a score of 0, when disease is present, and yet, the reproducibility of such assessment may be very high. Likewise, sites may be given a score of 2 after too heavy probing, when disease is either absent or minimal, and yet, reproducibility of such faulty assessment may be high.

In the studies presented by McClanahan et al. (2001), the magnitude of treatment differences observed by different experienced examiners between the groups ranged from 9.4% to 22.7% for mean GI in one cohort and from 13.8% to 39.2% for mean GI in another cohort. Moreover, the results for the number of bleeding sites exhibited substantial variation between examiners ranging from 21.5% to 34.7% in one cohort and from 34.9% to 84.6% in the second cohort. Although six examiners sequentially assessed each subject, the GI and bleeding percentage variation was completely at random with no apparent ordering effect. These substantial differences in the magnitude of the treatment effect were meaningless regarding the statistical outcomes where all examiners observed statistically significant differences for the GI and the percentage of bleeding sites. Hence, focusing on absolute treatment differences without understanding variance, confidence intervals, and examiner variability may be deceptive.

9.9   Inter- versus intra-examiner variability

In multicenter studies, multiple examiners are usually involved in assessing the same parameters. It is, therefore, a prerequisite to determine inter-examiner variability following standardization exercises, if results of the study are to be collapsed into one cohort, thereby increasing the statistical power of the study. Usually, calibration focuses on patient-based mean scores rather than single-site scores. It is understood that inter-examiner agreement is generally lower than intra-examiner agreement both for nonparametric indices (Shaw and Murray, 1977) as well as for continuous parameters (Kingman et al., 1991).

Determination of intra-examiner agreement has to follow standardization exercises prior to any clinical trial. Intra-examiner agreement procedures may be performed with patient-based scores or with site-based analysis. Both aspects may be of importance depending on the study planned. Obviously, intra-examiner agreement for patient-based mean scores is higher than that for site-based single scores. This is, again, the case for nonparametric indices (Shaw and Murray, 1977; Kingman, 1986) as well as for continuous measurements (Glavind and Löe, 1967; Kingman et al., 1991; Grossi et al., 1996).

9.10   Intra-examiner variability

In the ideal situation in which only one examiner performs all examinations, only intra-examiner variability has to be determined prior to the start of the clinical study.

It is understood that the determination of intra-examiner variability is only meaningful if the examiner has been properly trained and standardization assured before enrolling in calibration exercises.

9.10.1   Nonparametric indices

These include most of the parameters recommended to evaluate oral hygiene levels, gingival health status, plaque retentive factors, and assessment of stain.

Since these parameters are categorical, they may be best analyzed applying frequency analyses instead of only mean scores. However, for calibration exercises, patient-based evaluations may focus on representative mean scores for the dentition.

9.10.1.1   Patient-based parameters

Running a probe along the gingival margin, a requirement for proper assessment of the oral hygiene level at the gingival margin (PlI; Silness and Löe, 1964) may remove small plaque deposits, and therefore, repeat assessment of the oral hygiene level is most likely to result in lower plaque scores. This phenomenon has, indeed, been demonstrated in various calibration exercises (Shaw and Murray, 1975; 1977).

Similarly, repeated probing required for proper assessment of gingival conditions utilizing any index system with bleeding as a criterion (e.g., GI; Löe and Silness, 1963) may create gingival irritation and result in higher scores at subsequent examinations.

Hence, calibration exercises should aim at minimizing multiple passing at the same sites when determining examiner reproducibility.

To reduce the number of passes within a dentition and still obtain a representative mean for a subject, half-mouth assessments or even evaluations of representative teeth for the dentition may be recommended for calibration exercises (Gettinger et al., 1983; Goldberg et al., 1985; Dowsett et al., 2002).

For example, a mean score based on representative teeth of the mouth (Ramfjord, 1959, 1967) could be calculated for six patients with varying degrees of plaque and gingival health or disease. These six patients could be scored four times each, not consecutively, but in a random fashion. The first and the third scorings utilize exclusively the teeth proposed by Ramfjord (1959) (Teeth FDI No.: 16, 11, 24, 36, 31, 44; U.S.: 3, 9, 12, 19, 25, 28) as being representative of the dentition, while the second and fourth examinations utilize the contralateral teeth of Ramfjord (1959) (Teeth FDI No.: 14, 21, 26, 34, 41, 46; U.S.: 5, 8, 14, 21, 24, 30) as being representative of the dentition. All evaluations involve three buccal (mesio-buccal, buccal, and disto-buccal) and one lingual aspect.

A Student's t-test may be performed to verify that both groups of teeth would be representative for the whole dentition. Pending a positive outcome of no difference between the mean scores, the four scorings may be analyzed by an analysis of variance with—expectedly—no difference between the mean scores of the four assessments.

9.10.1.2   Site-based parameters

To determine the reproducibility of single-site scores, the clinical protocol and the results of the calibration exercise for mean PlI and GI may be used. However, the analysis will concentrate on the first and the third as well as on the second and fourth assessment of the sites. The reproducibility for the PlI and the GI will be determined applying κ statistics or percentage agreement.

Both the PlI and the GI are relatively subjective and nonparametric index systems as opposed to the measuring of millimeters using a probe.

When assessing plaque, the scores of PlI = 1 or 2 appear to be less reproducible than PlI = 0 and 3 scores. This is owing to the fact that the latter scores are easily recognizable. If PlI site scores are not identical at subsequent examinations, they are usually slightly lower (Birkeland and Jorkjend, 1975; Shaw and Murray, 1977) than at the preceding examination. It is likely that small amounts of plaque are removed during the first scoring as discussed above. Hence, a PlI = 1 score may have been converted to a PlI = 0 score.

When assessing gingival health, the lower GI scores (GI = 0 or 1) appear to be less reproducible than the higher GI scores of GI = 2 or 3. Bleeding on probing is the key feature of a GI = 2 score and is a more objective and easier to recognize feature than color, texture, and swelling characterizing a GI = 1. If GI site scores are not identical at subsequent examinations, they are usually higher (Birkeland and Jorkjend, 1975) than at the preceding examination. The running of the probe along the free gingival margin may disrupt the integrity of a slightly inflamed sulcus lining and, hence, convert a GI = 1 score to a GI $= 2$ score at a subsequent assessment. This has been established for examinations performed within 2 hours (Birkeland and Jorkjend, 1975; Müller and Barrieshi-Nusair, 2005).

9.10.2   Continuous parameters

The evaluation of periodontal pockets involves measuring probing depth and relating these measurements to a landmark, such as the cemento-enamel junction or the margin of a reconstruction in order to determine loss of connective tissue attachment (LA). Both parameters are expressed in millimeters, and hence, represent continuous parameters. Six aspects around a tooth or root are usually evaluated.

9.10.2.1   Patient-based parameters

For determining intra-examiner variability, it is proposed to examine either five patients five times, six patients four times, seven patients three times, or eight patients twice. The adequate number of subjects to be included in the calibration procedure depends on the specific margin of error in the examiner reliability estimates (Hill et al., 2006). Repeated probing of the same subject may severely compromise the well-being of that individual. Again, it is reasonable to limit the number of passing to two when determining intra-examiner variability. Therefore, the selection of a set of representative teeth (Ramfjord, 1959; 1967) and their contralateral counterparts as another set of representative teeth for the dentition has been advocated if patient-based outcomes are to be assessed.

As mentioned for the nonparametric indices, the first and third scorings will consider exclusively the teeth proposed by Ramfjord (1959) (Teeth FDI No.: 16, 11, 24, 36, 31, 44; U.S.: 3, 9, 12, 19, 25, 28) as being representative of the dentition. The second and fourth examinations, however, will consider only the contralateral teeth of Ramfjord (1959) (Teeth FDI No.: 14, 21, 26, 34, 41, 46; U.S.: 5, 8, 14, 21, 24, 30) as being representative of the dentition. The teeth are evaluated on three buccal (mesio-buccal, buccal, disto-buccal) and three lingual (mesio-lingual, lingual, distolingual) aspects.

If the mean values for PD and LA were generated with representative teeth and their contralateral counterparts, a Student's t-test may be performed to verify that both groups of teeth would be representative of the whole dentition. Pending a positive outcome of no difference between the mean scores, the four scorings may be analyzed by an analysis of variance with—expectedly—no difference between the mean scores for all assessments.

9.10.2.2   Site-based parameters

To determine the reproducibility of single-site measurements, the clinical protocol and the results of the calibration exercise for mean PD and LA may be used. However, the analysis will have to concentrate either on the first and the third or on the second and fourth assessments of the sites. The reproducibility for the PlI and the GI will be determined applying κ statistics or percentage agreement. Generally, the percentage agreement of single-site PD or LA measurements are higher than those obtained for nonparametric indices. Obviously, the assessment in millimeters is easier to perform than to assess thickness of plaque or early characteristics of inflammation. The intra-examiner variability for PD and LA has been identified to lie between 0.36–0.41 and 0.54 mm, respectively (Glavind and Löe,

1967; Ramfjord, 1974; Kingman et al., 1991). The calibration values for PD are normally slightly below than those for LA owing to the difficulties associated with identifying the cemento-enamel junction.

9.11   Statistical analysis of calibration data

When a duplicate set of observations on a group of subjects is available from either a single or multiple examiners, these may be characterized by coefficients of variation and interclass correlation coefficients for continuously distributed variables. For categorical variables, however, percentage agreement and associated κ statistics may summarize the set of observations.

9.11.1   Interclass correlation coefficients and analysis of variance

Inter- and intra-examiner reliability are assessed by using the interclass correlation coefficient. This coefficient is defined as the correlation between measurements made upon the same subject (Kingman, 1986).

Inter- and intra-examiner agreement should be evaluated for subject-based mean parameters. These include whole-mouth scorings for both continuous and categorical variables. Paired t-tests may be used to assess systematic bias between the first and the second subject-based mean scores or, in case of partial but representative recordings, between original and contralateral representative tooth mean scores. In case of multiple assessments, an analysis of variance to test the hypothesis of no difference between the assessments may be employed (Kingman, 1986).

9.11.2   Percentage agreement and κ statistics

When site-specific data are evaluated in a planned study, statistics on calibration results should be performed at the site level. Such evaluations for intra-examiner variability can be determined by either percent agreement scores after two passages and associated κ statistics for both continuous and categorical variables. Simple percentage agreement fails to adjust for chance agreement. Hence, the most useful statistical methods for assessing intra-examiner reliability are in descending order: the weighted κ, the correlation coefficient, the unweighted κ statistics, and the percentage agreement (Spolsky and Gornbein, 1996).

κ ≥ 0.75 corresponds to excellent agreement, 0.40 < κ < 0.75 reflects good agreement, and κ ≤ 0.40 represents poor agreement. For ordinal variables (e.g., PD/LA within a 1-mm increment), percentage agreement remains an option, but treats nonagreements equivalently. Alternatives include reporting agreement within 1 mm or weighted κ (κ_w). The latter, κ_w, differentially weights nonagreements based on their relative magnitude, while adjusting for chance agreement.

9.12   Needs for reporting

In most publications reporting on outcomes of clinical studies, it is mentioned that examiners were calibrated, but most often, information on how, when, and with what outcomes standardization exercises and calibration protocols have been performed is lacking. If quality control is to improve the standards of clinical studies (Imrey et al., 1994a, 1994b), such reporting is a prerequisite. Editors of journals and their editorial boards should insist that authors report these aspects. The Consolidated Standards of Reporting Trials (CONSORT) group was constituted to alleviate the problems arising from inadequate reporting of randomized controlled clinical trials (RCT). The CONSORT Statement (2001) is a minimum set of recommendations of reporting RCT, and a 22-point checklist is provided to authors facilitating their transparent and complete reporting. CONSORT is now widely recognized and endorsed by renowned medical and dental journals. Unfortunately, standardization and calibration exercises are not mentioned at all in this very influential document for quality control of clinical studies.

References

Abbas F, Hart AA, Oosting J, van der Velden U. 1982. Effect of training and probing force on the reproducibility of pocket depth measurements. *Journal of Periodontal Research* 17:226–234.

Aguero A, Garnick JJ, Keagle J, Steflik DE, Thompson WO. 1995. Histological location of a standardized periodontal probe in man. *Journal of Periodontology* 66:184–190.

Armitage GC, Svanberg GK, Löe H. 1977. Microscopic evaluation of clinical measurements of connective tissue attachment levels. *Journal of Clinical Periodontology* 4:173–190.

Badersten A, Nilvéus R, Egelberg J. 1984. Reproducibility of probing attachment level measurements. *Journal of Clinical Periodontology* 11:475–485.

Bergenholtz A, al-Harbi N, al-Hummayani FM, Anton P, al-Kahtani S. 2000. The accuracy of the Vivacare true pressure-sensitive periodontal probe system in terms of probing force. *Journal of Clinical Periodontology* 27:93–98.

Biesbrock AR, Bartizek RD. 2005. Plaque removal efficacy of a prototype power toothbrush compared to a control manual toothbrush. *American Journal of Dentistry* 18:116–120.

Birkeland JM, Jorkjend L. 1975. The influence of examination of the assessment of the intra-examiner error by using the plaque and gingival index systems. *Community Dentistry and Oral Epidemiology* 3:214–216.

Black GV. 1913. Something on the etiology and pathology of diseases of the periodontal membrane. *Dental Cosmos* 55:1219–1226.

Bollmer BW, Sturzenberger OP, Lehnhoff RW, Bosma ML, Lang NP, Mallatt ME, Meckel AH. 1986. A comparison of 3 clinical indices for measuring gingivitis. *Journal of Clinical Periodontology* 13:392–395.

Chaves ES, Wood RC, Jones AA, Newbold DA, Manwell MA, Kornman KS. 1993. Relationship of "bleeding on probing" and "gingival index bleeding" as clinical parameters of gingival inflammation. *Journal of Clinical Periodontology* 20:139–143.

Clark WB, Yang MC, Magnusson I. 1992. Measuring clinical attachment: reproducibility of relative measurements with an electronic probe. *Journal of Periodontology* 63:831–838.

CONSORT Group. 2001. *Consolidated Standards of Reporting Trials*. Consort statement. Available online at www.consort-statement.org.

Cullinan MP, Westerman B, Hamlet SM, Palmer JE, Faddy MJ, Seymour GJ. 2003. The effect of a triclosan-containing dentifrice on the progression of periodontal disease in an adult population. *Journal of Clinical Periodontology* 30:414–419.

Dowsett SA, Eckert GJ, Kowolik MJ. 2002. The applicability of half-mouth examination to periodontal disease assessment in untreated adult populations. *Journal of Periodontology* 73:975–981.

Fowler C, Garrett S, Crigger M, Egelberg J. 1982. Histologic probe position in treated and untreated human periodontal tissues. *Journal of Clinical Periodontology* 9:373–385.

Freed HK, Gapper RL, Kalkwarf KL. 1983. Evaluation of periodontal probing forces. *Journal of Periodontology* 54:488–492.

Gabathuler H, Hassel T. 1971. A pressure-sensitive periodontal probe. *Helvetica Odontologica Acta* 15:114–117.

Garnick JJ, Spray JR, Vernino DM, Klawitter JJ. 1980. Demonstration of probes in human periodontal pockets. *Journal of Periodontology* 51:563–570.

Gettinger G, Patters MR, Testa MA, Löe H, Anerud A, Boysen H, Robertson PB. 1983. The use of six selected teeth in population measures of periodontal status. *Journal of Periodontology* 54:155–159.

Gibbs CH, Hirschfeld JW, Lee JG, Low SB, Magnusson I, Thousand RR, Yerneni P, Clark WB. 1988. Description and clinical evaluation of a new computerized periodontal probe—the Florida probe. *Journal of Clinical Periodontology* 15:137–144.

Glavind L, Löe H. 1967. Errors in the clinical assessment of periodontal destruction. *Journal of Periodontal Research* 2:180–184.

Goldberg P, Matsson L, Anderson H. 1985. Partial recording of gingivitis and dental plaque in children of different ages and in young adults. *Community Dentistry and Oral Epidemiology* 13:44–46.

Greene JC, Vermillion JR. 1964. The simplified oral hygiene index. *Journal of the American Dental Association* 68:7–13.

Greenstein G, Caton J, Polson AM. 1981. Histologic characteristics associated with bleeding after probing and visual signs of inflammation. *Journal of Periodontology* 52:420–425.

Grossi SG, Dunford RG, Ho A, Koch G, Machtei EE, Genco RJ. 1996. Sources of error for periodontal probing measurements. *Journal of Periodontal Research* 31:330–336.

Fischman SL. 1986. Current status of indices of plaque. *Journal of Clinical Periodontology* 13:371–374, 379–380.

Haffajee AD, Socransky SS, Goodson JM. 1983. Comparison of different data analyses for detecting changes in attachment level. *Journal of Clinical Periodontology* 10:298–310.

Hassel TM, Germann MA, Saxer UP. 1973. Periodontal probing: investigator discrepancies and correlations between probing force and recorded depth. *Helvetica Odontologica Acta* 17:38–42.

Hill EG, Slate EH, Wiegand RE, Grossi SG, Salinas CF. 2006. Study design for calibration of clinical examiners measuring periodontal parameters. *Journal of Periodontology* 77:1129–1141.

Imrey PB, Chilton NW, Pihlstrom BL, Proskin HM, Kingman A, Listgarten MA, Zimmerman SO, Ciancio SG, Cohen ME, D'Agostino RB, Fine DH, Fischman SL, Fleiss JL, Gunsolley JC, Kent RL Jr., Killoy WJ, Laster LL, Marks RG, Verma AO. 1994a. Proposed guidelines for American Dental Association acceptance of products for professional, non-surgical treatment of adult periodontitis. Task Force on Design and Analysis in Dental and Oral Research. *Journal of Periodontal Research* 29:348–360.

Imrey PB, Chilton NW, Pihlstrom BL, Proskin HM, Kingman A, Listgarten MA, Zimmerman SO, Ciancio SG, Cohen ME, D'Agostino RB, Fine DH, Fischman SL, Fleiss JL, Gunsolley JC, Kent RL Jr., Killoy WJ, Laster LL, Marks RG, Verma AO. 1994b. Recommended revisions to American Dental Association guidelines for acceptance of chemotherapeutic products for gingivitis control. Report of the Task Force on Design and Analysis in Dental and Oral Research to the Council on Therapeutics of the American Dental Association. *Journal of Periodontal Research* 29:299–304.

Jeffcoat MK, Reddy MS. 1991. A comparison of probing and radiographic methods for detection of periodontal disease progression. *Current Opinions in Dentistry* 1:45–51.

Karayiannis A, Lang NP, Joss A, Nyman S. 1992. Bleeding on probing as it relates to probing pressure and gingival health in patients with a reduced but healthy periodontium. A clinical study. *Journal of Clinical Periodontology* 19:471–475.

Kingman A. 1986. A procedure for evaluating the reliability of a gingivitis index. *Journal of Clinical Periodontology* 13:385–391.

Kingman A. 1993. Statistical management of periodontal data. *Periodontology 2000* 2:46–56.

Kingman A, Löe H, Anerud A, Boysen H. 1991. Errors in measuring parameters associated with periodontal health and disease. *Journal of Periodontology* 62:477–486.

Lang NP, Cumming BR, Löe H. 1973. Toothbrushing frequency as it relates to plaque development and gingival health. *Journal of Periodontology* 44:396–405.

Lang NP, Joss A, Tonetti MS. 1996. Monitoring disease during supportive periodontal treatment by bleeding on probing. *Periodontology 2000* 12:44–48.

Lang NP, Nyman S, Senn C, Joss A. 1991. Bleeding on probing as it relates to probing pressure and gingival health. *Journal of Clinical Periodontology* 18:257–261.

Lang NP, Østergaard E, Löe H. 1972. A fluorescent plaque disclosing agent. *Journal of Periodontal Research* 7:59–67.

Listgarten MA, Mao R, Robinson PJ. 1976. Periodontal probing and the relationship of the probe tip to periodontal tissues. *Journal of Periodontology* 47:511–513.

Löe H, Silness J. 1963. Periodontal disease in pregnancy. I. Prevalence and severity. *Acta Odontologica Scandinavia* 21:533–551.

Löe H, Theilade E, Jensen SB. 1965. Experimental gingivitis in man. *Journal of Periodontology* 36:177–187.

Magnusson I, Listgarten MA. 1980. Histological evaluation of probing depth following periodontal treatment. *Journal of Clinical Periodontology* 7:26–31.

Mallatt M, Mankodi S, Bauroth K, Bsoul SA, Bartizek RD, He T. 2007. A controlled 6-month clinical trial to study the effects of a stannous fluoride dentifrice on gingivitis. *Journal of Clinical Periodontology* 34:762–767.

Marks RG, Low SB, Taylor M, Baggs R, Magnusson I, Clark WB. 1991. Reproducibility of attachment level measurements with two models of the Florida probe. *Journal of Clinical Periodontology* 18:780–784.

McClanahan SF, Bartizek RD, Biesbrock AR. 2001. Identification and consequences of distinct Löe–Silness gingival index examiner styles for the clinical assessment of gingivitis. *Journal of Periodontology* 72:383–392.

Mombelli A. 2005. Clinical parameters: biological validity and clinical utility. *Periodontology 2000*, 39:30–39.

Mombelli A, Graf H. 1986. Depth–force-patterns in periodontal probing. *Journal of Clinical Periodontology* 13:126–130.

Mombelli A, Mühle T, Brägger U, Lang NP, Bürgin WB. 1997. Comparison of periodontal and peri-implant probing by depth–force pattern analysis. *Clinical Oral Implants Research* 8:448–454.

Mombelli A, Mühle T, Frigg R. 1992. Depth–force patterns of periodontal probing. Attachment-gain in relation to probing force. *Journal of Clinical Periodontology* 19:295–300.

Mombelli A, Nicopoulou-Karayianni K, Lang NP. 1990. Local differences in the newly formed crevicular microbiota. *Schweizerische Monatsschrift für Zahnmedizin* 100:154–158.

Müller HP, Barrieshi-Nusair KM. 2005. Gingival bleeding on repeat probing after different time intervals in plaque-induced gingivitis. *Clinical Oral Investigations* 9:278–283.

Osborn J, Stoltenberg J, Huso B, Aeppli D, Pihlstrom B. 1990. Comparison of measurement variability using a standard and constant force periodontal probe. *Journal of Periodontology* 61:497–503.

Osborn JB, Stoltenberg JL, Huso BA, Aeppli DM, Pihlstrom BL. 1992. Comparison of measurement variability in subjects with moderate periodontitis using a conventional and constant force periodontal probe. *Journal of Periodontology* 63:283–289.

Page RC, Kornman KS. 1997. The pathogenesis of human periodontitis: an introduction. *Periodontology 2000*, 14:9–11.

Pihlstrom BL. 1992. Measurement of attachment level in clinical trials: probing methods. *Journal of Periodontology* 63(Suppl. 12):1072–1077.

Quigley GA, Hein JW. 1962. Comparative cleansing efficiency of manual and power brushing. *Journal of the American Dental Association* 65:26–29.

Ramfjord SP. 1959. Indices for prevalence and incidence of periodontal disease. *Journal of Periodontology* 30:51–59.

Ramfjord SP. 1967. The periodontal disease index (PDI). *Journal of Periodontology* 38:602–610.

Ramfjord SP. 1974. Design of studies or clinical trials to evaluate the effectiveness of agents or procedures for the prevention, or treatment, of loss of the periodontium. *Journal of Periodontal Research* 9(Suppl. 14):78–93.

Seymour GJ. 1991. Importance of the host response in the periodontium. *Journal of Clinical Periodontology* 18:421–426.

Seymour GJ, Gemmell E, Westerman B, Cullinan M. 1996. Periodontics into the 21st century. *Annals of the Royal Australasian College of Dental Surgeons* 13:71–78.

Shaw L, Murray JJ. 1975. Inter-examiner and intra-examiner reproducibility in clinical and radiographic diagnosis. *International Dental Journal* 25:280–288.

Shaw L, Murray JJ. 1977. Diagnostic reproducibility of periodontal indices. *Journal of Periodontal Research* 12:141–147.

Silness J, Löe H. 1964. Periodontal disease in pregnancy. II. Correlation between oral hygiene and periodontal condition. *Acta Odontologica Scandinavia* 22:121–135.

Spolsky VW, Gornbein JA. 1996. Comparing measures of reliability for indices of gingivitis and plaque. *Journal of Periodontology* 67:853–859.

Sturzenberger OP, Lehnhoff RW, Bollmer BW. 1985. A clinical procedure for determining the proficiency of gingivitis examiners. *Journal of Clinical Periodontology* 12:756–761.

Turesky S, Gilmore ND, Glickman I. 1970. Reduced plaque formation by the chloromethyl analogue of victamine C. *Journal of Periodontology* 41:41–43.

Van Der Weijden GA, Timmerman MF, Nijboer A, Reijerse E, Van Der Velden U. 1994. Comparison of different approaches to assess bleeding on probing as indicators of gingivitis. *Journal of Clinical Periodontology* 21:589–594.

Vartoukian SR, Palmer RM, Wilson RF. 2004. Evaluation of a new periodontal probe tip design. A clinical and *in vitro* study. *Journal of Clinical Periodontology* 31:918–925.

Walsh TF, Saxby MS. 1989. Inter- and intra-examiner variability using standard and constant force periodontal probes. *Journal of Clinical Periodontology* 16:140–143.

Watts T. 1987. Constant force probing with and without a stent in untreated periodontal disease: the clinical reproducibility problem and possible sources of error. *Journal of Clinical Periodontology* 14:407–411.

Watts TL. 1989. Probing site configuration in patients with untreated periodontitis. A study of horizontal positional error. *Journal of Clinical Periodontology* 16:529–533.

10

Observational studies in oral health research

Hal Morgenstern, PhD, **and Woosung Sohn,** DDS, MS, PhD, DrPH

10.1   Introduction

The empirical investigation of oral health involves the study of disease occurrence and health indicators in human populations. An important focus of this research, as in other areas of applied epidemiology, is to test hypotheses and make causal inferences about the net effects of specific exposures or treatments on the development or course of disease. This objective is achieved by making comparisons between groups or within groups over time. Not only do the findings from such studies provide insights about the causes of disease and other health outcomes, but they also enhance our ability to translate basic science knowledge into clinical and public health practice.

There are three types of general research strategies for conducting population-based research. They are defined by two criteria regarding how the investigator deals with the exposure or treatment of primary interest (Kleinbaum et al., 1982). First, does the investigator manipulate the exposure or treatment, that is, does the investigator determine which subjects get exposed to an intervention and which do not get exposed? Second, if manipulation is used, is it done randomly, that is, are subjects randomly assigned (randomized) to different treatment groups? As shown in Table 10.1, these two criteria define three types of research: experiments, quasi experiments, and observational studies.

Experiments involve randomization of subjects to treatment groups. For example, in a standard two-group randomized clinical trial, subjects in the experimental group are assigned to receive the treatment under study, and subjects in the control group are assigned to receive no treatment, a placebo or sham treatment, or a standard treatment. All subjects are followed for changes in the outcome variable. With a sufficient number of subjects,

Table 10.1   Three types of studies for conducting research in human populations, by two criteria for dealing with the primary exposure or treatment variable.

Manipulation of exposure/treatment?	Randomization?	
	Yes	No
Yes	Experiment	Quasi experiment
No	—	Observational study

randomization helps to ensure *comparability* among treatment groups (no confounding); that is, in the absence of treatment in any group, we expect the distribution of the outcome variable to be the same in all assigned groups (though differences may occur by chance). Although we cannot observe this condition directly, we can observe its manifestation in our data: all groups will have, on average, similar distributions of extraneous factors (potential confounders) that also affect the outcome—even those factors that are unmeasured or unknown.

Quasi experiments involve manipulation of the treatment by the investigator but without randomization. There are two approaches for conducting a quasi experiment: a multiple-group design in which the groups differ with respect to the intervention under study (analogous to an experiment), and a one-group design in which the outcome is compared for subjects before and after the intervention begins.

In an *observational study*, the investigator does not manipulate the exposure/treatment variable; rather, exposure status of each unit of observation (e.g., subject) is simply observed or recorded. In this type of study, the exposure variable may be defined more broadly than in experiments or quasi experiments, for example, as an environmental exposure or condition, an individual characteristic or behavior, or an intervention performed by others.

The purpose of this chapter is to describe specific observational designs used in oral health research with examples and to point out important methodologic issues and challenges. First, however, we discuss the rationale and value of observational studies and highlight the concepts, principles, and methods that underlie this type of research.

10.2   Rationale and value of observational studies

Observational studies are often criticized and even ignored in clinical research under the belief that causal effects cannot be observed in these studies, but they can be observed in experiments. This belief is misguided because, as discussed in the next section, causal effects cannot be observed in any type of study. Furthermore, despite the important advantage of experiments to control for confounding when assessing a specific causal hypothesis, randomized studies have several methodologic problems that limit causal inference. Because experiments are often conducted in small restricted samples of volunteers, the precision of effect estimation and the power of statistical tests are low and the generalizability of results to the target population is compromised. Experiments also have several potential sources of bias due to noncompliance with assigned treatment protocols, loss to follow-up, poor outcome measures based on self reports or unreliable assays, and lack of double blinding. In addition, randomization is often not ethical, feasible, or allowable by participating institutions or clinicians.

In light of these limitations of experiments, observational studies have considerable value in clinical research. First, they can often be done more quickly and inexpensively than experiments, and they require less cooperation from subjects, making them more feasible and practical. Second, observational studies can often be conducted in large populations that closely reflect the target population of interest to the investigator, thereby enhancing precision, power, and generalizability. Third, observational studies can more readily be used to assess multiple hypotheses involving different exposures or interventions in the same study. Fourth, findings from observational studies are often used by researchers to generate new hypotheses and to justify and plan randomized clinical trials.

10.3   Concepts, principles, and methods

Population researchers operate on two levels: understanding and intervention. At the understanding level, we plan and implement scientific investigations to acquire knowledge about disease occurrence in specific populations. The focus is causal inference for individuals. At the intervention level, we develop and evaluate clinical practices, health programs, and policies to prevent disease, promote health, and reduce health disparities. The focus at this level is decision making for populations. There is a dynamic interplay between these two levels, which gains importance with increased attention to translational research and evidence-based clinical practice.

As shown in Figure 10.1, both levels may be conceived as a set of connections among four stages in the natural history of disease: the start of causal action, the occurrence of disease (often not observable), the time when disease is clinically detectable (onset of signs and symptoms), and change in disease status (e.g., clinical improvement, recovery, or death). At the understanding level, the natural history of disease is seen as three sequential processes or periods linking the four stages: induction (before disease occurrence), latency (preclinical period), and course of disease (clinical period). At the intervention level, the natural history of disease is seen as three strategies of prevention: primary (preventing disease occurrence), secondary (early detection and treatment), and tertiary (treatment and rehabilitation).

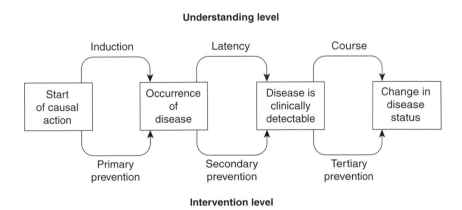

Figure 10.1 The natural history of disease: understanding versus intervention levels.

10.3.1   Population measures

There is a close connection between the design of a study and the types of quantitative measures that we can estimate in that study.

10.3.1.1   Measures of disease frequency

Measures of disease frequency reflect how common the disease is in a particular population relative to the size of the population, and they serve as the foundation for most epidemiologic analyses. Different measures are used to quantify *incidence* (new case occurrences), *prevalence* (existing cases), and *mortality* (deaths from one or more diseases). Prevalence is the probability of being a case at a "point" in time, and it is computed as the proportion of persons in the population that have the disease at that time.

Disease incidence and mortality can be measured in two ways: as a *risk*, that is, the probability of becoming a case or dying during a given period (a cumulative measure), and as a *rate*, that is, the instantaneous occurrence of disease or death per unit of time (Morgenstern et al., 1980; Kleinbaum et al., 1982; Rothman et al., 2008). The average risk in a population may be computed as the proportion of persons initially at risk who become cases during the subsequent follow-up period (assuming no loss to follow-up), and the average incidence rate or incidence density (per unit of time) is computed as the number of new cases divided by the amount of person-time experienced by the population at risk during the follow-up period. For example, if 13 people at risk are followed for 2 years without loss and one case occurs at the midpoint of the 2-year period, the 2-year risk is 1/13 = 0.077 (7.7%). The number of person-years at risk is 12×2 (for noncases) $+ 1 \times 1$ (for the case) $= 25$; therefore, the average incidence rate for the 2-year period is 1/25 = 0.040/year.

10.3.1.2   Measures of effect

The net causal effect of an exposure on disease occurrence in a particular population is expressed as a *counterfactual* contrast between different exposure conditions (Maldonado and Greenland, 2002). Suppose, for example, that 100 exposed persons at risk are followed for 10 years during which 10 incident cases occur. The causal question is how many of those 100 exposed persons would have become cases if they had not been exposed (counter to fact). If the number of cases in the absence of exposure would be different from 10, we say that there was a net effect in the population; thus, the exposure is a *risk factor*—either causal or preventive—for the disease in that population.

Because we cannot observe the number of cases in the absence of exposure, we must rely on the epidemiologic method to estimate effect. That is, we compare disease incidence in the exposed group with incidence in another unexposed (reference) group; this quantitative comparison is a measure of association (see below). Finding that disease risk is different for the exposed and unexposed groups is consistent with a net effect of the exposure, but this interpretation depends on a key assumption that the risk in the unexposed group is equal to what the risk in the exposed group would have been in the absence of exposure. This assumption is another way of saying that the exposure groups are comparable or that the observed comparison is not confounded. Unfortunately, we cannot observe directly from our data whether the comparability assumption holds, so that we must use an indirect approach to assess and control for confounding in observational studies (see "Estimation Error").

10.3.1.3   Measures of association

Measures of association reflect the magnitude of a statistical relation between two variables such as an exposure and disease. While effect measures reflect counterfactual (unobservable) contrasts between exposure conditions, association measures reflect observable contrasts between exposure groups.

Four types of association measures are used when the outcome is a dichotomous variable or event: ratios of disease frequency, comparing exposed and unexposed groups (e.g., the risk ratio (relative risk) or incidence rate ratio); differences in disease frequency between exposed and unexposed groups (e.g., the risk or rate difference); regression coefficients (slopes) estimated from fitted prediction models, which can usually be interpreted as ratio or difference measures; and correlation coefficients. When exposure groups are comparable, ratios or differences of disease risk or incidence rates can be interpreted as effect measures (assuming no other sources of bias). Other ratio measures, such as odds ratios (the odds of being or becoming a case in the exposed group, divided by the odds of being or becoming a case in the unexposed group) and prevalence ratios (disease prevalence in the exposed group divided by disease prevalence in the unexposed group), require additional assumptions to be interpreted as effect measures (Rothman et al., 2008). Correlation coefficients can never be interpreted as effect measures because they are based on variances (noncausal information that depends on selection decisions) (Greenland et al., 1986, 1991).

10.3.2   Elements of statistical analysis

Every statistical analysis involves two fundamental elements: statistical testing and parameter estimation. Statistical testing is done because we recognize that our findings are influenced by random sampling error (chance). The usual purpose of testing is to determine the extent to which the null hypothesis of no association in the source population is compatible with our observed results. To achieve this objective, we compute from the data a test statistic with a known probability distribution and derive from it a p value. The p value is the probability of obtaining the observed result or a more extreme value if the null hypothesis were true. The smaller the p value, the less compatible is the null hypothesis with the observed results.

Overreliance on p values for making causal inferences is common among researchers, probably because p values are often misinterpreted. It is important to recognize that a p value is not the probability that the null hypothesis is true or that the result was due to chance. Reporting p values without effect estimates can be very misleading because the p value reflects both the size of the study and the magnitude of the association. Even more misleading is the common practice of interpreting p values as "significant" (usually $p < 0.05$) or "not significant" ($p > 0.05$). In fact, this cutoff value for the accepted probability of a type I error is entirely arbitrary and has no scientific value for making causal inferences. Thus, for example, concluding that there is no association or no effect because the p value is greater than 0.05 is incorrect and often misleading, especially when the sample size is small. Furthermore, this practice, which is now strongly discouraged by many statisticians and epidemiologists, ignores possible biases in effect estimation (e.g., Poole, 1987; Savitz, 2003; Jewell, 2004; Rothman et al., 2008). These warnings notwithstanding, p values are still informative when reported with effect estimates, especially when testing dose–response associations or interactions between exposures.

Interpretation of statistical findings, therefore, should focus primarily on the magnitude of associations and their confidence intervals that reflect the precision with which the associations are estimated (see "Estimation Error"). It is tempting, however, to misinterpret confidence intervals in the same way as significance testing (Poole, 1987). In particular, researchers often interpret associations as "significant" or "not significant" according to whether the 95% confidence interval around the estimate excludes or includes the null value (e.g., a risk ratio of one). In principle, therefore, statistical results do not tell us whether there is, or whether there is not, an effect; rather, they convey a continuum of information that we use along with prior knowledge and logic to make causal inferences.

10.3.3   Estimation error

Our ability to make inferences about possible effects is limited in practice by the error with which effects are estimated. Estimation error may be classified into two types: random and nonrandom (systematic). *Precision* refers to the relative lack of random error. A precise estimate is one that has a relatively small variance and therefore a relatively narrow confidence interval. In general, imprecise estimation is due to small sample sizes, rare outcomes or exposures, the need to adjust for too many covariates (potential confounders), or strong associations between the exposure and those covariates (collinearity).

Internal validity (or simply validity) refers to the lack of systematic error of estimation—called *bias* in epidemiology. A valid effect estimate is one that is expected to represent perfectly, aside from random error, the value of the effect parameter in the entire population of interest (including members who are not selected or observed). Assessing validity and correcting for bias is a complex, multifaceted process, particularly in observational studies.

A popular framework for assessing estimation validity in population studies is to distinguish among three sources of bias: confounding, selection bias, and information bias (e.g., Kleinbaum et al., 1982; Rothman et al., 2008). *Confounding*, as defined earlier, is lack of comparability between exposure groups, and it can occur in any type of study. Particularly in observational studies, confounding is always possible, regardless of the sample size, and the direction of the bias might be to overestimate or underestimate the effect. *Selection bias* occurs when subject selection, participation, or loss to follow-up is affected by exposure status and/or disease status. As discussed later, the threat of selection bias varies considerably for different types of observational studies. *Information bias* occurs when data are incomplete or missing or when variables are measured with error, for example, when exposed persons are misclassified as unexposed or vice versa. If misclassification of each variable is independent of other variables and independent of other errors, effects will typically be underestimated (i.e., "bias toward the null").

10.3.3.1   Confounders and confounder control

Because comparability between exposure groups cannot be observed directly, researchers attempt to identify and control for empirical manifestations of confounding. This is done by searching for differences between exposure groups in the distribution of extraneous risk factors—called *confounders*. To be confounder, a covariate must be (1) a risk factor for the disease in the unexposed population; (2) associated with the exposure in the total population; and (3) the latter association cannot be due entirely to the effect of the exposure on the covariate, for example, as an *intermediate variable* in the causal pathway between exposure and disease.

In observational studies, it is critical for the investigator to identify potential confounders and to control for their biasing influence on effect estimation. Such control can be achieved by certain procedures in the design of the study or in the data analysis. In the design phase, confounder control can be done by selecting exposed and unexposed groups that are appear to be comparable (called a "natural experiment," which is uncommon), restricting subject eligibility according to known risk factors (i.e., making exposed and unexposed subjects similar with respect to the distribution of certain potential confounders), or matching unexposed subjects to exposed subjects (or noncases to cases) on known risk factors. In the analysis phase, confounder control can be achieved by measuring potential confounders, then adjusting for their biasing effect by examining the exposure-disease association within categories of the confounders (*stratified analysis*) or by fitting to the data a mathematical model that includes both the exposure and confounders as predictors of the outcome.

10.3.4   Model fitting in practice

Measures of association and confidence intervals can be derived from fitted models, and the type of model determines which type of measure is readily estimated. Four types of models are commonly used in epidemiologic analysis (Kalbfleisch and Prentice, 2002; Jewell, 2004; Woodward, 2005; Rothman et al., 2008). *Linear models* are typically used when the outcome variable is continuous. Fitted results yield an estimate of the difference in outcome mean for each predictor (e.g., comparing exposed and unexposed subjects), which is adjusted for all other predictors in the model. *Logistic models* are used when the outcome is dichotomous (e.g., case vs. noncase), and fitted results yield an estimate of the adjusted odds ratio for each predictor. *Poisson models* are used when the outcome is the number of events observed during a certain amount of person-time at risk within each joint category of the predictors; fitted results yield an estimate of the adjusted rate ratio for each predictor. *Proportional hazards models* (Cox regression) are used when the outcome is time to an event, and fitted results yield an estimate of the adjusted rate (hazard) ratio for each predictor. This latter method allows for predictors to be treated as time dependent, that is, their measured values for individual subjects can change during the same period that outcome events are detected.

In oral health research, as in other research areas, special model-fitting procedures are often needed to deal with special design features and challenging estimation issues. Several of these procedures are highlighted below:

1. *Correlated data*: In studies of dental caries or periodontal disease, the analysis must usually take into consideration observations that are not independent, for example, when observing repeated outcome measures over time in the same individuals, when observing different teeth or sites in the same individuals, or when observing individuals from different dental practices. For example, we would expect greater correlation between the attachment losses at different sites of the same person than between different sites of different persons. Two statistical methods are frequently used to deal with these types of correlated (clustered) data: *generalized estimating equations*, and *survey regression models* developed to analyze data from complex sample designs (e.g., using SUDAAN) (Zeger and Liang, 1992; Liang and Zeger, 1993; Beck et al., 1997b).

2. *Multilevel data and estimation of contextual effects*: There is a growing interest in oral health research, as in other fields of population health, in the effects of

macrolevel (ecologic) factors, such as characteristics of dental practices or neighborhoods, on the risk of disease in individuals (Holst et al., 2001; Malikaew et al., 2003; Newton and Bower, 2005; Gilbert et al., 2006). Methods for estimating such contextual effects must usually involve variables measured at different levels of organization (e.g., tooth, individual, and dental practice). A general method for estimating these effects, which takes into consideration within-level clustering of outcomes, is *multilevel modeling* (also called hierarchical regression and mixed-effects modeling) (Albandar and Goldstein, 1992; Raudenbush and Bryk, 2002; Goldstein, 2003).

3. *Time-dependent confounders*: If a time-varying risk factor can affect exposure status and be affected by exposure status, that risk factor can be both a confounder of the estimated exposure effect and an intermediate variable in the causal pathway between exposure and disease. Standard methods of analysis, even those treating the predictors as time dependent, can yield biased estimates of the exposure effect even when there are no unmeasured confounders. To obtain unbiased estimates, special causal modeling techniques are required, such as *marginal structural models* using inverse-probability-of-treatment weighted estimation (Robins et al., 2000; Hernán et al., 2001) or *structural nested models* using G estimation (Robins, 1998).

4. *Unmeasured confounders*: In observational studies, it can be difficult to identify and measure accurately all important confounders. This problem is particularly relevant in clinical research where we wish to estimate the effect of a new clinical treatment by comparing it with a standard treatment or no treatment. The problem is that the indication for using the new treatment is typically a poor prognosis, that is, the new treatment is given to patients whose condition is most severe or nonresponsive to standard treatments (Miettinen, 1983). The resulting bias, called *confounding by indication*, is difficult to control because the investigator must be able to identify and measure the specific confounders responsible for the bias. One approach to control for unmeasured confounders in an observational study is the method of instrumental variables (Angrist et al., 1996; Greenland, 2000; Hernán and Robins, 2006). An instrument is a variable that affects exposure status but not the outcome independent of the exposure and that is not associated with the unmeasured confounders.

5. *Missing data*: When data are missing on key variables, restricting the analysis to only those subjects with complete data has two problems: the sample size may be reduced substantially, thereby losing estimation precision, and the loss of subjects is likely to produce bias unless the data are "missing completely at random." One approach for dealing with this problem is to impute the values of missing variables, based on their associations with other variables that are not missing. The best application of this method, which takes into account imputation variability, is called *multiple imputation* (Little and Rubin, 2002; Molenberghs and Kenward, 2007).

6. *Longitudinal analysis of periodontal disease*: Longitudinal studies of periodontal disease typically involve measurements of attachment level at different sites in each subject's mouth and at multiple exams during follow-up (where attachment

level is pocket depth plus gingival recession, in mm). In order to focus attention on the effects of individual-level and macrolevel exposures (rather than site-specific exposures) on the development and course of periodontal disease, Beck et al. (1994, 1997a, 1997b) and Beck and Elter (2000) recommend what they call the "incidence density" method for dealing with recurrent outcome events and the loss of teeth and subjects during follow-up. The outcome event in their method is an increase in attachment level (attachment loss) at a given site of at least 3 mm between successive exams. The incidence density (rate) of attachment loss for each subject can be estimated by aggregating events across sites (and possibly exams) and dividing by the total amount of site-time at risk (analogous to person-time). These rate estimates can then be modeled as a function of desired predictors, using Poisson regression and generalized estimating equations to deal with correlated data across exams.

10.4   Types of observational study designs

The types of observational studies that are commonly used in oral health research can be grouped into four general designs: cohort studies, cross-sectional studies, case-control studies, and ecologic studies. Each study design described in this section is accompanied by a figure depicting basic features of that design, where both the exposure and disease are diagrammed as dichotomous variables (see the Key to Symbols in Figures 10.2–10.9).

Key to Symbols in Figures 10.2–10.9

N   **Population** from which subjects are selected; subscripts (1, 2,...,k) indicate subgroups of the population or the population observed at different times

E/ Ē   **Exposed/unexposed** subjects

C/ C̄   **Prevalent**   cases/noncases (at risk of becoming cases)

D/ D̄   **Incident**   cases/noncases, or deaths/survivors

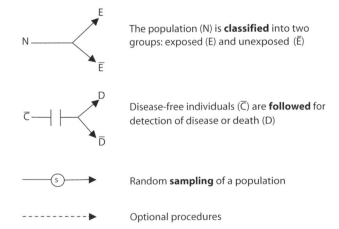

The population (N) is **classified** into two groups: exposed (E) and unexposed (Ē)

Disease-free individuals (C̄) are **followed** for detection of disease or death (D)

Random **sampling** of a population

Optional procedures

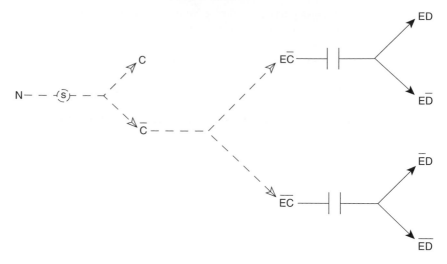

Figure 10.2 Cohort study design.

10.4.1   Cohort studies

A cohort study is a longitudinal design of a particular population at risk, which is followed for a given period to detect the first occurrences of an incident event (D), death, or other changes in health status (Figure 10.2). Prevalent cases (C) identified at baseline that are not at risk are excluded from the study population. Exposure status and covariates are measured at baseline (start of follow-up), and the outcome risk or rate during follow-up is compared for different levels of exposure (e.g., exposed (E) vs. unexposed ($\bar{\text{E}}$) groups in Figure 10.2), adjusting for the confounding effects of the covariates. In a *prospective* cohort study, both current exposure status and disease status are observed during the course of the investigation. In a *retrospective* cohort study, previous exposure status and disease status before the start of the study are obtained from the subjects' recall of past events or conditions or from abstracted records that were created for other purposes; thus, the follow-up period precedes the period during which the study is conducted.

Example 10.1. DeStefano et al. (1993) analyzed data from a prospective cohort study to estimate the effect of dental disease on the rate of coronary heart disease (CHD). A national sample of 9,760 adults, aged 25–74 years at baseline, who participated in the first National Health and Examination Survey (NHANES I), were followed from 1971–1974 to 1987. Outcome events were first hospital admissions for CHD or deaths in which CHD was listed as the underlying cause of death on the death certificate. The investigators used two baseline measures of dental disease: a periodontal index reflecting gingivitis and periodontitis, and an oral hygiene index reflecting the degree of debris and calculus. Using proportional hazards analysis, they found that both baseline indices were positively associated with the CHD rate, adjusting for several demographic, behavioral, and clinical risk factors for CHD. These associations were strongest for men under 50 years of age at baseline. The authors were cautious about making a causal inference, however, because they were not able to control for health practices and health care access that might have confounded the results.

As noted in the previous section, the analysis of data from cohort studies becomes more complicated when taking into account predictors that change during follow-up, repeated outcome measures or recurrent outcome events in the same person, and other types of correlated data (see Example 10.2).

Example 10.2. Beck et al. (1997a) analyzed data from the Piedmont 65+ Dental Study in North Carolina to examine trends and identify risk factors for attachment loss among 540 older adults followed for 5 years—with dental examinations at baseline, 18, 36, and 60 months. Outcome events—observed at each site in each subject at each exam—were increases in attachment level of 3 mm or more since the previous exam. Using their "incidence density" method (see Model Fitting in Practice, #6) with SUDAAN to handle sampling weights and correlated outcome within persons and primary sampling units, the investigators estimated the overall incidence rate of attachment loss to be 0.0206/year. They found that this rate was greater for blacks than for whites, men than for women, subjects with less than a high-school education than for subjects with more education, and smokers than for nonsmokers.

One advantage of the cohort design relative to other observational designs is that exposure status is measured before disease is detected. Thus, we usually know that the exposure preceded disease occurrence, which is a requirement for making causal inferences; that is, *temporal ambiguity* is not usually a problem in cohort studies. Another relative advantage of cohort designs is that subjects are selected before disease is detected so that the outcome cannot generally influence the selection of subjects. Therefore, certain forms of selection bias that threaten other observational designs are not likely to bias the results of cohort studies.

A practical limitation of cohort designs, especially prospective studies, is that they tend to be time consuming and expensive. Furthermore, cohort studies are inefficient for studying rare outcome events because large sample sizes are needed to yield precise estimates of effect. Another limitation is loss to follow-up, which not only reduces the effective sample size (and estimation precision) but can also lead to estimation bias because subject loss does not occur randomly.

10.4.2   Cross-sectional studies

In a basic cross-sectional study, one set of observations is made on each subject at a single time (Figure 10.3). Thus, the outcome in this type of study is disease prevalence (C vs. C̄ in Figure 10.3) or current health status in a study population. Random (probability) sampling (s) is used to select subjects when the investigator wishes to estimate disease prevalence in a large source population (N) within definable limits of sampling error without observing everyone in that source population. The major reason for random sampling, therefore, is to make the study population representative of the larger source population. (Note that random sampling is different from randomization, which is done to achieve comparability between exposure and treatment groups.) Cross-sectional designs are often used to study clinical or biological characteristics that are measured on a continuous or ordinal scale or nonfatal, chronic conditions (e.g., attachment loss or periodontitis).

Example 10.3. Bower et al. (2007) conducted a cross-sectional study to estimate the effect of "area deprivation" on oral health among 632 adults living in 346 households in 31 postcode sectors in Scotland. They measured three outcomes, including periodontal pocketing of at least 4 mm in one or more teeth. An index of area deprivation for each postcode sector was based on four factors: level of household overcrowding, male unemployment rate, proportion of the population in (low) social classes IV or V, and proportion

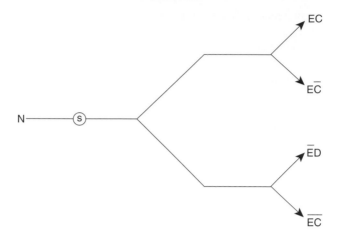

Figure 10.3 Basic cross-sectional study design.

of persons living in a private household with no car. This index was categorized into five ordinal groups. The investigators used multilevel logistic regression to estimate the effect of area deprivation on periodontal pocketing, adjusting for several sociodemographic factors measured at the individual and household levels. Although they found evidence for a positive association, odds ratios were imprecisely estimated and there was not a consistent dose–response association observed across area-deprivation categories. The authors also noted the limitations of their cross-sectional design (see below).

The main advantage of a cross-sectional design, relative to a cohort design, is that it tends to be less time consuming and expensive because there is no follow-up period. Descriptive results from cross-sectional studies also assist health planners and policy makers because they provide valuable information about the health needs of large populations.

Nonetheless, cross-sectional studies have several methodologic limitations for making causal inferences. First, because we seldom know when the disease occurred in prevalent cases, we often cannot determine whether the exposure preceded the disease; that is, there may be temporal ambiguity, especially when the disease can influence exposure status or when exposure is not measured retrospectively. Second, because prevalent cases first occurred before the study is started, disease status can influence which eligible persons get selected or which selected persons agree to participate. If selection or participation is also affected by exposure status, the estimated exposure effect will usually be biased (Greenland, 2003). This selection bias tends to occur, for example, when eligibility is restricted to patients who have sought care or been referred to certain providers or facilities. Third, because disease prevalence depends on both disease incidence and duration, we may not be able to distinguish the effects of exposures on disease occurrence from their effects on disease outcome; that is, the effects of risk factors from the effects of *prognostic factors* (see Figure 10.1).

10.4.2.1   Nested cross-sectional study

Sometimes a cross-sectional study of disease prevalence is conducted after the start of follow-up in a cohort study that was designed to investigate other outcomes (Figure 10.4).

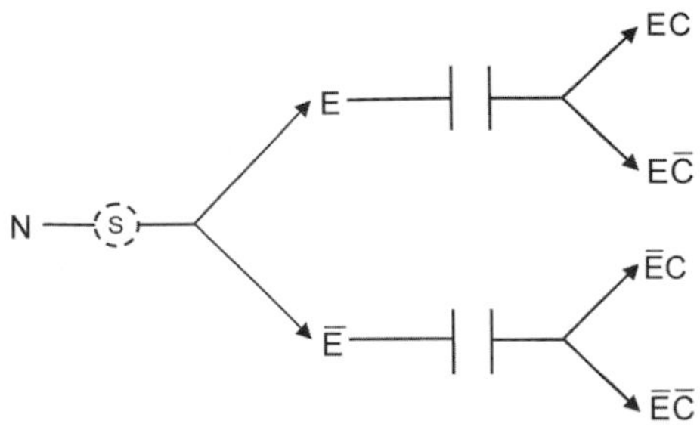

Figure 10.4 Nested cross-sectional study design.

That is, the study population for the cross-sectional study is those subjects from the original cohort who are not lost to follow-up and who agree to participate in the new study. The advantage of this nested cross-sectional study, relative to a basic cross-sectional study, is that exposure and covariate data are available from the original cohort. Thus, the data on past exposures and covariates are likely to be more complete and measured more accurately than would retrospective measurement in a basic design, and temporal ambiguity may be less problematic. On the other hand, the nested design has the same potential for selection bias because the investigator does not know disease status at the start of follow-up and subjects from the original cohort are lost to follow-up. In addition, results from the nested design might not be able to distinguish the effects of risk factors from the effects of prognostic factors.

Example 10.4. Thomson et al. (2004) used a "life-course" approach to estimate the effects of childhood factors on oral health at age 26 among residents of Dunedin, New Zealand, who had been followed since birth in 1972–1973. One of their outcomes was the presence of periodontitis at age 26 (i.e., an attachment level of at least 4 mm at one or more sites). Early childhood socioeconomic status (SES) was based on parental occupations and was dichotomized into low and high groups. Using logistic regression, the authors found that childhood SES was inversely associated with periodontitis prevalence at age 26, adjusting for sex, smoking at ages 21 and 26, dental visiting pattern, and number of dental caries at age 5. The prevalence of periodontitis was highest for subjects who were classified as low SES in early childhood and at age 26. Despite the nested cross-sectional design, the results of this study may approximate the results of a cohort study because only 24% of the cohort at age 3 was lost by age 26, and it is reasonable to assume that these subjects were free of peridontitis in early childhood.

10.4.2.2 Repeated cross-sectional study

In a repeated cross-sectional study, two or more similar cross-sectional studies of the same outcome are conducted in the same geographically defined (dynamic) population at different times (N_1 and N_2 in Figure 10.5). Because the samples at different times do not generally involve the same subjects, we do not observe individual changes in outcome status (incidence) but rather changes in outcome prevalence over time. This design is used to examine trends in disease prevalence, sometimes before versus after the start of a population intervention, and to understand the extent to which the change in prevalence was attributable to changes in other factors measured at different times (e.g., changes in

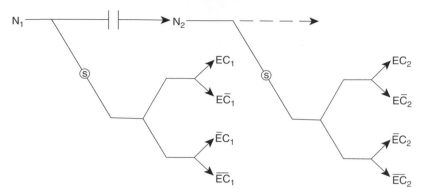

Figure 10.5 Repeated cross-sectional study design.

risk factors). Each cross-sectional study used alone, however, has the same limitations as mentioned earlier for making causal inferences about risk-factor effects.

Example 10.5. Using data from two national surveys, NHANES I (1971–1974) and NHANES III (1988–1994), Brown et al. (1999) examined the trend in dental-caries prevalence among children, aged 6–18 years. The main outcome of their analyses was the number of untreated carious permanent teeth per child. The authors found that the mean outcome decreased by 77% between NHANES I and NHANES III. They also found that the disparity in mean outcome between blacks and whites and between low- and high-income families decreased during the same period. The authors interpreted these findings as consistent with the shift from restorative to preventive dental services. This interpretation assumes that the change in outcome reflects predominantly a decrease in the incidence rate of dental caries, rather than an increase in the rate at which caries are filled or extracted.

10.4.3   Case-control studies

In a case-control study, the investigator selects subjects by stratifying on the outcome; that is, persons with the outcome (cases) and persons without the outcome (controls) are selected separately and typically come from different populations (N' and N in Figure 10.6). Thus, the ratio of controls to cases is fixed by the investigator. Case-control studies may be cross-sectional, involving prevalent cases (C), or longitudinal, involving incident cases (D, in practice, newly diagnosed cases as depicted in Figure 10.6). In longitudinal designs, there are two methods for selecting controls: cumulative sampling, where all controls are noncases at the end of the follow-up period during which cases are identified; and density sampling (more common), where one or more controls (noncases) are selected at the time of each case occurrence. In all types of case-control designs, controls are frequently matched to cases on known risk factors that are potential confounders. Exposure and covariate information is then obtained for cases and controls, and logistic regression is typically used to estimate their associations with disease (measured as odds ratios). To make causal inferences, the underlying assumption of this design is that controls ($\bar{C}$) are representative of the population at risk (N') from which the study cases (D) arose (see Figure 10.6). For time-varying exposures, the investigator will usually measure those variables retrospectively (before cases occurred) to reduce temporal ambiguity.

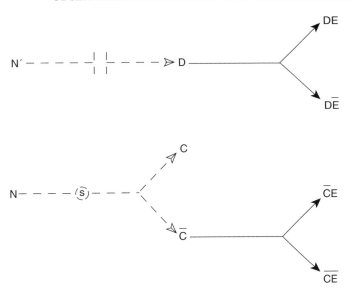

Figure 10.6 Basic case-control study design (longitudinal).

Example 10.6. Stotowski et al. (1995) conducted a case-control study to estimate the effect of fluoride exposure from water and toothpaste on dental fluorosis among children, aged 8–17 years, who had attended a dental clinic in 1991. The presence of fluorosis was determined from dental exams, and study cases were those children who were observed to have the most severe and extensive fluorosis. Fifty-four (54) controls (without any fluorosis) were matched to 54 cases on age and sex. Information on fluoride exposure during the first 8 years of life and other factors was obtained by questionnaire from the subjects' parents. Using multiple logistic regression, the authors found a positive association between fluoride exposure and the prevalence of fluorosis, adjusting for potential confounders. These results should be interpreted cautiously because of possible information bias due to error in measuring fluoride exposure and possible selection bias. The latter bias would occur if both fluorosis status and fluoride exposure were associated with use of the dental clinic from which subjects were selected (see "Estimation Error"). In addition, the investigators' method of comparing the most severe cases with noncases complicates the interpretation of effect estimates. The problem is that the observed exposure-disease association might reflect the effect of fluoride exposure as a risk factor on the occurrence of fluorosis or as a prognostic factor on the course of disease (because some, but not all, incident cases eventually become severe).

10.4.3.1 Population-based case-control study

The best approach for doing a case-control study is called a population-based case-control design (Figure 10.7). Ideally, this type of study is done by identifying all incident cases (D) that occur in a well-defined population at risk during a given period (N in Figure 10.7) and by randomly selecting controls ($\bar{C}$) from that population (excluding prevalent cases, C). In this way, we make the controls representative of the population that gave rise to the cases,

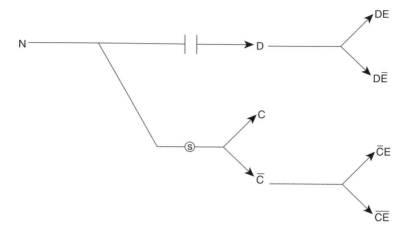

Figure 10.7 Population-based case-control study design.

thereby preventing selection bias. This design is feasible when there is a disease registry or surveillance system operating in a particular population or when the case-control study is nested within a cohort study. Exposure and covariate information is collected from cases and controls, as described for the basic design.

Example 10.7. Hashibe et al. (2006) conducted a population-based case-control study to estimate the effects of marijuana use on the risks of several smoking-related cancers, including oral cancer, among adults, aged 18–62 years, living in Los Angeles County between 1999 and 2004. Three hundred and three (303) histologically confirmed incident cases of oral cancer were identified and located through the Cancer Surveillance Program for Los Angeles County. The participation rate among eligible cases was 54% due to refusals, inability to contact, and death. Controls were selected from eligible noncases in the same residential population and were matched to cases on age, sex, and residential neighborhood. Detailed information on lifetime marijuana use and other factors was obtained from face-to-face interviews with all subjects. Using logistic regression, the investigators found a crude (unadjusted) dose–response association between lifetime use of marijuana (measured in joint-years) and the incidence of oral cancer; that is, the greater the exposure to marijuana, the higher the rate of oral cancer. When adjusted for smoking, alcohol use, and other risk factors, however, the association with marijuana use disappeared. Despite the potential for selection bias due to the low participation rate among cases, the authors concluded that the effect of marijuana use—even long-term heavy use—was not strong and may be below practically detectable limits.

10.4.4   Ecologic studies

An ecologic study is one in which the units of analysis are groups, rather than individuals (Morgenstern, 1998, 2008). The groups are often geographic areas such as counties or states, but they may also be families, schools, clinical practices, or other clusters possibly observed at different times. The key feature of an ecologic study is that data are missing on the joint distribution of the exposure and disease at the individual level within each group; thus, we know the proportion exposed and the disease frequency in each group, but we do not

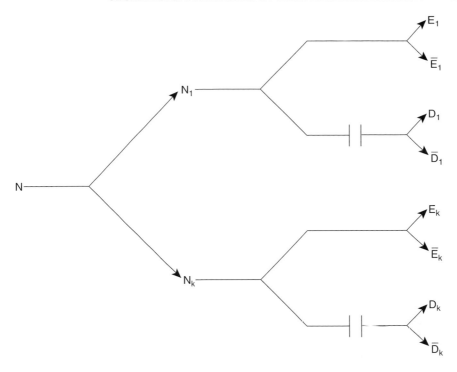

Figure 10.8 Multiple-group ecologic study design (k groups).

know the proportions of exposed cases, unexposed cases, exposed noncases, and unexposed noncases. The outcome variable in an ecologic study may involve incidence, mortality, or prevalence. The exposure variable may be an aggregate measure such as the proportion of smokers in each group, an environmental measure such as average air pollution level in each group (which has an analog at the individual level), or a global measure such as income inequality in a group (which does not have an analog at the individual level).

There are three types of ecologic studies used to examine associations between exposures and disease; they differ according to how groups are distinguished. In a *multiple-group* ecologic study, groups are distinguished by place, for example, people living in different counties or states (Figure 10.8, where only two groups are shown, N_1 and N_k). The objective is to examine the ecologic association between the average exposure level or frequency and the rate or prevalence of disease among many groups. This is the ecologic design used most often, especially in oral health research. In a *time-trend* study, groups are distinguished by time, for example, Michigan residents in 1995, 2000, and 2005 (Figure 10.9). The objective is to examine the ecologic association between change in average exposure level or frequency and change in the rate or prevalence of disease in one geographically defined population (shown as N_1 and N_2 at different times in Figure 10.9). This design is often used to evaluate the effect of a population intervention on the rate or prevalence of disease. In a *mixed* ecologic study, groups are distinguished by a combination of place and time. The objective is to examine the ecologic association between change in average exposure level or frequency and change in the rate or prevalence of disease among many groups.

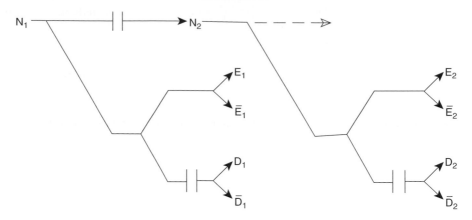

Figure 10.9 Time-trend ecologic study design.

10.4.4.1   Ecologic analysis: multiple-group study

Because of the missing data in ecologic studies, we cannot make a direct comparison of the disease rate between exposed and unexposed segments of each group in a multiple-group design, as we would in a cohort study. Instead, we regress the group-specific disease rates on the group-specific exposure and covariate frequencies (e.g., the proportion exposed or mean exposure level in each group), typically by fitting a linear model. From the fitted model, we can predict the rates of disease in hypothetical groups that are entirely exposed and entirely unexposed. Then we compare those predicted rates in the form of a ratio or difference to estimate the rate ratio or rate difference, the same measures that we would have estimated if the study had been conducted at the individual level (Morgenstern, 1998, 2008).

Example 10.8. Muirhead and Marcenes (2004) conducted a multiple-group ecologic study to examine the associations between two ecologic measures—mean social deprivation and mean school performance—and mean dental-caries prevalence among 5-year-old children attending 55 state primary schools (units of analysis) in one borough of London. Caries data were obtained from an oral health survey, and the outcome variable was the mean number of decayed, missing, and filled teeth (dmft) per child for all 5-year-olds in each school. Social deprivation was measured as an index based on the school's address and as the proportion of children in each school in receipt of free school meals. School performance was measured as the mean scores on English, mathematics, and literacy tests for 5-year-olds in each school. Using multiple linear regression, the investigators found that the mean dmft score was positively associated with the proportion of children receiving free school meals and inversely associated with mean school performance, especially the literacy score. The authors concluded that these ecologic variables were good indicators of caries prevalence in each school, but they did not attempt to make causal inferences from their findings.

The main advantage of ecologic studies over other observational designs is that they can be done quickly and inexpensively by linking different sources of available data at the group level. Thus, ecologic measures of the exposure, disease, and covariates can be obtained from different data sets and combined into one data set to be used for the ecologic analysis. Of course, certain individual data that would be desired in a study might not be available in aggregate form, such as medical and dental histories or health-related behaviors.

Ecologic studies share most of the methodologic limitations discussed for other observational designs, including confounding, information bias, and temporal ambiguity. In addition, causal inferences are further limited by a type of bias—*ecologic bias* (also called the *ecological fallacy*)—that is unique to this design (Morgenstern, 1998, 2008). The underlying problem is that groups are not entirely homogeneous with respect to the exposure and covariates; for example, most groups contain a mixture of exposed and unexposed persons. Consequently, it is possible—often likely—that ecologic associations will differ from associations between the same variables measured at the individual level in the same population. For example, in Example 10.8, just because we observe a positive association between the proportion of children receiving free meals and the mean dmft score of each school does not necessarily imply that children receiving free meals (from low-income families) are the ones in that school with more dental caries (high dmft scores). It may be the children from high-income families who have more dental caries in schools with children from predominantly low-income families. Under these conditions, the ecologic measure of an association would be a biased estimate of the exposure effect on outcome risk at the individual level.

Unfortunately, it is not possible for the investigator to identify or correct for ecologic bias when data are missing at the individual level. Furthermore, it is not necessarily true that a better fitting model, which explains a higher proportion of the outcome variance, will yield effect estimates that are less biased than a poorer fitting model. The best approach for preventing ecologic bias is to combine ecologic data with individual-level data—that is, a multilevel design and analysis—as in Example 10.3 (Morgenstern, 1998, 2008).

10.5   Final comments

There are several types of observational designs that can be used to address a variety of questions about population health, and no one design is always preferable to others or can be always expected to produce the most informative results. The choice in a particular investigation depends on several factors, including the objectives of the study, the quality of data expected, the cost of conducting the study, and ethical considerations concerning informed consent, confidentiality, and conflicts of interest. Observational studies are valuable in oral health research for describing health outcomes in large populations, for avoiding the ethical and practical constraints of conducting interventions and randomizing subjects, for studying complex processes that vary over time and among individuals, for combining information at different levels, for generating new hypotheses, and for justifying and planning randomized clinical trials. To achieve these objectives, however, observational studies must be designed, conducted, and interpreted carefully to minimize bias, avoid misinterpretations, and enhance generalizability.

Acknowledgment

All figures except Figure 10.4 are reproduced (Figure 10.1 with modification) with permission from Kleinbaum et al. (1982).

References

Albandar JM, Goldstein H. 1992. Multi-level statistical models in studies of periodontal diseases. *Journal of Periodontology* 63:690–695.

Angrist JD, Imbens GW, Rubin DB. 1996. Identification of causal effects using instrumental variables. *Journal of the American Statistical Association* 91:444–455.

Beck JD, Cusmano L, Green-Helms W, Koch GG, Offenbacher S. 1997a. A 5-year study of attachment loss in community-dwelling older adults: incidence density. *Journal of Periodontal Research* 32:506–515.

Beck JD, Elter JR. 2000. Analysis strategies for longitudinal attachment loss data. *Community Dentistry and Oral Epidemiology* 28:1–9.

Beck JD, Koch GG, Offenbacher S. 1994. Attachment loss trends over 3 years in community-dwelling older adults. *Journal of Periodontology* 65:737–743.

Beck JD, Lawrence HP, Koch GG. 1997b. Analytic approaches to longitudinal caries data in adults. *Community Dentistry and Oral Epidemiology* 25:42–51.

Bower E, Guilliford M, Steele J, Newton T. 2007. Area deprivation and oral health in Scottish adults: a multilevel study. *Community Dentistry and Oral Epidemiology* 35:118–129.

Brown LJ, Wall TP, Lazar V. 1999. Trends in untreated caries in permanent teeth of children 6 to 18 years old. *Journal of the American Dental Association* 130:1637–1644.

DeStefano F, Anda RF, Kahn HS, Williamson DF, Russell CM. 1993. Dental disease and risk of coronary heart disease and mortality. *BMJ: British Medical Association* 306:688–691.

Gilbert GH, Shewchuk RM, Litaker MS. 2006. Effect of dental practice characteristics on racial disparities in patient-specific tooth loss. *Medical Care* 44:414–420.

Goldstein H. 2003. *Multilevel Statistical Models*. New York: Oxford University Press.

Greenland S. 2000. An introduction to instrumental variables for epidemiologists. *International Journal of Epidemiology* 29:722–729.

Greenland S. 2003. Quantifying biases in causal models: classical confounding *vs* collider-stratification bias. *Epidemiology* 14:300–306.

Greenland S, Maclure M, Schlesselman JJ, Poole C, Morgenstern H. 1991. Standardized regression coefficients: a further critique and review of some alternatives. *Epidemiology* 2:383–386.

Greenland S, Schlesselman JJ, Criqui MH. 1986. The fallacy of employing standardized regression coefficients and correlations as measures of effect. *American Journal of Epidemiology* 123:203–208.

Hashibe M, Morgenstern H, Cui Y, Tashkin DP, Zhang ZF, Cozen W, Mack TM, Greenland S. 2006. Marijuana use and the risk of lung and upper aerodigestive tract cancers: results of a population-based case-control study. *Cancer Epidemiology, Biomarkers and Prevention* 15:1829–1834.

Hernán MA, Brumback B, Robins JM. 2001. Marginal structural models to estimate the joint causal effect of nonrandomized treatments. *Journal of the American Statistical Association* 96:440–448.

Hernán MA, Robins JM. 2006. Instruments for causal inference: an epidemiologist's dream? *Epidemiology* 17:360–372.

Holst D, Schuller AA, Aleksejuniené J, Eriksen HM. 2001. Cariers in populations—a theoretical, causal approach. *European Journal of Oral Sciences* 109:143–148.

Jewell NP. 2004. *Statistics for Epidemiology*. Boca Raton, FL: Chapman & Hall/CRC.

Kalbfleisch JK, Prentice RL. 2002. *The Statistical Analysis of Failure Time Data*. Hoboken, NJ: Wiley.

Kleinbaum DG, Kupper LL, Morgenstern H. 1982. *Epidemiologic Research: Principles and Quantitative Methods*. New York: Van Nostrand Reinhold.

Liang K-Y, Zeger SL. 1993. Regression analysis for correlated data. *Annual Review of Public Health* 14:43–68.

Little RJA, Rubin DB. 2002. *Statistical Analysis with Missing Data*. Hoboken, NJ: Wiley.

Maldonado G, Greenland S. 2002. Estimating causal effects. *International Journal of Epidemiology* 31:422–429.

Malikaew P, Watt RG, Sheiham A. 2003. Associations between school environments and childhood traumatic dental injuries. *Oral Health and Preventive Dentistry* 1:255–266.

Miettinen OS. 1983. The need for randomization in the study of intended effects. *Statistics in Medicine* 2:267–271.

Molenberghs G, Kenward MG. 2007. *Missing Data in Clinical Studies*. Chichester: Wiley.

Morgenstern H. 1998. Ecologic study. In: Armitage P, Colton T (eds). *Encyclopedia of Biostatistics*, Vol. 2. Chichester: Wiley, pp. 1255–1276.

Morgenstern H. 2008. Ecologic studies. In: Rothman KJ, Greenland S, Lash T (eds). *Modern Epidemiology*, 3rd edn. Philadelphia, PA: Lippincott Williams & Wilkins, pp. 511–531.

Morgenstern H, Kleinbaum DG, Kupper LL. 1980. Measures of disease incidence used in epidemiologic research. *International Journal of Epidemiology* 9:97–104.

Muirhead V, Marcenes W. 2004. An ecological study of caries experience, school performance and material deprivation in 5-year-old state primary school children. *Community Dentistry and Oral Epidemiology* 32:265–270.

Newton JT, Bower EJ. 2005. The social determinants of oral health: new approaches to conceptualizing and researching complex networks. *Community Dentistry and Oral Epidemiology* 33:25–34.

Poole C. 1987. Beyond the confidence interval. *American Journal of Public Health* 77:195–199.

Raudenbush SW, Bryk AS. 2002. *Hierarchical Linear Models: Applications and Data Analysis Methods*. Thousand Oaks, CA: Sage Publications.

Robins JM. 1998. Structural nested failure time models. In: Armitage P, Colton T (eds). *The Encyclopedia of Biostatistics*. Chichester: Wiley.

Robins JM, Hernán MA, Brumback B. 2000. Marginal structural models and causal inference in epidemiology. *Epidemiology* 11:550–560.

Rothman KJ, Greenland S, Lash TL. 2008. *Modern Epidemiology*, 3rd edn. Philadelphia, PA: Lippincott Williams & Wilkins.

Savitz DA. 2003. *Interpreting Epidemiologic Evidence: Strategies for Study Design and Analysis*. New York: Oxford University Press.

Stotowski MC, Hunt RJ, Levy SM. 1995. Risk factors for dental fluorosis in pediatric dental patients. *Journal of Public Health Dentistry* 55:154–159.

Thomson WM, Poulton R, Milne BJ, Caspi A, Broughton JR, Ayers KMS. 2004. Socioeconomic inequalities in oral health in childhood and adulthood in a birth cohort. *Community Dentistry and Oral Epidemiology* 32:345–353.

Woodward M. 2005. *Epidemiology: Study Design and Data Analysis*, 2nd edn. Boca Raton, FL: Chapman & Hall/CRC.

Zeger SL, Liang K-Y. 1992. An overview of methods for the analysis of longitudinal data. *Statistics in Medicine* 11:1825–1839.

11

Initial clinical trials allow assessment of safety, dosing, and preliminary efficacy prior to large randomized controlled pivotal studies

Jules T. Mitchel, MBA, PhD, **Glen Park,** PharmD, **Mark Citron,** MS, **Russ Pagano,** PhD, **Leslie Wisner-Lynch,** DDS, DMSc, **and Samuel E. Lynch,** DMD, DMSc

11.1   Introduction

Before launching into the expensive and lengthy pivotal clinical trials that are needed to establish effectiveness and safety of a new therapeutic, the decision to initiate human testing requires thoughtful consideration and rational design of early clinical trials (see also Chapter 1 on clinical and translational research). In order to identify a potentially beneficial dose regimen to be used later in the pivotal clinical trials for the disease under investigation, phase 1 and phase 2 clinical trials are required when evaluating new molecular entities and novel delivery systems for approved products. The goals of the early phase 1 clinical trials, usually performed in normal volunteers, are most often to characterize the pharmacodynamics and pharmacokinetics of the investigational product. The goals of phase 2 clinical trials are to identify early safety signals of concern and to establish effectiveness in patients with the disease of interest. The purpose of this chapter is to outline the objectives and designs of phase 1 and 2 clinical trials for new therapeutics, whether they be drugs, biologics, or combination products using devices plus active drug substances, and for comparable early stage studies for medical or dental devices.

11.2   Phase 1 clinical trials—drugs

After a new therapeutic agent is studied in nonclinical *in vivo* and *in vitro* models of safety and effectiveness, and after the original investigational new drug application (IND) is submitted and cleared/approved by the U.S. Food and Drug Administration (FDA), an investigational drug can be given for the first time to a human in a phase 1 clinical trial. Phase 1 studies are designed to determine the pharmacodynamic and pharmacologic actions, pharmacokinetic characteristics, and initial signals of adverse effects with increasing doses of an investigational drug in humans. During the phase 1 program, sufficient information about the drug's pharmacokinetics, pharmacological effects, and safety in both males and females should be obtained to permit the design of well-controlled, scientifically valid, phase 2 dose ranging and proof of concept studies in patients with the disease of interest. Phase 1 studies are performed under good clinical practices (GCP), which defines on a global basis the procedures to execute clinical trials and to minimize risk to clinical trial participants. These procedures are described in detail in the Guidance for Industry, E6 Good Clinical Practice: Consolidated Guidance (1996). Investigational products to support an IND must also be manufactured in compliance with current good manufacturing practices (cGMP) as described in the Guidance for Industry, INDs—Approaches to Complying with cGMP During Phase 1 (2005). Good manufacturing practices define on a global basis the methods and procedures to be followed to meet the quality standards in the manufacturing of drugs, devices, and biologics.

Phase 1 studies in healthy volunteers develop new knowledge about the drug, primarily in terms of basic science and safety, with no clinical benefit to the volunteer subjects (Table 11.1). A healthy volunteer is a subject with no known significant health problems who participates in a clinical research program. The advantage of using healthy volunteers for the initial safety studies is that in patients, underlying disease can obscure adverse effects signals of the drug, while a sign or symptom of a disease (e.g., hypertension) would not be expected in a healthy normal volunteer. The total number of subjects included in phase 1 studies varies with the drug, but is generally in the range of 20–80 subjects.

"First in Man," phase 1 studies may also be conducted in patients in certain circumstances. Cytotoxic drugs that are used in the treatment of cancer are always studied in diseased patients because it is not ethical to expose healthy subjects to potentially toxic drugs. In phase 1 oncology studies, study patients often have failed other proven therapies and participate in the phase 1 clinical trial with the understanding that the information found in the study may not necessarily help them, though it is possible, but may help others.

Safety in phase 1 trials is evaluated by observing adverse events, looking for changes in clinical laboratory test results, electrocardiograms, vital signs, and physical examinations. Special attention is given to changes in liver and renal function tests and to any clinical chemistry changes observed in the animal studies. Other special safety measures may be included as part of the phase 1 program, such as development of antibodies, if the drug is a potentially immunogenic molecule such as a peptide or monoclonal antibody.

Table 11.1   Phase 1 and phase 2 study designs.

Phase of development	Design	Subjects	Number of subjects	Goal
Phase 1	Single dose	Healthy volunteers[a]	20–40	Pharmacokinetics, pharmacodynamics, safety
	Dose escalation Placebo-controlled randomized Blinding to treatment			
	Multiple dose	Healthy volunteers[a]	20–60	Steady state, pharmacokinetics, pharmacodynamics, phase 2 dosing, safety
	Dose escalation Placebo-controlled randomized Blinding to treatment			
Phase 2				
2a	Randomized Double blind	Patients	40–80	Dose ranging, safety
2b	Randomized Double blind	Patients	60–200	Expanded efficacy, safety
Phase 3	Randomized Double blind Placebo controlled Active controlled	Patients	100–10,000	Confirmatory efficacy, safety
Phase 4	Randomized Double blind Placebo controlled Active controlled Open label	Patients	100–10,000	Meet postmarketing commitments, expanded knowledge of product

[1] Except for toxic drugs used for oncology.

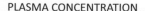

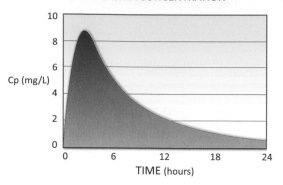

Figure 11.1 Plasma concentration.

Safety in phase 1 studies may also be evaluated via pharmacokinetics, mechanism of action, and depending on the drug, structure–activity relationships. Pharmacokinetic studies involve collecting blood samples at specified times after dosing in order to analyze the drug concentration using specific and validated assays (Figure 11.1). These studies allow the determination of the following key pharmacokinetic parameters including (1) the biological half-life of the drug that assists in determining the frequency of dosing, (2) the maximum concentration of the drug after each dose, and (3) the time it takes for the drug to reach its maximum concentration, each of which assists in assessing the risk associated with circulating levels of drug in the blood. In addition, the area under the concentration–time curve (AUC), which integrates the concentration and time course of the drug in the blood, is calculated. The AUC is a key parameter for describing the total exposure to the drug, and allows for the comparison of the safety results in animals and of the comparison of different dose regimens. Pharmacokinetic analyses also provide information on linearity, that is, as the dose is increased, do the pharmacokinetics of the drug change proportionally to the dose with a linear response, or is there nonlinearity with disproportionately higher exposure as the dose increases. Also, in some cases, higher doses show a disproportionately lower exposure because of such factors as saturation of absorption.

The selection of the initial dose in the initial phase 1 study is based on the results of studies in animal models of toxicity, animal toxicokinetics (pharmacokinetics in toxicology studies), and animal models of efficacy. The initial dose is often one-tenth the dose that shows no adverse effect in animal studies. Animal toxicokinetics results are used to design the human phase 1 pharmacokinetic study. The animal studies also assist in the determination of the number of blood samples to be collected for the pharmacokinetic analyses.

The first few volunteer subjects receive low doses of the investigational drug to see how well the drug is initially tolerated. The next groups of volunteers receive larger amounts of the drug until a nontolerated dose is reached. However, it is not the goal of these studies to produce overt toxicity, but to identify an upper dose level that shows a clear effect without putting the subjects at risk. As part of the study design, placebo is given to a certain number of volunteers in phase 1. Placebos are harmless, inactive substances made to resemble the appearance of the investigational drug used in the clinical trial. The use of a placebo treatment arm allows the clinical research team to learn whether the investigational drug has an acceptable safety profile compared to "no treatment."

Subjects in phase 1 studies are often blinded or masked to treatment. In single-blind studies, the study participants do not know which medicine they are receiving. Double-blind studies are designed to prevent anyone (doctors, nurses, or patients) from knowing the treatment. This allows the investigator to avoid bias and draw what is considered to be a higher level of scientifically accurate conclusions. However, in an emergency, it is always possible to identify what drug the subject is taking. If a placebo is part of a study, the study subject is always informed in the informed consent form that they may receive an inactive substance ("sugar pill" or water).

All the clinical research is affected by the "placebo effect"—the real or apparent improvement in a patient's condition due to being part of a clinical trial or a belief that the medication will provide a benefit. Methods to address the placebo effect involve randomization, single-blind, or double-blind studies, and the use of a placebo or control treatment group in the clinical trial. A control group is one that is used as a comparator to the treatment group. Randomization is when the drugs are selected by chance and not by choice. Thus, the highest scientific standard is nominally considered to be a randomized controlled clinical trial or RCT study.

After the maximum tolerated dose and initial pharmacokinetic studies are determined in single-dose studies, multiple-dose studies can be carried out depending on how the new therapeutic is to be delivered for disease treatment. Multiple-dose studies are generally conducted over a 7-day period depending on the pharmacokinetic determinations in the single-dose study. If the drug has a long half-life, the duration of the multiple-dose study will be longer than for a drug with a shorter half-life. The goals of the multiple-dose study are to determine pharmacokinetic and safety data at steady state, where just as much drug is taken in as is excreted. This is done to make sure that the drug is not accumulating in the body over time to potentially dangerous levels. Similar safety data are also collected as were collected in the single-dose studies.

There are special studies that can be performed under an exploratory IND based on the Guidance for Industry, Investigators, and Reviewers—Exploratory IND Studies (2006). Exploratory IND studies are conducted early in phase 1, involve very limited human exposure of the drug, and have no therapeutic or diagnostic intent (e.g., screening studies, microdose studies). These studies are usually performed to determine whether the investigational molecule binds to the target receptor, for example, or shows the intended distribution in the body. These types of exploratory IND studies are conducted prior to the traditional dose escalation, safety, and tolerance studies that ordinarily initiate a clinical drug development program. The duration of dosing in an exploratory IND study is expected to be limited (e.g., no more than 7 days).

11.3 Medical devices—pilot and prepivotal studies

After a new therapeutic agent is studied in nonclinical *in vivo* and *in vitro* models of safety and effectiveness, and after the original investigational device exemption (IDE) application is submitted and cleared/approved by the FDA, an investigational device can be used for the first time to a human in a pilot or pivotal clinical trial (see also Chapter 4). Often, a pre-IDE meeting is held with FDA prior to the IDE submission to discuss product development planning. These meetings are based on the guidance entitled Early Collaboration Meetings Under the FDA Modernization Act (FDAMA); Final Guidance for Industry and for CDRH Staff (2001). See also Chapter 4 on regulatory aspects of clinical studies.

Clinical trials of medical devices fall into three categories: pilot or prepivotal studies, pivotal trials of safety and effectiveness, and postapproval studies (PAS). Pilot studies, also known as feasibility studies, are somewhat similar to phase 1 studies with drugs, in that they are conducted to obtain preliminary information on safety and effectiveness of a device before a larger scale pivotal study is initiated. Pilot studies are often, but not always, conducted at a single center and involve a small number of patients. Pilot studies are conducted when the device is being used for the first time in man or with limited experience in people, or if specific feasibility testing is required before initiating the pivotal trial. Unlike the larger pivotal trials, pilot studies usually are designed to obtain preliminary safety data in small numbers of patients, usually no more than 20, in order to design the pivotal trial or design device modifications that cannot be done in an animal model. Biocompatibility studies performed *in vitro* and in animals are required to support the clinical trial. For medical devices, the biocompatibility requirements usually required to obtain an IDE are described in the ISO 10993 standards. Pilot device studies include subjects with the disease of interest and are designed to identify clinical endpoints as well as unanticipated adverse events. Like phase 1 studies for drugs, device pilot studies are performed under GCP and incorporate procedures to minimize risk to the study participants. A fundamental difference between early drug and device studies is that drug studies undergoing phase 1 evaluation are generally true 'First in Man' assessments, whereas devices are often incremental improvements in product design or materials. The device pilot studies often focus on the device design characteristics using patients who are undergoing treatment versus normal healthy volunteers used in phase 1 drug studies. Thus, pilot studies for devices can provide both preliminary safety and design (effectiveness) information. This effectiveness information is then utilized to create the statistical hypothesis and sample size calculation needed to show effectiveness in the pivotal trial.

11.4   Phase 2 clinical trials—drugs

The fundamental goals of phase 2 clinical trials are to obtain sufficient information about a drug's safety and effectiveness, in order to improve the likelihood for the success of the larger pivotal phase 3 clinical trials. In phase 3 clinical trials, the drug's effectiveness and safety are established, and they serve as the primary basis for marketing approval. Therefore, in order to establish a successful design of phase 3 studies to evidence the efficacy and safety in patients with the target disease, key factors that need to be learned from phase 2 studies include (1) selection of the optimal dosing regimen, and (2) the choice of the optimal clinical endpoint to demonstrate the benefit of the new therapeutic (i.e., the primary endpoint).

Once the initial single-dose and multiple-dose safety studies have been completed in the phase 1 clinical trial program, and the pharmacokinetics and pharmacodynamics of the drug have been established to assist in the determination of the dosing schedule, the phase 2 clinical trial program can be designed and implemented. Phase 2 studies are performed in patients with the target disease, and in contrast with most phase 1 studies, patient volunteers may benefit from treatment in a phase 2 study. Phase 2 studies are sometimes divided into

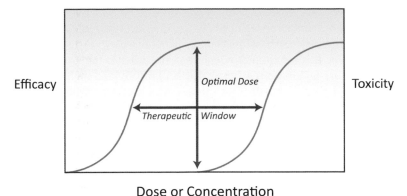

Efficacy   *Optimal Dose*   Toxicity

Therapeutic | *Window*

Dose or Concentration

Figure 11.2 Dose or concentration.

phase 2a and phase 2b. While the distinction between these two phases is often somewhat arbitrary, in general, phase 2a studies are specifically designed to assess dosing requirements (how much drug should be given and how often), whereas phase 2b studies are specifically designed to study efficacy (how well the drug works at prescribed doses).

Generally speaking, there are two main objectives of the phase 2 program: (1) determination of the optimal dose(s), and (2) proof of concept of effectiveness. The first objective is to test a range of doses in patients to assess safety and efficacy in patients with the disease of interest. Knowledge of the relationship between the dose of the drug and its efficacy and safety allows for the safe and effective use of medications. What this means is that as the dose of a drug is increased, there should be an increase in efficacy until a plateau is reached, where adding more drug does not increase effectiveness. Similarly, there is a dose response for safety. Safety is monitored extensively by looking at changes in clinical chemistry test results, changes in physical examination and vital signs, changes in medications taken by the patient, and adverse events. At lower doses, there are usually few safety signals, but as the dose increases, there is usually an increase in the frequency and severity of adverse events. It is the intersection of the dose response for safety and efficacy that the ideal dose is determined (Figure 11.2). There may be exceptions to this rule, where the ratio of benefit to risk justifies a higher dose even with an increased risk for adverse events, or vice versa, when a lower than optimally effective dose may be used, when the potential adverse events may be life threatening. It may also be necessary to evaluate dosing frequency in phase 2 to obtain the optimal dosing regimen. For example, a drug with a short half-life may be present in the blood for only a few hours and may require multiple daily doses to achieve the intended clinical response. This would be true for a drug that shows a good correlation between the pharmacokinetics and pharmacodynamics, that is, the concentration of the drug in the blood predicts the magnitude of the pharmacodynamic effect.

If the mechanism of action of the drug requires the movement of the drug into a tissue compartment, the concentration of the drug in the plasma may not predict the pharmacodynamic effect. For example, the drug imiglucerase is an enzyme similar to the native enzyme glucocerebrosidase and is used as an enzyme replacement therapy for a rare genetic defect resulting in Gaucher disease. Gaucher disease, the most prevalent lysosomal storage disorder, is caused by mutations in the human glucocerebrosidase gene (GCD). While imiglucerase has a short half-life of approximately 10 minutes, the enzyme needs to be administered only every 2 weeks. This is presumed to be because the enzyme is taken up by the target monocyte/macrophage cells where imiglucerase reduces the accumulation of substrate glucocerebroside, the hallmark of Gaucher disease.

In phase 2 studies, it is important to determine the onset of the drug effect so that the initial response occurs within a time frame that is clinically acceptable. For example, in mucositis, a quick response is required as mucositis can be acutely quite debilitating. On the other hand, periodontal disease can be managed clinically while waiting for a drug response that either acts directly on the causative organism or on bone regrowth.

If three to four dose concentrations of the investigational drug are to be studied in phase 2, it may be adequate to initially study 10–12 patients per group plus placebo, to identify the apparent minimum and maximum effective doses. It is not necessary in these studies to prove that one dose is statistically better than another. Rather, a trend in dose response is usually sufficient.

Clinical trials using double-blind, parallel, randomized, fixed-dose groups are considered the gold standard for dose-response studies. However, in examining dose response for long-term outcomes, fixed-dose trials may have limitations, including having suboptimal doses or having a dose with unacceptable side effects. These results may be exacerbated by the individual to individual variations in pharmacokinetic and pharmacodynamic results. On the other hand, flexible-dose trials may be better at simulating clinical practice and better reflect risk/benefit considerations; with a flexible design, doses may be changed based on individual patient response.

While determination of preliminary safety is a main objective of the phase 2 study program, the second objective of phase 2 studies is to obtain a "proof of concept" for the desired clinical effect in the target patient population. The goal of a proof of concept study is to provide evidence of clinical effectiveness to the degree that phase 3 studies can be designed with a high degree of confidence that they will be successful. Proof of concept should be assessed with the primary clinical endpoint to be used in the phase 3 studies, so that information about the primary endpoint, such as time to onset, the magnitude, and the variability of the clinical effect, can be obtained to support the clinical and statistical design of the phase 3 studies. However, in order to complete the phase 2 program in a practical time frame, it may be preferable to also identify and evaluate multiple endpoints that do not necessarily require the same study duration that may be required for phase 3, but provide a high level of confidence for the investigational drug's safety and effectiveness.

Depending on the indications for use, a phase 2 program may last from several months to a year or more, and can involve up to several hundred patients. Longer term studies may be required for chronic diseases such as rheumatoid arthritis and osteoporosis. Use of biomarkers, pharmacodynamic or surrogate endpoints may reduce the duration of the phase 2 program, while at the same time provide a high enough level of confidence that the phase 3 program will have a positive outcome. For example, in osteoporosis, the desired clinical outcome is to demonstrate a reduction in risk of bone fractures, which may require studies of 2–3 years in duration. Improvement in, or preservation of, bone density may serve as a surrogate endpoint, but may still require a 1-year study. However, a biomarker of bone turnover may provide the information needed in phase 2 to assess dose response as well as proof of concept. A note of caution—the biomarker or surrogate endpoint chosen must have sufficient previous scientific and clinical information to support its use to ensure that it will predict the clinical endpoint required for phase 3. Furthermore, it can be beneficial to include exploratory endpoints in phase 2, particularly for indications that have not been well established historically. By doing this, it could lead to the use of a different primary endpoint in phase 3 than previously anticipated.

Selection of the patient population for inclusion in phase 2 studies is very important. In order to reduce the variability in response phase 2 studies, the inclusion criteria for the target disease state is usually much more stringent than for phase 3 studies. This may allow for the demonstration of efficacy with a fewer number of patients. In phase 3, in contrast, the patient selection criteria should more closely match the desired patient population that will be included in the eventual labeling for the investigational product. Phase 2 studies usually also have more exclusions criteria in order to select a patient population with only the disease of interest, but without the presence of other diseases or conditions that may confound the assessment of safety and/or efficacy. Certain characteristics of the disease may also be controlled, such as severity or duration of disease, particularly for the initial dose–response studies. It should be kept in mind that the results of the phase 2 efficacy studies may also be useful in identifying subpopulations that demonstrate a higher rate of response than the total population, and may represent the true population of interest for phase 3 (see also Chapter 12 on Phase 3 trials).

11.5 Sample study designs

11.5.1 Phase 1 normal volunteers

Mucositis is an acute painful inflammation and ulceration of the mucous membranes lining the digestive tract, usually as an adverse effect of chemotherapy and radiotherapy treatment for cancer. The following is a summary of a phase 1 study designed for the evaluation of a drug to be used as an oral rinse to treat mucositis. This drug was to be further studied for the treatment of oral mucositis secondary to conditioning for hematopoietic stem cell transplants. The study was a single-center, dose-escalating, randomized, double-blind, placebo-controlled phase 1 clinical trial to determine the safety and pharmacokinetic profile of a drug when used as an oral rinse in healthy volunteers. The placebo group was included as a negative control for the preliminary comparison of the safety results (i.e., to improve the assessment of drug-related adverse events). The relationship of adverse events to study medication was determined by the investigator based in part on the temporal relationship of the onset of the adverse event relative to the administration of the medication. The comparison between the placebo and active treatment groups was exploratory in nature to help establish the design of future studies.

To be included in the study, volunteers had to be healthy, nontobacco using ($\geq$ 6 months), males or females of any race, and $\geq$18 years of age. Female subjects had to be using a medically acceptable form of birth control during the study. Acceptable birth control measures were abstinence, hormonal contraceptives (oral and implant), barrier contraceptives (condom, diaphragm with spermicide), IUD, surgical (hysterectomy, tubal ligation, vasectomy partner), or natural menopausal. Subjects had to be informed of the nature of the study and provide written informed consent prior to receiving study medication. Subjects had to weigh at least 45 kg and had to be within the average weight for their gender and height as determined by the Metropolitan Life Insurance Company Weight Tables. There was to be no significant diseases or clinically significant abnormal laboratory values during the screening medical history, physical examination, EKG, or laboratory evaluations.

All subjects and investigators were blinded as to the identity of the study solutions. Each dose cohort of 12 subjects had 9 active and 3 placebo-treated subjects. For each of the three dose levels, subjects were randomized either to active treatment or placebo control, at a ratio of 9 (active) to 3 (placebo). Subjects were randomized to either active drug or placebo treatment starting with the dose level 1. Assignment to treatment was determined by a randomization scheme that was provided to the center's research pharmacy. After the first dose, 5 mL blood samples were taken at 0.25, 0.5, 1, 2, 3, 4, 6, 8, 12, 18, and 24 hours after dosing. In addition, 24-hour and 48-hour urine samples were taken to measure drug excretion and 48-hour blood samples were obtained for clinical laboratory, CBC with differential and urinalysis testing. Preparing a schedule of events as found in Table 11.2 facilitates the understanding of the work flow of a phase 1 study.

After the initial dose group completed treatment, and prior to treating any subject at the second dose level, there was an interim review of the safety data (clinical laboratory tests, vital signs, adverse events) and plasma concentrations of the drug from all 12 subjects. The safety review of data from the first group of patients was used to decide whether to proceed with the next dose level. If any subject experienced a serious adverse event, that in the judgment of the investigator and managing physician was life threatening and definitely related to study medication, the study was to be stopped. Additionally, there was no dose escalation if subjects at any dosage level experienced moderate or severe nausea, vomiting, diarrhea, blood pressure changes, or other emergent AE according to a standard toxicity criteria table that defined the severity of an event as mild, moderate, or severe. If 6 of the 12 subjects experienced a moderate AE, no dose escalation would occur. If 3 of the 12 subjects experienced a severe AE, no dose escalation would occur.

11.5.2   Phase 2—patients with mucositis

This was a single-center, dose-finding, randomized, double-blind, placebo-controlled, phase 2 clinical trial to determine the safety and pharmacokinetic profile of a drug when administered as an oral rinse solution in patients undergoing hematopoietic stem cell transplantation. The patients were randomly assigned to either active drug or placebo treatment at a ratio of 7:3 (active:placebo). Patients received one of three escalating level treatments starting with the dose level 1. Assignment to treatment was determined by a randomization scheme that was provided to the center's research pharmacy. After the initial group completed dosing at level 1, and prior to any subject being treated with the second dose level, an interim review of the safety data (clinical laboratory tests, vital signs, adverse events) and plasma concentration level of the drug was performed for all 10 patients. Escalation to the next level of study medication was based on safety assessments and pharmacokinetic data. For subsequent higher dose treatment groups, randomization was performed only if eight patients in the previous group completed the treatment period. There was no dose escalation if 6 of 10 patients experienced severe nausea or vomiting and could not adequately manage to rinse the study medication or were unable/unwilling to rinse due to intolerable taste of the study medication.

Patients were dosed beginning on the first day of conditioning and extending through day 14 posttransplantation. The specific analyses of safety data were carried out relative to the number of days of exposure to the investigational agent. Patients who received total body irradiation (TBI) could be started on study drug 1 day prior to the first day of conditioning to accommodate the TBI schedule and the PK sample blood draws. Patients

Table 11.2   Detailed flow chart.

Procedure study day		Day 1									Day 2	Day 3
Time (hour relative to study drug administration)	Predose	:00	:15	:30	1:00	2:00	3:00	4:00	8:00	12:00	24:00	48:00
Admitted to unit—discharge from unit	X											X
Administration of study drug		X										
Review entry criteria	X											
Physical examination	X											
Vital signs (BP/pulse: supine)	X					X		X	X		X	X
12 lead ECG	X					X			X		X	
Hematology, coagulation, clinical chemistry (safety) tests	X									X	X	X
ESR test											X	
Urinalysis test											X	
Fractionated urine sampling for PK	X							X		X	X	X
Blood sampling for PK	X		X	X	X	X	X	X	X	X	X	X
Adverse event recording			X	X	X	X	X	X	X	X	X	X
Prior/concomitant medication	X		X	X	X	X	X	X	X	X	X	X

209

received chemotherapeutics, busulfan (or dilantin), 1 hour prior to taking study drug. The study medication was to be administered at approximately 8:00 AM, 12:00 PM, 4:00 PM, and 8:00 PM (at the earliest, or before bedtime). The study drug had to be taken as follows:

Immediately prior to study drug administration, the patients were to rinse their mouth with water and expectorate. For dose level 1, the patients were to swallow the study drug after swishing. Due to the inability of most patients to swallow the drug, the study was amended to eliminate the swallowing of the drug.

The patients were not to eat, drink, or rinse for $\frac{1}{2}$ hour after dosing.

Oral mucositis scores were assessed three times per week (Monday, Wednesday, Friday ± 1 day) throughout the study administration period. The time of assessment was standardized for each patient. Oral cavity assessment was performed using OMI and NCI CTC stomatitis scale recording. Oropharyngeal pain was to be assessed 6 days/week throughout the study administration period. The time of assessment was standardized. Patient self-assessment was scored using a 10-point scale that measured oral pain and throat pain.

11.5.3   Prepivotal device trial—patients with periodontal disease

An example of a prepivotal device program in periodontal disease can be illustrated by a study performed with recombinant human platelet derived growth factor BB (rhPDGF-BB) delivered in bone allograft for the treatment of advanced periodontal bone defects. The purpose of this trial was to evaluate the clinical and histological response to localized treatment of advanced periodontal bone defects using a combination product consisting of a biologic (rhPDGF) and a device component (bone allograft). Nine adult patients (15 sites) were studied with advanced periodontitis exhibiting at least one tooth requiring extraction due to an extensive interproximal intrabony, and/or molar class II furcation defects (Camelo et al., 2003; Nevins et al., 2003). Eleven defects were randomly selected to receive treatment with the device. Following full-thickness flap reflection and initial debridement, the tooth roots were notched at the apical extent of the calculus, the osseous defects were thoroughly debrided, and the tooth root(s) were planed/prepared. The osseous defects were then filled with bone allograft and saturated with one of three concentrations of rhPDGF-BB. Concurrently, four interproximal defects were treated with a well-accepted commercially available graft (anorganic bovine bone in collagen, ABB-C) and a bilayer collagen membrane. Radiographs, clinical probing depths, and attachment levels were obtained preoperatively (at baseline) and 9 months later. At 9 months postoperatively, the study teeth and surrounding tissues were removed en bloc and studied histologically. Clinical and radiographic data were analyzed for change from baseline by defect type and PDGF concentration. This trial design allowed for a detailed assessment of the study device in a relatively small number of patients. The tissue response to the implant was assessed on a histologic level for biocompatibility, safety, and evidence of its intended therapeutic benefit prior to initiation of larger trials that would expose greater number of patients to the test device. Since in this example the test device contained an active biological agent, different doses of the biologic were also tested in combination with the osteoconductive scaffold. Multiple-dose groups would not be necessary in a traditional device trial, unless the device is intended to be implanted multiple times in which case multiple implantations could be tested.

11.6   Summary and conclusion

Phase 3 clinical trials in drugs and pivotal trials in devices serve as the primary basis for marketing approval, where effectiveness and safety are established (see Chapter 12). The biggest mistake that researchers and developers of investigational products can make is to rush into large, expensive pivotal clinical trials exposing large number of patients to the test agent with the wrong dosing regimen or lack of clear evidence that the investigational product has the intended effect in the target patient population. Phase 1 and pilot programs tell us about the pharmacokinetics, pharmacodynamics, and preliminary safety of investigational products. Phase 2 is one of the most critical stages of drug development as it bridges phase 1 and phase 3. While there is a temptation to "jump" to the pivotal trials as quickly as possible, solid pilot, phase 1 and phase 2 programs will significantly reduce the likelihood of failure in the pivotal trials. If an investigational product fails, it should occur early in development when the investigational product is discovered not to be efficacious or to have unacceptable adverse effects. Well-designed early programs can assure high likelihood of success in pivotal trials as well as early elimination of investigational products that do not work.

References

Camelo M, Nevins ML, Schenk RK, Lynch SE, Nevins M. 2003. Periodontal regeneration in human class II furcations using purified recombinant human platelet-derived growth factor-BB (rhPDGF-BB) with bone allograft. *International Journal of Periodontics and Restorative Dentistry* 23(3): 213–225.

Early Collaboration Meetings Under the FDA Modernization Act (FDAMA); Final Guidance for Industry and for CDRH Staff. 2001. U.S. Department of Health and Human Services, Food and Drug Administration, Center for Devices and Radiological Health (CDRH).

Guidance for Industry, INDs—Approaches to Complying with cGMP During Phase 1. 2005. U.S. Department of Health and Human Services, Food and Drug Administration, Center for Drug Evaluation and Research (CDER).

Guidance for Industry, E6 Good Clinical Practice: Consolidated Guidance. 1996. U.S. Department of Health and Human Services, Food and Drug Administration, Center for Drug Evaluation and Research (CDER)

Guidance for Industry, Investigators, and Reviewers—Exploratory IND Studies. 2006. U.S. Department of Health and Human Services, Food and Drug Administration, Center for Drug Evaluation and Research (CDER).

Nevins M, Camelo M, Nevins ML, Schenk RK, Lynch SE. 2003. Periodontal regeneration in humans using recombinant human platelet-derived growth factor-BB (rhPDGF-BB) and allogenic bone. *Journal of Periodontology* 74(9):1282–1292.

12

Phase III pivotal clinical trials: clinical decision making

Norman S. Braveman, PhD, and Bryan S. Michalowicz, DDS, MS

Phase III clinical trials are the foundation upon which most of what is done in clinical practice is based. Well-designed and well-conducted phase III clinical trials can provide clinicians with the best information about the safety, efficacy, and effectiveness of the preventive regimens, diagnostic tests, or treatments in use or planned for use. In short, information from phase III trials can let us know whether or not an intervention benefits patients by improving the quality of their health and/or prolonging life. As noted by Begg et al. (1996), "the randomized controlled trial (RCT), more than any other methodology, can have a powerful and immediate impact on patient care..."

While phase III trials can be and have been used to generate new knowledge about disease processes and the interventions, a more common use is to provide information required by the Food and Drug Administration (FDA) before a new intervention can be brought to market and used in the general population. It is beyond the scope of this chapter to detail the FDA's approval process. Our aim is to present information that will help oral health researchers understand the major issues in the design and conduct of phase III clinical trials, which, in turn, may be helpful in the FDA approval process.

This is not a "do-it-yourself" chapter. Phase III trials are complex and require experienced, diverse, and collaborative teams to conduct them. This chapter introduces the complexities of phase III trials and raises questions and issues that need to be addressed during their design and conduct. Details about the actual implementation of these principles can be found in many excellent textbooks on clinical trials (Meinert, 1986; Friedman et al., 1998; Piantodosi, 2005).

12.1   Where do phase III trials fit into the grand scheme?

Phase III trials are a type of *clinical research*, that is, any research involving humans, their cells, tissues, organs, organ systems, or behaviors. There are many types of clinical research, each one provides different types of information and has a different level of validity and/or reliability. Clinical research can be observational (describing the disease), mechanistic (describing its biological and behavioral causes) or interventional (trying to reduce the disease burden by manipulating mechanisms, influencing the conditions that cause it, or both).

According to *ClinicalTrials.gov,* a clinical trial is a biomedical or health-related research study in human beings that follows a predefined protocol. Trials themselves can be interventional or observational. In *interventional studies*, investigators assign participants to interventions and measure the impact of the intervention on the disease or condition using some well-defined and previously specified outcome. *Observational studies* are those in which the intervention is applied, individuals are observed, and their outcomes are measured by the investigators, most often but not always according to a predetermined plan or for a predetermined amount of time. Assignment of individuals in observational studies may or may not be according to some predefined plan, and occasionally the outcomes and length of follow-up may be determined after the intervention is introduced and changed as the study progresses. *The essential difference between an interventional and observational study is whether or not the investigator proactively assigns individuals to one intervention or another in a predetermined manner and for a prescribed amount of time.*

12.1.1   Clinical research: levels of evidence

Not all data from clinical research are equal in the strength of evidence they provide. As the accompanying text box (Text box 12.1) indicates, there is a continuum of evidence generated from clinical studies with that from clinical anecdotes providing the lowest level while evidence from prospective randomized controlled clinical trials, such a phase III trials, providing the highest level of evidence.

The strength of evidence generated by the various approaches is determined by the degree to which data collection is systematic and unbiased. For example, *while*

Text box 12.1   Levels of evidence (from Koch and Paquette (1997).

Prospective randomized controlled clinical trials	Highest level of evidence
Prospective longitudinal studies	—
Retrospective cohort studies	—
Case–control studies	—
Cross-sectional studies	—
Case histories	—
Clinical observations	—
Anecdotes	Lowest level of evidence

cross-sectional, case-controlled, and retrospective cohort studies may be large and may have detailed descriptions of the data collection methods, as pointed out by Koch and Paquette (1997), "... takes place during a single point (or brief interval) in time ... a patient's experience prior to that time is only partially available either through historical records which may be incomplete, or through patient recollections which may be unreliable." This is not to imply that we should not conduct such studies. They may be the only approaches that can be ethically otherwise justified in a given situation. However, their limitations impact the conclusions that can be drawn. Phase III clinical trials are the gold standard because they are systematic, prospective, large, unbiased through the use of randomization, and involve the use of control or comparison groups.

12.1.2   Efficacy and effectiveness

The purpose of clinical trials in general, and phase III trials in particular, is to systematically document the *safety, efficacy,* and *effectiveness* of a preventive or diagnostic method or treatment. In medicine, the term *efficacy* refers to the therapeutic effect of a treatment. The efficacy of an intervention is typically assessed in a clinical trial by comparing the impact of one treatment on a given disease or condition with the impact of another. Because of ethical and experimental design considerations, comparisons of an active intervention with no intervention occurs infrequently, if, at all. Efficacy can also refer to preventive regimens, that is, those that have been demonstrated by phase III trials as preventing, lessening, or otherwise ameliorating a disease or condition. Similarly, an efficacious diagnostic is one that accurately detects the presence of a given trait.

Effectiveness refers to the impact of one intervention in comparison to another. The essential difference between *efficacy* and *effectiveness* is if an intervention is said to be effective, it generally means that it has been assessed in a broader context. An intervention is said to be efficacious after testing it under ideal conditions while the same intervention may be viewed as effective only after it is tested under conditions that are more like those that exist in "real life" clinical situations. As we will note later, the efficacy of a treatment is typically assessed in a phase III clinical trial while the treatment's effectiveness is typically assessed in what is termed a demonstration and education study or a phase IV trial (see Chapter 13).

12.2   Clinical trial or not: a decision-making overview

12.2.1   What is the justification for conducting the trial?

Often the decision to conduct a phase III is driven by regulatory requirements. Even so, clinical trials are justified for reasons other than the need to bring a product to the market. Levine and Dennison (1997) state the issue in the following way:

> Ethical justification for beginning an RCT (*randomized clinical trial*) requires at a minimum, that the investigators be able to make an honest statement of no difference; that is, a statement that there is no scientifically validated reason to predict that therapy A will be superior to therapy B. Further there must be no therapy C known to be superior to either A or B unless there is good cause to reject therapy C... (italics ours)

There must be a state of clinical equipoise, a disagreement, or ambiguity in the clinical community as to the appropriateness of various treatment options. From this perspective, the clinical trial must be designed in a way that will resolve the disagreement or remove the uncertainty.

It is important to keep in mind that clinical trials are research and the decision whether to conduct a clinical trial must include an assessment of the risks to participants inherent in conducting research. The risks may be out of the direct control of the investigators, for example, a trial participant being injured or killed while driving to the trial site. On the other hand, the risks of increased morbidity or mortality may be directly linked either to the experimental or control intervention even though the research team takes every precaution possible to protect participants from injury. The key point is that participation in a clinical trial has risks and, before deciding that a clinical trial should be done, investigators must carefully weigh the risks against the expected or potential benefits to participants. The potential benefits must be judged to outweigh the risks inherent in exposing participants to the experimental intervention. Ideally, the risk–benefit assessment will be carried out by a totally independent individual or group that includes bioethicists and input from patients or patient representatives. If it is found that the risks do not outweigh the benefits, investigators should look for alternative ways to assess the safety, effectiveness, or efficacy of the intervention.

Even if investigators could eliminate all risks (an impossible proposition), there are still questions that need to be answered before deciding that a trial is needed and/or justified. Is the clinical trial simply an intellectual exercise or will its outcome influences how patients and clinicians approach the prevention, diagnosis, and/or treatment of the disease? Does the current state of the science allow for honest disagreement or uncertainty about existing therapies (i.e., is there *equipoise*)?

We might ask what the research literature tells us about whether or how a current intervention affects the etiology and pathogenesis of a disease. Do we know enough about either or both of these aspects of the disease to justify a modification in the current approach(es) to preventing, diagnosing, or treating it? Has new information been added to the scientific or clinical literature that would lead us to look for a new approach? This question is particularly critical in the current era of molecular biomedicine as we learn about normal and abnormal biological functioning. Newly gained knowledge about the molecular basis of disease can give us an entirely different picture of disease, its prevention, etiology, pathogenesis, diagnosis, and treatment, providing a strong justification for testing new and more precisely targeted interventions.

We should also ask questions about the current state of knowledge about the intervention(s) currently in use. Based on what we now know about a disease, is the new approach likely to be less taxing on the patient or more successful? Is the intervention already being used "off-label"? That is, is the new intervention already in use without the benefit of a systematic review of the research literature or even a clinical trial? There are numerous preventative regimens, treatments, and diagnostic procedures that are in use without the benefit of definitive phase III clinical trials (Brownlee, 2007).

If there have been previous studies using the intervention in question, are the studies published in peer-reviewed journals? Has a meta-analysis of the published literature been conducted and published? If so, what does it show? Is it possible that a meta-analysis could answer the questions raised about the new intervention and, thus, serve as the basis for or even substitute for a proposed clinical trial? What are the economic ramifications of the new intervention? Will the intervention be so costly that it will be deemed impractical?

There are many resources available to the clinical researcher for reviews of studies on specific interventions. One in particular, The Cochrane Collaboration (http://www.cochrane.org/) provides systematic reviews of the effects of health care interventions including those involving oral health. The collaboration consists of a global network of volunteers who have expertise in various areas of health care research. The *oral health group* (http://www.ohg.cochrane.org/), one of approximately 50 groups, maintains and disseminates systematic reviews of randomized controlled clinical trials in oral health (see also Chapter 18).

12.3   Clinical trials and their phases

Text box 12.2 summarizes the various phases of clinical trials. Also see Chapters 1 and 4 for a more general overview of the stepwise phases of clinical trials.

Text box 12.2   Phases of clinical trials.

Phase I dose ranging or safety trial:

- Intervention is administered to a small group of people (approximately 20–80).

- Used to determine safe dose range and identify side effects.

- Typically, the first research done on humans after animal studies has shown the intervention not to be toxic or otherwise injurious.

- Look for the physiological effects of the intervention (i.e., how the body responds biologically) . . . typically many laboratory studies.

- May or may not use control groups.

- Proceed very slowly and are done in groups called cohorts; cohorts may be used repeatedly in dose escalation study.

Phase II safety and intervention tolerance trial:

- Begins to determine whether or not the intervention produces the desired effect on the disease.

- Number of participants typically in the range of 100–300[2].

- Control groups may be used for comparison.

- Can also serve to determine what pitfalls might be faced in mounting a large multicenter phase III trial, particularly with regard to issues of participant availability, enrollment, and follow-up as well as about other logistic and organizational aspects of the larger phase III trial.

Phase III trial:

- Involves very large groups of individuals, typically 1,000–3,000[2] or more.

- Used to obtain a definitive answer as to whether or not the intervention, as used in clinical practice, is effective *under ideal conditions*.

- Continue to monitor side effects and other aspects of the intervention related to safety and more broadly general health effects.

- May continue to collect data about biological or physiological changes resulting from the intervention.

Phase IV trials:

- Typically conducted after a new intervention has been marketed; also known as postmarketing studies.

- Continue to study the intervention in new populations or subgroups of individual not included or included in small numbers in the phase III trial.

- Look for adverse effects over a long time period.

- Study the *efficacy* of the intervention in "demonstration and evaluation (D&E)" study carried out on a community or institutional basis; unit of analysis can be the "practice" or "community" or "interventional site" as opposed to the individual participant.

- D&E trials determine whether or not an intervention can be delivered in a safe and effective way in a more broadly based setting and under more "real life" set of conditions.

While there is overlap and some redundancy among various phases of clinical trials, in general, the major differences among them are in the kind of question(s) being asked and the size of the test group involved. The number of individuals used in the different phases of clinical trials is determined by several factors including statistical considerations as well as compliance with the requirements of regulatory or funding agencies. In the end, the goal is to be able to draw statistically and clinically meaningful conclusions about the intervention being tested. In addition, it is important that enough participants be included in the phase III or phase IV trial so that the results are generalizable. The numbers cited in Text box 12.2 of this chapter are taken from the FDA Consumer Magazine, Volume 37, Number 5, September–October 2003, and are provided only as guidelines.

Phase III and IV clinical trials typically share several characteristics. They both involve at least one *control* group. Typically, but not always, the new intervention is compared to one that is considered to be the current state of the art in clinical practice. Both are also *prospective* (i.e., individuals are assigned to various treatment groups after their eligibility is determined), involve *randomization* of some kind (i.e., the chances of an individual being assigned to the test intervention are the same as assignment to the control intervention), are *masked* (i.e., either the participants or the researchers or both are kept from knowing whether they are receiving the test intervention or the control intervention), and typically they involve very *complex organizational structures*. In addition, phase III and IV trials, like other trials, require *prior review* by an Institutional Review Board (IRB) and *continual*

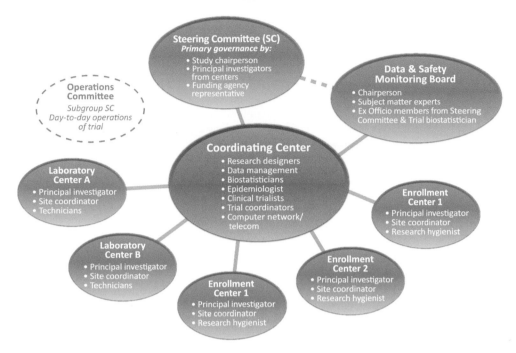

Figure 12.1   Hypothetical organizational structure of a phase III clinical trial.

oversight by an independent group throughout the conduct of the trial (typically referred to as a Data and Safety Monitoring Committee or Board).

12.4   Phase III trials: organizational complexity

Phase III clinical trials are large and complex because the sample size requirements often dictate the need for multiple enrollment centers. Figure 12.1 illustrates the organizational components of a hypothetical phase III clinical trial.

As the figure implies, many people are needed to carry out a phase III trial. In most cases, certainly in cases involving multiple centers, the coordinating center serves as the organizational linchpin for the trial. The Bypass Angioplasty Revascularization Investigation (BARI) trial is a useful example for illustrating many issues related to the organization of a large trial. BARI was a multicenter clinical trial designed to assess the long-term safety and efficacy of coronary bypass graft surgery (CABG) or percutaneous transluminal coronary angioplasty (PTCA) in patients with multivessel coronary artery disease requiring revascularization (Naydeck et al., 1996). The trial involved 14 primary enrollment centers, 4 satellite sites, a clinical coordinating center, and separate ECG, and radiographic central laboratories. Once the participating centers were identified, it took 1 year to plan the trial. Over a 3-year period, more than 25,000 patients were screened, more than 1,800 patients randomized, and more than 2,400 entered into a registry. Participants were followed for 8 years.

In discussing the organizational aspects of the BARI trial, Naydeck et al. (1996) state that:

> The challenge in designing a (*Phase III*) clinical trial is to successfully integrate the control possible in a simple structure with the volume achieved in a machine bureaucracy without sacrificing professional creativity. . . .*O*(o)rganizational design of a trial. . .(*is*) as important as the experimental design. . .organizational structure (*should*) take shape after consideration of the needs of the individual trial and its participating investigators. . .many clinical trial investigators are medical professionals or academicians without in-depth expertise in administrative management. From the design phase to protocol implementation, reporting of results to study closeout, effective communications, and the establishment of administrative routine are the keys to a well functioning trial. (italics ours)

There are many ways to organize a complex trial. Most importantly, the structure should facilitate effective and timely communication between all trial components, which can include the clinical sites (some of which were outside of the continental United States in the BARI trial), the central analytic laboratories, the clinical coordinating center, the funding agency, and the independent monitoring groups. Any organizational structure should ensure that those involved in the conduct of the trial have well-defined roles, know where their roles fit into the grand scheme of things, and are viewed and feel as valued contributors to the overall goals of the trial. In this regard, a major role of the coordinating center is to facilitate communication through collaboration rather than by directive. The BARI trial did this through regularly scheduled conference calls between the coordinating center and each component, completion and distribution of sequentially numbered operation memos through site coordinators, a dedicated telephone line referred to as the BARI hotline to handle questions from the clinical sites, a patient newsletter, and a communication plan within the coordinating center to deal with data management/programming issues, correspondence, data analysis, and publication of manuscripts.

Recent developments involving the use of the internet have facilitated communications among components (e.g., Marks et al., 2001a, 2001b; Formica et al., 2004; Marks, 2004). Internet-based trials have tools that can facilitate almost instantaneous communication. These tools alone, however, should not drive the organizational structure of the trial, nor should they replace periodic one-on-one communication. Several commercial vendors provide software that can help manage phase III trials. These software packages are flexible and can aid in recruitment, tracking a participant's flow through the trial, workload planning, internal communications, and data entry. Internet-based programs can also assist in identifying potential enrollment sites and/or analytic laboratories. Potential enrollment sites may be asked to provide information about characteristics of patient populations, the number of individuals treated in a given period, past clinical trial experience, and other qualifications that can help the organizers of the trial decide whether to include a particular clinical site.

12.4.1   Who's who in a phase III trial?

Even though there is a tool kit containing a variety of resources, each trial still needs people with varied skills to ensure its success. The key is for the trial leadership to put people into roles that will allow them to maximize their skills. The accompanying text box (Text box 12.3) provides a list and description of the expertise necessary for a phase III trial. The list

---

Text box 12.3   Who's who in a clinical trial.

Experienced clinician-scientists—Ask the initial question, develop the clinical protocol, administer intervention(s) in a way that mirrors clinical practice, and provide
overall leadership.

Research designers/biostatisticians or epidemiologists—Work closely, *from the start*,
with clinician-scientists in the experimental design of the trial; develop the experimental design (e.g., number and types of groups and subgroups; number of
participants; develop randomization procedure; develop/implement data capture,
distribution, and analysis schemes; often the only one within the study group that
tracks the endpoints throughout a trial even in one that is masked).

Research assistants/nurses/dental hygienists—Enroll and follow participants; make
sure that each participant is where she or he should be at the right time; often
fulfill the role of data collector including for demographic and health event data;
oversees implementation of treatment and randomization schemes; in some cases
may administer the intervention(s).

Data collectors—Typically research assistants, nurses, or hygienists; trained to collect data in the same way from all participants across centers.

Data analyzers—Biostatistical assistants who carry out the proscribed statistical
analysis including data checks and data cleanup.

Clinical trialists/methodologists—Provide guidance, oversight, advice, and leadership; often an individual with a background in biostatistics or epidemiology; often
in charge of the organizational activities of trial (e.g., regular meetings of the
investigators, research assistants, individual site personnel in charge of gathering,
and distributing data).

Site coordinators—Manage the operations of each site and who are responsible for
reporting to the site scientific/clinical director and/or coordinating center; could
be a clinical trialist.

Bioethicists/participant advocates—Provide and protect the participant's perspective; they help balance the interests of the participants with those of the scientific
interests of the research team.

Participants—Without whom there would be no trial.

---

is not intended to be comprehensive, and the exact mix or numbers are determined by the
subject matter, complexity, and size of the trial.

There are other models available in the literature including those involving periodontal
(Polson, 1997) and caries clinical trials (Proceedings of the ICW–CCT, 2004). *Once again,
it is (are) the goal(s) and purpose(s) of the trial that should determine the mix of individuals
involved in the trial and their respective responsibilities . . . not vice versa.*

12.5   Key elements of a phase III clinical trial

As described earlier, phase III trials are *systematic, prospective,* and *randomized* studies that compare the effect and value of a preventive, diagnostic, or treatment against a *control.* Next, we examine each descriptor in more detail.

12.5.1   Phase III trials are systematic: the manual of procedures

Phase III clinical trials are *conducted according to a carefully devised written formal plan,* which is documented in the trial's Manual of Procedures (MOP). The MOP *spells out in detail ALL of the procedures followed in the trial.* The MOP also serves as the historical record of the trial. A trial's MOP should enable independent groups to replicate the trial based solely on procedures described in the MOP alone.

The MOP is organized in chapters, each of which corresponds to a different aspect of the trial. The MOP should standardize how various steps in the trial are carried out, designate who carries them out, provide a timeline for when they are done, and specify what is done if procedural deviations occur. Adherence to procedures and specifications is one of the single most important ways to reduce "error variance," that is, variability in the outcome that arises from factors other than inherent participant-related individual differences. Minimizing variance is important because it can mask the effect of an otherwise effective intervention.

Typically, MOPs are modified throughout the course of a phase III trial. Constructing the MOP as a loose-leaf notebook allows amendments to be added easily. If electronic versions are used, changes must be clearly identified. Modifications also must be reviewed and approved by designated individuals who should sign and date the change(s). The modification process itself should be detailed in the MOP. While these processes may seem bureaucratic and burdensome, they are important in multicenter trials to ensure that all centers are performing study tasks in the same manner and sequence. Changes must also be communicated to all trial personnel, who should be monitored regularly to ensure they are aware of and comply with these changes. Again, this is particularly important in multisite trials. Since the MOP can also serve as the historical record of the trial, it is important to retain all original pages as they provide documentation of procedures followed throughout the trial.

Participant recruitment strategies outlined in MOP are commonly modified for trials that are unable to recruit participants as originally planned. MOP may also be modified if data forms are altered or added.

Among the information contained in the MOP, the following are listed:

Justification for the trial. This section addresses the questions: "Why is this trial being done?" and "How will information from the trial be used?" This section typically includes a discussion of the scientific literature supporting the need for a trial.

Trial design. The details of the experimental design, including power calculations, provide the research team with a general overview of the trial. This section describes the trial groups and interventions, sample sizes, the stratification of participants, if needed, and the major trial endpoint(s).

Trial timeline. The timeline provides important milestones, including those related to study enrollment, provision of interventions, and data collection and analysis. This information is used by the research team *and* external groups such as the trial's Steering Committee

(SC) and Data and Safety Monitoring Committee. These milestones allow all interested parties to gauge the trial's progress, which often occurs slower than planned. Start-up or organizational issues (particularly if the trial involves multiple enrollment centers) and participant recruitment and randomization typically take longer than planned as does data analysis and paper preparation. Although some delays may be inevitable, others can be avoided with careful organizational preparation and planning. Using experienced research teams also help reduce delays in meeting trial milestones.

Organizational structure. Specifying the organizational structure of the trial (i.e., the roles and responsibilities of all team members) helps ensure a trial, particularly a multicenter one, is conducted in a systematic and efficient manner. This section should also include a description of the Data and Safety Monitoring Board (DSMB), their meeting schedule, responsibilities, and processes by which they are selected and replaced if necessary. This section should also refer to role(s) of the Institutional Review Board(s) and any other oversight groups in the trial.

Regulatory requirements. A separate section outlining the various regulatory requirements is advisable. This section's focus should be on the forms that need to be completed, when they need to be submitted, and to whom and by whom. The specific adverse event reporting protocol should be described here. Adverse events are discussed in more detail later in this chapter.

Recruitment of participants. This section describes the recruitment approach(es)/ procedure(s) used, and should include a detailed description of the recruitment staff, and methods (e.g., direct contact, newspaper or radio/TV ads), the sources of participants, and the timetable for recruitment. If the trial involves a stratified sample, it is important to specify the subpopulations from which the individuals in the various strata will be selected, their characteristics, where they can be found, special approach(es) that are used to recruit them, and the proportions in each stratum. Forms used to track the recruitment process should be included in this section.

Participant enrollment criteria. This section defines who is and who is not eligible to participate in the trial and how eligibility is determined. This section should also include any forms used in the process.

Randomization procedure(s). Randomization involves assignment of participants to one of two or more study groups. There are various schemes for randomizing participants. Some involve using a table of random numbers, others may use a computer program or web-based process, and still others may be accomplished using a presorted, computer-generated list. The randomization procedure should be specified in detail and be invariable. A Data or Statistical Coordinating Center typically designs and manages randomization schemes. Several issues related to randomization are described later in this chapter.

Informed consent procedure. Informed consent refers both to a document and to a process that begins before a person agrees to become involved in the trial and ends after they have completed the trial. A sample document along with a helpful series of FAQ about informed consent is available at www.clinicaltrials.gov.

The intent of informed consent is to equalize the decision-making relationship between the participant and trial staff. It helps to ensure that nothing can be done to a participant without his or her full knowledge, understanding, and approval. Participants must understand what is going to happen to them, when and where it will happen, who will be involved in administering the intervention, and their rights and responsibilities.

All risks and potential benefits of participation are explained in the informed consent documents.

The informed consent document is not a binding contract. It must state that individuals are free to withdraw from the trial at any time without any adverse consequences to them. The document is read by the participant in the presence of a trial official and, upon signing it, a copy is provided to the participant and the original kept in a secure file. Each participant should have all their questions answered at any time during the trial but in particular during the initial informed consent visit. In short, the informed consent process helps participants decide whether or not initially they want to become involved in the trial and then whether or not they want to continue as the trial progresses.

A copy of the approved informed consent document and instructions for its administration should be included in the MOP. A list of frequently asked questions and suggested answers should be included and updated regularly. Questions can be gleaned from the pretest of the informed consent as well as from participants during the conduct of the trial itself. As new questions or answers are added, trial staff must be informed and this section of the MOP must be changed. Training in the administration of the informed consent is essential to ensure consistency.

Clinical protocol. This is one of the most important parts of the MOP. It specifies what will be done in the experimental treatment group(s) and control group(s), how it will be done, in what order, who will do it, and how protocol deviations will be handled. A detailed protocol helps ensure the clinical procedures are administered and tracked consistently across centers. All study forms directly related to the clinical protocol should also be included. These forms can include baseline measurements of specific as well as general physiological functions, a procedure checklist, as well as forms that describe deviations from the protocol or unusual events that may have occurred during the delivery of the protocol.

There are several consequences of not standardizing delivery of the interventions. Protocol deviations not only introduce unwanted variability in outcome measures—which can mask intervention effects or create artificial differences between groups—but they also make it inappropriate to combine endpoint data from individuals who were treated differently. Neither of these possibilities is desirable insofar as they can bias the outcome of the trial. A third possibility is that slight variations in administration of the intervention in order to adapt to participant needs may mask very important limitations of a new intervention. Finally, it is imperative that deviations in administration of the intervention, unintentional or otherwise, be documented fully and considered in the data analysis.

It is not sufficient simply to specify the intervention protocol in the MOP. Therapists should be trained and assessed against some "standard," certified by an independent judge or panel of judges. Training and examination should occur at various times throughout the trial to guard against "operator drift," which happens when an operator becomes increasingly proficient with the protocol as the study progresses. Retraining guards against changes in the way the operator delivers the intervention. Retraining and examination also helps ensure that modifications of the protocol are being adhered to by all staff. The schedule for training should be prespecified and included in the MOP.

Masking procedure(s). Masking procedures prevent participants and/or investigators from determining whether a participant received an experimental or control treatment. Masking, also referred to as "blinding," is used to reduce bias resulting from preconceived ideas about the safety, effectiveness, or efficacy of the intervention under study. In some studies, only the participant is unaware of which treatment she or he received. These are referred to as *single-masked* studies. *Double-masked* studies are those in which neither the participant nor the investigator is aware of the treatment received by the participant. *Triple-masking* can refer to trials in which participants, investigators, *and* biostatisticians remained masked until after the data are analyzed. A more common use of the term, however, refers to the situation in which neither the participant, the investigator, nor the committee(s) monitoring the trial (e.g., DSMB) is aware of the treatment administered to any participants.

In some instances, it is neither necessary nor possible to mask the participant or the investigator. These are referred to as *open label or unmasked studies* and typically occur in surgical or lifestyle intervention trials in which the intervention is obvious. For example, in studying a new restorative material, it would be difficult to mask the person doing the restoration while the participant could potentially identify which one she or he received by simply looking in a mirror. Similarly, in a trial testing the effect of a particular diet on oral health, it would be difficult to mask either the participant or the investigator who presumably would have access to the dietary advice given to participants. On the other hand, and depending on the specific dietary intervention of interest, it may be possible to put the essential dietary constituents into pill form so that its content is not apparent to the participant or even the trial staff providing the pill. Regardless, it is imperative that participants be informed during the informed consent process if a masking procedure will be used to prevent identification of the intervention.

Trials of dental procedures are typically inherently (therapist) unmasked (i.e., single masked) and are at times difficult to mask from the fully conscious participant. It is possible to address this issue by masking individuals who collect endpoint data, as was done in safety trials of dental amalgam in children (DeRouen et al., 2002; McKinlay et al., 2003). In these trials, eligible participants were randomized to restoration with composite or dental amalgam. Clearly, the operator and participants (or their parents) knew or could determine what restorative material the participant child had received. In both trials, however, the major endpoints and biospecimens were collected and analyzed by individuals who were masked to the dental treatment. With the exception of one-on-one assessments (e.g., behavioral, cognitive, or neurological), evaluators also had no contact with the participants. As part of the protocol, individuals conducting the one-on-one tests were instructed to not look into the children's mouths and complied with this request.

In any masked trial, participants, investigators, and even trial monitors may try to guess which treatment a participant received. While studies have shown that their overall accuracy is around 50%, one should be mindful of the effects of "expectations" or "placebo effects" on endpoint outcomes. If a participant is convinced that she or he has received an active intervention, there is a very high likelihood that she or he will show a positive effect of that intervention, particularly if she or he believes the intervention to be beneficial.

Placebo effects are well documented (Braunholtz et al., 2001) and should not be discounted. So-called inert treatments can cause the same or very similar physiological responses as active ones. A striking example of this is seen in studies of osteoarthritic knees, which have repeatedly documented that sham surgery can provide similar pain relief when compared to full arthroscopic surgery (Moseley et al., 2002). The interested reader is referred to Wager and Nitschke (2005) for a more in-depth discussion of the placebo effect. The placebo effect can have profound effects on trial's outcomes, and in some instances completely obscure true differences between a new treatment and a control.

Trial endpoint(s). An *endpoint* is an objective measurement that reflects the impact or effect of the intervention. Other terms used in place of endpoint are *outcome measure* and *response variable.* The *primary endpoint* is the one prespecified indicator that tells us how the new intervention compares to the control intervention. Because of normal physiological and psychological variability among participants, the interventions can have slightly different effects on participants. This will be reflected in the variability in the endpoint measure, which is assumed to be normal in both the biological and statistical sense. An estimate of variability in the endpoint is used to estimate the sample size needed to detect a prespecified difference between the experimental and control groups. Use of multiple primary endpoints is not recommended, in part because it reflects uncertainty about the way in which a new treatment may influence the course of disease, and if there is that level of uncertainty then it is doubtful that the trial should be done in the first place. Further, it allows for the possibility that one endpoint can support the hypothesis while another does not, making it impossible to determine the true meaning of the trial outcome.

A primary endpoint may consist of a single event or of a combination of endpoints, termed a *composite endpoint.* For example, the Children's Amalgam Trial (DeRouen et al., 2002) used a composite neurobehavioral endpoint, which consisted of measures of memory, attention/concentration, and motor/visual motor skills.

A *secondary endpoint* is one that, while of interest, will not be used to determine whether or not the intervention is effective or safe. It is not used to determine the sample size of the trial. Many secondary endpoints are biological in nature and can provide important information about the mechanism(s) of action of the intervention on the disease. While it is tempting to include many secondary endpoints in order to better understand the way(s) in which the intervention works, incorporating too many procedures or tests in the protocol can adversely affect participant recruitment and retention, unnecessarily complicate the trial protocol, tax study personnel, and reduce the quality of the data.

When biological samples are to be sent to a central laboratory for analysis, the MOP should include a complete description and timetable for sample collection, storage, and shipment. Packing and handling instructions, laboratory and site contact information, and follow-up procedures should be documented carefully. The MOP should detail all steps in the process, even if samples are to be collected and analyzed on site. The laboratory procedures should be tested thoroughly beforehand to ensure they yield reliable and valid results.

The MOP also describes in detail how the endpoint(s) will be measured/assessed. As with the interventions, detailed descriptions of endpoint assessments can help standardize the procedures for collecting data and, in so doing, reduce variability between sites and examiners. The MOP should specify who assesses the endpoints, when and how it will be done, and, if it involves biological samples, how those samples will be handled and stored. Also included in the MOP are instructions about how, when, and where information will be entered into the trial's databases. Copies of any forms that may need to be completed in the data collection process should be included in the MOP.

A major consideration in designing a trial is whether measurements used in clinical practice are appropriate or even possible to be used as endpoints. For example, the main interest in clinical periodontology is the prevention of tooth loss. It makes intuitive sense to use tooth loss, an objective, unambiguous and binary (yes/no) measure, as the primary endpoint in periodontal trials. Depending on the population from which the sample is selected, however, tooth loss from periodontal disease may be relatively rare and occur over years or even decades, which may be too long to feasibly evaluate a new intervention. Increasing the trial's sample size can partially offset the problem of infrequent endpoints (in this case tooth loss), although the related cost increase may make the trial prohibitively expensive or scientifically unwarranted.

It is, however, possible to use another measure in place of an endpoint of real interest (e.g., tooth loss in the example above). These are referred to as *surrogate measures* or *endpoints*. Fleming and DeMets (1996) define a surrogate endpoint as a laboratory measurement or physical sign that is used as a substitute for a clinically meaningful endpoint. According to Fleming (2005), surrogate endpoints themselves do not predict that the individual will derive symptom relief or prolongation of life from the intervention. However, because they are associated with the disease condition, changes in the surrogate resulting from the intervention can predict the effect of the intervention on the clinical endpoint of interest.

Importantly, surrogates are indicators of risk for the disease and are not causes. As such, surrogates must be more than statistically correlated with a primary endpoint to be valid. The effects of an intervention on a surrogate marker must reliably predict the intervention's effect on the true endpoint of interest. Depth of gingival pockets in periodontal trials, for example, is typically used as a surrogate measure in trials of periodontal therapy. It is an appropriate surrogate to the extent that change in pocket depth reflects a change in the potential for tooth loss.

Fleming (2005) has suggested a hierarchy for outcome measures:

Level 1: A measure that indicates the true benefit of the intervention to the individual.
Level 2: A validated surrogate measure that may not directly assess the direct clinical benefit of the intervention to the individual but can reliably predict the levels of such benefit.
Level 3: Measures that reflect the likelihood of clinical benefit, typically based on the accumulated statistical evidence (e.g., risk ratios) and clinical knowledge about the condition for which the treatment is designed.
Level 4: A measure that is correlated with the underlying biological activity of the intervention but for which there is no validation at a higher level.

In selecting surrogate endpoint(s) for a trial, it is imperative to obtain input from biostatisticians and clinicians. Several nonstatistical questions should be considered in making the final determination. These include the following:

1. Is the surrogate endpoint valid?
2. Can it be assessed and used widely in clinical practice?
3. Will clinicians accept changes in the endpoint as evidence of the new treatment's safety, efficacy, or effectiveness?
4. Is the surrogate the best or most appropriate one in terms of reflecting benefit to the patient?

It is important to keep in mind limitations when using surrogate endpoints for phase III trials. As noted by Fleming and DeMets (1996):

Surrogate end points can be useful in phase 2 screening trials for identifying whether a new intervention is biologically active and for guiding decisions about whether the intervention is promising enough to justify a large definitive trial with clinically meaningful outcomes. In definitive phase 3 trials, except for rare circumstances in which the validity of the surrogate end point has already been rigorously established, the primary end point should be the true clinical outcome.

Stopping rule. A stopping rule specifies the conditions under which a trial will be stopped before its planned completion (Whitehead, 2004). A trial's stopping rule should be clearly specified in the MOP along with the process by which the trial is stopped and the team's subsequent responsibilities to trial participants.

Trials can be stopped early for two main reasons; both are based on assessments of the benefits to society weighed against the risks faced by the participants. The first is based on whether a statistical criterion has been or can be met. A trial may be stopped if a monitoring board determines that additional data collection will not change the interim inference about the new intervention. That is, a trial can be stopped if it is determined that no additional data collection or testing will change the conclusion that the test intervention is either equivalent to, better than, or worse than the control treatment.

Being able to determine if a statistical criterion has been reached before all participants are enrolled and/or tested requires that the endpoints are tracked at regular intervals throughout the trial. Typically, this is done by the trial biostatistician who is and should be the only person unmasked in an otherwise masked trial.

Trials can also be stopped out of concern for the safety of participants. A notable example of early stopping of a trial is illustrated by the Cardiac Arrhythmia Suppression Trial (CAST) in which three antiarrhythmia drugs were tested against a placebo (CAST Investigators, 1989). During a 10-month follow-up, deaths from arrhythmia and nonfatal cardiac arrests occurred more frequently in patients receiving encainide or flecainide when compared to those receiving placebo. It was because of these findings that the part of the trial involving these drugs was discontinued. There are many other similar examples in the literature.

In general, the responsibility for stopping a trial lies with the Data and Safety Monitoring Board or some other similar group. Monitoring boards are discussed in more detail later in this chapter.

Data collection, entry, and distribution. Clinical trial's data must be collected, entered, and distributed in a standardized, accurate, and timely manner. Typically, data-related protocols are developed by the data coordinating center. This section or these sections of the MOP provide the who, what, when, where, and why of data collection, entry, and distribution. Two key issues in data collection, entry, and distribution are *accuracy of the data* and *privacy of participants*. Procedures for ensuring both accuracy and privacy must be specified in the MOP along with detailed instructions, protocols, and forms (even if hard-copy data forms are not used) for data collection, entry, and distribution. It is essential that data be entered and distributed from enrollment or data collection centers to the coordinating center in a timely manner and in accordance with all of the steps and timing spelled out in the MOP.

Data sharing plan. If the trial is funded by the U.S. government, there are requirements that unidentified data be shared or otherwise made available for secondary data analysis. Specific steps involved in this plan, including a timeline and trial personnel responsibilities, should be included in the MOP and be consistent with agency requirements.

Data analysis plan. The design, specific statistical analysis, method for carrying it out (e.g., SAS or other program), staff involved, timeline, and related matters should be provided in the MOP.

Sample collection, analysis, storage, and/or distribution. All procedures including quality control for collecting, storing, and, if necessary, distributing biological samples are included in the MOP.

Writing timetable, responsibilities, and authorships. In order to avoid later misunderstandings, the order of authorship should be determined before the trial begins and be included in the MOP. In addition, a list of manuscripts planned for publication, the timing of their preparation and submission, and the internal process of review and submission should be included. It is not uncommon for secondary data analysis to lead to publications that were not anticipated prior to the start of the trial. At the same time, however, it is possible to anticipate publications involving the primary endpoint(s) and these should be provided in the MOP.

Training and monitoring schedule. Also included in the MOP should be a written plan and schedule for training and retraining trial staff as well as for regular review of updates in the MOP. Also regular checks of whether trial staff at all levels, particularly those who carry out the intervention(s), should be included so as to make sure that all procedures and processes are being carried out in the prescribed manner.

Changing the MOP. Procedures for changes in the MOP should be specified in the MOP. This includes all aspects of changes, including any forms that must be filled out, the approval track for changes, along with the review, approval, and communication process. As we have indicated, it is important to communicate changes in the MOP to all trial personnel in a timely manner. One way to facilitate this is with a web-based MOP as was done in the OPT trial (Michalowicz et al., 2006). The MOP is available at http://www.biostat.umn.edu/OPT/. While access to the MOP using the internet is immediate, it is important to ensure that the site and information are secure and can only be changed by one individual and through a process that is specified in the MOP.

Pretesting the MOP. Because of the complexity and level of detail, the MOP should be field tested in its entirety before the trial begins. Some investigators have used a planning or run-in phase to the trial so that data from individuals used to determine whether the procedures described in the MOP work in practice. The decision about whether these data should or can be included in the overall data analysis and the process for doing this should be determined beforehand with input from the biostatistician.

12.5.2   Phase III trials are prospective

Phase III trials are prospective in that they plan for the selection and assignment of participants and for the collection, analysis, and reporting of outcome data. In contrast to retrospective case–control studies or case series, data in phase III are collected forward in time. The clinical researcher specifies beforehand who will be recruited for the phase III trial and intentionally assigns interventions or treatments to participants with well-specified eligibility characteristics.

As noted earlier, phase III trials carefully and explicitly define certain characteristics of the individuals that will be included in the study including their demographics and health status. Specifying eligibility criteria is critical in that it defines the population(s) to which the results of the trial may be generalized.

Other differences between retrospective and prospective studies may also impact on our ability to interpret the findings of a phase III trial. One is in the uniformity of the population from which the participants come. In a prospective study, if the research team specifies completely and accurately the characteristics of the individuals recruited for the study and is able to provide data to show that there are no differences in these characteristics between those enrolled and randomized in the study and those who are not, then the population to which the findings of the trial can be generalized is clearly delineated.

In contrast, subject characterization in retrospective studies may be incomplete or unknown. It is also possible that limits may not be placed on how far in the past one can go and still include patient records. The consequences of this are important insofar as diagnostic accuracy or criteria for treating a patient with the intervention under study may have changed over time. As a result, patients whose records are older may not be comparable to patients whose records are more recent. In addition, the condition being treated may have changed over time so that an intervention that was once effective may now have become less so in treating a disease that has changed and become more difficult to treat. Similarly, with the passage of time, there may have been improvements in the ability of clinicians to use the intervention so that more recently treated patients may have benefited more from the intervention that those treated earlier. Also, there is no guarantee that patients from various time periods were treated for the same amount of time. In a prospective study, these factors are all controlled since all participants are enrolled in the study for a proscribed and equivalent period of time. As a result, the impact of these and other *time-dependent factors* are the same for all participants in the study; they are known, and they can be factored into our conclusions about the intervention tested in the trial.

12.5.3   Phase III trials involve control groups

Phase III trials include control groups, which, more than any other feature, makes them the gold standard for interventional clinical research. In a scientific experiment, we use controls to manage variables that can have an influence on the outcome of the experiment. These are also termed extraneous variables. By controlling for these variables, investigators can better isolate and assess the effect of an intervention on a *primary endpoint*. Without controls, we can only say that if intervention A leads to a particular outcome, there is a *correlation* between the intervention and outcome. There is no guarantee that it was the introduction of the specific intervention that *caused* the specific result we have observed. *While correlation is a necessary condition for establishing causation, it is not sufficient.* Participants must be prospectively and randomly assigned to an experimental group to be able to infer a causal relationship between an intervention and an outcome.

There are several ways to satisfy the requirement that experimental and control groups are alike in all ways except for the specific intervention being tested. One is by matching groups on all variables known to be associated with the endpoint of interest. It is never possible, however, to assess or even know all the variables that may be related to the primary endpoint, and incomplete matching can introduce systematic bias into a trial's results.

Alternatively, by *randomly assigning participants* to intervention and control groups, it is assumed that extraneous variables are randomly distributed among groups and thus have no *systematic* effect on the outcome. While randomization can produce "unbalanced" groups, it is assumed that when done often enough, randomization will yield "equivalent" groups. It is incumbent, however, on those conducting the trial to collect, analyze, and report data on all extraneous or randomized variables thought to influence the outcome of the intervention to determine the extent to which the groups are in fact equivalent.

As mentioned earlier, control groups are necessary to establish causal relationships between an intervention and an outcome. A number of issues related to the selection of controls are discussed below:

No-treatment, placebo, and standard of care controls. There are three essential types of control groups: no-treatment, placebo control, and the current standard of care. The *no-treatment control* is not an option either ethically or from an experimental design perspective. Withholding treatment from an individual in need is unethical. Even if the trial intervention does not involve treatment, for example, studies of prevention interventions or diagnostic procedures, a no-intervention control violates the basic principle of experimental design that all conditions between the experimental and control group are the same except for the provision of the experimental intervention. Individuals in a no-treatment group do not experience the interaction with individuals involved in the study team, for example, in receiving informed consent, and there is evidence that contact with study team members alone can have measurable therapeutic effects, also termed the Hawthorne or hello–goodbye effect (DiAmici et al., 2000).

Individuals in a *placebo control* group receive what is presumed to be an inert intervention instead of the experimental intervention. The placebo itself should be the same in all respects (e.g., taste, appearance, method of administration) as the experimental intervention except that the active or physiological part of the experimental intervention is absent. Once again, there are ethical issues about knowingly using an intervention that does not contain a physiologically active therapeutic ingredient in it, even if there is a chance that the placebo may produce an appropriate physiological response. The ethical issue has been discussed in relationship to a range of trials but most notably during the late 1990s with regard to a trial of zidovudine versus placebo in disrupting vertical transmission of HIV from pregnant African women to their newborns (Angell, 1997; Annas & Grodin, 1998; Bayer, 1998; Karim, 1998). While the focus of this debate was around the issue of exploitation of individuals who had no other access to care, the issues apply well beyond these individuals and the time period of those trials. Moreover, as noted by Annas and Grodin (1998) participants ". . . should not be drawn from populations who are especially vulnerable (e.g., the poor, children or mentally impaired persons) unless the population is the only group in which research can be conducted and the group itself will derive benefits from the research. Even when these conditions are met, informed consent must be obtained" *and be appropriate for the population.* (italics ours)

The *current standard of care* for a given condition or the *currently recommended practice*, as in the case of preventive interventions or diagnostics, is generally the most appropriate and ethically defensible control intervention in a trial. Comparisons between individuals randomized to receive the current standard of care and those randomized to receive the experimental intervention enable investigators to determine if the experimental intervention is equivalent or superior to the one that is currently in use. If there are multiple interventions that are in current use, with appropriate justification and sufficient resources, they all can be included as comparison groups in the trial. As a general guide, the highest standards should be applied in all research situations. If there is a treatment available that constitutes the current standard of care, it should be the basis for comparison for any new intervention.

Concurrent and nonconcurrent control groups. Friedman et al. (1998) and others distinguish between several types of control procedures. We have already referred to the *concurrent randomized control procedure*, one in which a group of individuals are selected from a pool of individuals, all of whom share a well-defined set of characteristics, and for whom, the probability of being assigned to one of several treatment conditions or groups is the same as their being assigned to any other group. A second type of control procedure is referred to as the *nonrandomized concurrent control*. Using this approach, outcome data collected from participants who are being treated with the standard of care or some other intervention (control) are compared with those who received the intervention being tested (experimental). Those in the so-called control group may have been treated by their dentist or physician in a particular way without any thought of using an alternative treatment, particularly an unproven or experimental one. This decision may have been made because the dentist or physician could have ethical misgivings about randomizing an individual in need of care. A third type of control is referred to as the *historical control procedure*. Historical controls are both nonrandom and nonconcurrent. They typically have received the "control" intervention prior to the administration of the experimental intervention.

There are limitations inherent in the use of nonrandom and/or nonconcurrent controls. For example, changes over time in the diagnostic criteria, the severity or characteristics of the disease being treated, the experience of the clinicians treating the disease, and the demographic characteristics and associated general health status or behavioral patterns of the populations from different geographical areas may all introduce extraneous variables that can bias the outcome of a trial and lead to incorrect conclusions.

Crossover or withdrawal controls. Crossover and *withdrawal controls* both require only one group of participants. The *withdrawal control* involves assessing the response to withdrawal or reduction of an experimental intervention. That is, individuals entering into a withdrawal trial first receive an intervention and their response to it is measured. This can be a drug, a diet, an exercise regimen, a behavioral treatment, or any intervention that *is not permanent*. After a prescribed period of time with the intervention, the intervention is withdrawn or reduced and the effect on the outcome measure is noted. This can be done repeatedly to ensure that it is the introduction and removal of the intervention per se that is responsible for the change in the outcome measurement. This approach is typically used in phase II studies with reversible interventions (e.g., drugs, exercise, diet) and is typically used for individuals with a chronic condition.

The *crossover control* involves shifting individuals from one intervention (A) to another (B). The interventions can both be new, or one can be the current standard of care or a placebo. The simplest case is what is referred to as a *two-period crossover,* in which individuals receive intervention A then B or B then A, the specific order being determined by random allocation. More complex arrangements can be used as well depending on the needs of the trial and the specific conclusions about the intervention(s) that are sought. A key point in this type of control is the *"wash-out" period* between the two interventions. Sufficient time should be allowed so that the effects of an intervention are not present before beginning the next intervention. This of course limits the use of the crossover to situations in which a period without intervention does not have untoward health effects. It is also limited to those interventions that do not cause permanent or very long-range changes. At the same time, however, a crossover control can be very useful in making direct comparisons of multiple interventions on the same individuals.

A unique and very creative application of the crossover design was employed by Burns and Elswick (2001) in a prospective, randomized trial on implant overdenture treatments. While not a phase III trial, this illustrates the point that even though the crossover procedure used to control for bias is typically said to be useful only for treatments that are reversible, or that at least do not cause permanent or long-lasting effects, it is possible to apply the approach in a wide variety of situations. In this trial, a four-period crossover design was employed to examine the efficacy of three overdenture treatments: (A) two-implant independently attached (O-ring) treatment; (B) two-implant, bar/clip-attached treatment; and (C) four-implant, bar/clip-attached treatment. Each participant had four implants placed into the anterior mandible and new dentures fabricated. After successful implant/tissue integration, participants were randomly assigned to one of six sequences of treatments as follows: A-B-C-C; A-C-B-B; B-A-C-C; B-C-A-A; C-A-B-B; C-B-A-A. The fourth period in each sequence allowed estimation of the carryover effect separate from any treatment effect. Participants were followed for at least 12 months before the mandibular denture was modified to incorporate the next treatment in the predefined treatment sequence. Outcome measures included prosthesis retention and stability using force measures, supporting and peri-implant tissue response using a criterion-based scoring system, participant satisfaction/preference and treatment complications/failures. While not typically used in phase III trials because of regulatory requirements, the crossover control can be useful in many instances when it is not possible to use independent experimental and control groups as in the instance when doing a clinical trial on rare or low-frequency diseases or when one of the other control procedures is not feasible.

12.5.4   Phase III trials are randomized

Random allocation of participants to treatment groups was derived from R. A. Fisher's work in agriculture in the 1940s. Randomized clinical trial designs have several important advantages over nonrandomized designs (Friedman et al., 1998). First, randomization removes the potential bias in the allocation of participants to groups. That is, it eliminates the possibility that a trial's outcome results from the assignment of participants to intervention groups in a biased or preferential manner and not from the effect of the intervention. Second, randomization tends to balance groups in terms of measured and unmeasured risk and prognostic factors for the disease. Third, the validity of the statistical tests of significance is guaranteed when subjects are randomly assigned to groups. This validity is independent of how well prognostic factors are balanced between groups (Friedman et al., 1998). Nonrandomized trials require that imbalances be managed post hoc and in ways that may be difficult to validate. Accidental biases occur when groups are not balanced for important covariates, and are more likely to affect small rather than large randomized trials:

Participant selection and randomization. It is important in clinical trials research to consider the characteristics of both the participants who are selected to participate in the trial and who complete the trial. A guiding principle here is that *we can only generalize results of a phase III trial to the population that shares the same characteristics as the group that completes the trial.* There are some exceptions to this generalization and design approaches that can be used (e.g., the intent-to-treat design). However, in general, it is important to at least keep the principle in mind and to adhere to it.

In selecting study populations, investigators should take into consideration not only gender, age, ethnicity, race, and socioeconomic status, but also the entire breadth of health/disease characteristics of individuals for whom a specific preventive regimen, diagnostic, or treatment might be used. The next logical question then is: How many variables should one include in order to generalize findings broadly? There is no simple answer to this question. Part of the answer depends on how much is known about the distribution, etiology, and pathogenesis of the disease for which the intervention is designed. The answer also depends on how much is known about the site(s) and mode(s) of action of the intervention. The more that is known about the disease, its prevention, diagnosis, and/or treatment, the more likely it is that the variables important in influencing the clinical outcome can be identified.

Participant selection and randomization can influence the generalizability of the trial's results. We can illustrate this by tracking how a sample is derived from the population for inclusion in the trial. Once the disease or condition is determined, the next step is to identify who with the disease will and will not be eligible to participate. In general, the more that is known about a disease's etiology, pathogenesis, and aims of current treatments, the more refined the selection criteria will be. Investigators may exclude patients with significant comorbid conditions, very early or late-stage disease, or those who have been treated previously for the same condition. In general, phase III trials should be more rather than less inclusive in order to maximize generalizability and facilitate recruitment.

Once the target population is defined, potential participants are recruited, screened, and consented into the trial. It is important to characterize in detail the trial's recruitment and final sample populations. Screening failures and the reasons for failure should be recorded. Baseline information should be collected and maintained from individuals who are deemed eligible but later refuse to participate in the trial. Comparisons between this group and the final sample can determine if the trial population was highly self-selected in terms of important disease risk or prognostic factors. If it is, conclusions about the efficacy of the intervention must be tempered and limited only to those who share characteristics with the study sample.

Many scientific journals require that clinical trials reports include a flow diagram to enable the reader to quickly assess the relative efficiency of the screening process, common reasons that patients were ineligible, and the fraction of randomized subjects for whom outcome data was collected (see, e.g., www.consort-statement.org). Figure 12.2 depicts the flow of participants in a phase III oral health-related clinical trial, the obstetrics and periodontal therapy (OPT) trial (Michalowicz et al., 2006). For example, in the OPT trial, roughly 3,500 patients were screened in obstetrics clinics. Obstetricians and clinic staff were asked to refer all patients to study personnel, particularly if either the physician or staff noticed signs of gingival inflammation or the patient reported signs or symptoms of periodontal disease. Of these, 929 appeared to meet the study's eligibility criteria in terms of age, medical history, estimated gestational age, and extent and severity of periodontitis. These patients were referred for comprehensive baseline examinations. From the figure, one can readily determine that the final study sample represents only a fraction of pregnant women who sought prenatal care before 17 weeks of gestation.

Following the baseline examination, an additional 119 women did not meet the trial's eligibility criteria. Eight hundred and twenty-three women were randomized using a process that was stratified by enrollment site and managed by the trial's data coordinating center.

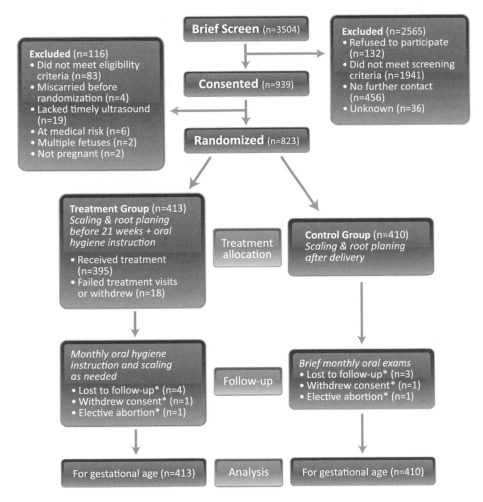

Figure 12.2   Participant selection and randomization in the obstetrics and periodontal therapy (OPT) trial. Source: Michalowicz et al. (2006).

Randomization and stratification. Randomization in multicenter phase III trials should be stratified by enrollment site to help maintain balance across centers. Enrollment success is often skewed across centers, with some centers randomizing large numbers of subjects and others relatively few. Patient characteristics, including the severity and extent of disease, and therapist experience and efficiency may also vary among sites. In some instances, investigators may stratify randomization based on important baseline characteristics that affect susceptibility to disease (risk factors) or are known to affect the response to treatment (prognostic factors).

In large clinical trials, randomization tends to balance measured and unmeasured risk and prognostic factors (Friedman et al., 1998). For smaller trials, however, stratification by select baseline characteristics can help protect against imbalances. For example, in testing a treatment for a disease in which prevalence differs by gender and treatment response by smoking status, eligible participants are first grouped into strata (female smokers, female nonsmokers, male smokers, male nonsmokers) and randomized to treatment groups within these strata. Stratifying the randomization process increases the chance that the treatment groups will be balanced in terms of the selected risk and prognostic factors. In smaller trials, stratification should be limited to only the most important factors because of the difficulty in recruiting sufficient numbers of subjects into each substratum. Because of their size, phase III clinical trials generally do not use stratified randomization schemes.

Patient and operator reluctance to participate in a randomized clinical trial. While a randomized trial design is appealing in many ways to investigators, it may not be to patients or clinicians. Patients who are recruited for a clinical trial are often ill and are seeking treatment for their illness. When faced with the notion that interventions will be allocated by chance alone, patients may refuse to participate if they can be assured of receiving a relatively untested but perceived state-of-the-art treatment outside of the trial. A patient's interest in a trial may depend on the length of treatment, the severity of their condition, the urgency of the need for treatment, the known effectiveness of nonexperimental interventions, and other factors. Offering all participants access to the most effective treatment after the trial is completed may mitigate a patient's reluctance to enroll in the trial. However, this must not be used to coerce participation and the potential risks as well as benefits of randomization to an experimental treatment must be clearly presented to potential participants. Guarantees must also be in place to ensure that a patient's refusal to participate in the trial will not affect their relationship with their care provider or the institution.

Participants are randomized after they are deemed eligible for and committed to the trial. Biases that plague nonrandomized trials may also affect randomized trials if a participant's willingness to participate depends on his or her assignment to a particular treatment group. Consider, for example, a single-masked trial designed to compare a minimally invasive restorative procedure to a remineralization protocol for the treatment of incipient dental caries. Concerns about the study results may arise if patients who were randomized to the restorative group were less likely to undergo this care because of their desire to receive the more conservative remineralization treatment. Potential problems associated with patient treatment preferences are circumvented in double-masked clinical trials, in which neither the participant nor the individual administering the treatment is aware of which treatment the participant receives.

Clinicians may be reluctant to participate in clinical trials because their patients may receive what is later shown to be an ineffective therapy. Also, clinicians may prefer one intervention over another, which can create a bias, recognized or not, in favor of their preferred treatment. The issue of clinician preferences within the randomized clinical trial has been addressed by Korn and Baumrind (1991) who proposed an experimental design that takes into account clinician preferences. In their approach, each eligible participant is assessed by a panel of clinicians. If the panel agrees on a preferred course of treatment (i.e., clinical equipoise exists for those patients), that patient is not randomized into the trial. Participants not vetted at this stage are assessed by a second panel of clinicians who are willing and able to treat the patient. If the panel disagrees about what constitutes preferred treatment (i.e., clinical equipoise does not exist), the patient is consented and randomized into the trial. The patient is then assigned to a clinician who initially favored the treatment to which the patient was subsequently and randomly assigned.

There are limitations to this approach including that it may take longer and be more costly to get to the stage of randomization than in the more typical design, it can only be used when participants have no preexisting relationship with participating clinicians, it takes more work on the part of participating clinicians in that they must be willing to screen all potential participants, the design may not be appropriate for those diseases that require immediate treatment, interactions between clinician preference and the treatment used may make interpretation of results difficult, and objective screening criteria may not be adequate. Finally, results from such trials may also not be accepted by the Food and Drug Administration.

Randomization of enrollment centers. While the allocation of patients to study groups is random, the selection of enrollment centers is not. Enrollment centers are often selected based on their proven ability to enroll sufficient numbers of participants, adhere to study protocols, and collect complete and accurate data. Successful enrollment centers may serve populations that are highly motivated to participate in research, are less sick, or both. Such characteristics can have profound effects on the outcome of a trial. For example, if a site's clinic population tends to have less severe disease or is otherwise healthy, a test intervention may appear more effective than it would be when used in a less healthy population or in patients with complex medical needs. Although the trial may find important clinical differences between test and control groups, it may not be appropriate to generalize findings from the trial to the general population that is likely to be more heterogeneous. Presumably, phase IV trials, in which the treatment is tested in general clinical practice, will detect these subtle differences or inconsistencies among groups.

12.5.5 Participant selection and randomization: to whom are findings generalizable?

Done correctly, phase III trials allow us to generalize findings from a relatively small group to entire populations. However, we are always faced with the question as to whether the group that completes the trial is representative of the population to which we would like to make generalizations about the efficacy of the intervention? In any trial, there are those who are enrolled but never get randomized, those who get randomized but never treated, and those who begin treatment but do not finish. These "dropouts" play a critical role in defining the characteristics of the sample that completes the entire trial and hence the population to whom results of the trial are applicable.

It does not end there either. Among those who stay enrolled in a trial, there are individuals who do not comply with the protocol for any of a number of reasons (e.g., they do not understand what they are supposed to do; they are using the trial for their health care and only do those things that they feel will help; they do not get randomized to the treatment of their choice). Beyond that, there are a variety of factors that can introduce bias into a trial. These factors include *participant motivation* (e.g., motivation to enroll, comply with the protocol, complete the trail), *demographics* (e.g., SES, ethnic/race/culture/nationality, neighborhood of residence, age, gender, social mobility), and *medical/dental history* (e.g., severity of illness, presence of comorbid conditions). Other potential biasing factors stem from the fact that many phase III trials are conducted at academic health centers. One could question whether or not patients who go to *academic health centers* for care, and in doing so are most likely to be given the opportunity to enroll in a phase III trial, are representative of the entire patient population for any given disease. Even within a trial, it is unlikely that individuals at multiple sites are all the same. As we will discuss in the next section, there are other factors that may further limit the generalizations that we are able to make because they place additional constraints on the heterogeneity of the group that completes a trial.

In the face of all of these potential biasing factors, we assume that random assignment will distribute them evenly among the treatment groups. That is to say, they would not have more of an effect on one group within the trial than among others. And, as we have pointed out, the use of an "intent-to-treat design can lessen the impact of biasing factors on the outcome of the trial." The intent to treat approach, however, does not help us deal with selection bias that influences the characteristics of the individuals who complete the trial. And it is these characteristics that determine the population to which the results can be generalized.

As noted by Begg et al. (1996), ". . . the report *(of the trial)* . . . needs to convey to the reader relevant information concerning the design, conduct, analysis and generalizability of the trial. This information should provide . . . the ability to make informed judgments regarding the internal and external validity of the trial. . ." (emphasis ours)

12.6   Recruitment and retention of participants in phase III trials

Phase III trials typically involve multiple enrollment centers for several reasons. Because phase III trials are large, it is unlikely that enough participants would be available at a single center. The inclusion of multiple enrollment centers also helps to ensure the sample population is diverse and the results are generalizable. Phase III trials must also maximize participant retention because losses to follow-up introduces a bias that cannot be fully quantified or managed.

Participant recruitment. For intervention trials, the sample should be representative of clinic populations in terms of demographics and disease extent and severity. Strategies for successful recruitment are population specific (e.g., Milgrom et al., 1997; MacEntee et al., 2002). Trust in researchers (e.g., Katz et al., 2003, 2008), views about health and healthy behavior (Atchison and Fagan, 2003), variations in the clinical manifestations of the disease (e.g., Barrow et al., 2003; Craig et al., 2003; Cruz et al., 2003; Linke et al., 2003), age- and ethnicity-appropriateness of the approach used in recruitment (MacEntee et al., 2002), and changes in the incidence of the disease or condition among groups (e.g., Dasanayake et al., 2003; Leathers et al., 2003) can all affect recruitment success. Whatever the reason(s), recruitment plans must be sufficiently broad and flexible to ensure that individuals from all at-risk populations have an opportunity to participate.

Milgrom et al. (1997) have suggested that study design can play an important role in enhancing or interfering with recruitment. Narrowly defined, entry criteria can have a negative effect on recruitment. The use of a "run-in" or pretreatment period can help expand the pool of eligible participants and can also possibly identify individuals who are likely to drop out of the trial or be poor compliers with the protocol. Conversely, Data and Safety Monitoring Board can have a positive effect on recruitment by requiring the study team to regularly report recruitment progress. This motivational aspect of the DSMB is important and can be enhanced if the trial team sets recruitment goals at the start of the trial by using visual or graphical representations to depict planned and actual enrollment.

Participant retention. Another key to the successful phase III clinical trial is preventing participant dropout. On the one hand, the informed consent should make it clear that individuals are free to discontinue their participation in a trial without any negative consequences at any time during the trial. It should also be made clear that their decision to not participate in the trial at any time will in no way affect their ability to be treated for their condition. At the same time, much can be learned about the test intervention from individuals who drop out. It is imperative to collect health status and demographic information from those who refuse to enter the trial as well as those who drop out. This will not only tell us whether those who drop out are comparable to those who stay in the trial until the end, but it may also provide insight into the type of person for whom the intervention is best suited. For example, individuals will drop out if the protocol is too onerous (e.g., the intervention is painful, takes too much time, takes too long, has a heavy response burden) or if it conflicts with their beliefs about health and healthy behaviors.

The issue of response burden on participants is an important one and totally within the control of the clinical trial team. There is always a reason for collecting one more behavioral or biological sample. It goes something like this: "[W]e might as well get another _____ sample (*you fill in the blank*) as long as the participants are here." Decisions about adding an additional sample should be made very carefully as they could add enough to the response burden to make individuals feel that the requirements of the trial are too great causing them to drop out of the trial or, if they do stay, to follow the protocol as intended by the study. To guard against the tendency to add many additional tests, keep in mind that the primary purpose for doing a phase III trial is to test the safety, efficacy, or effectiveness of a given intervention. Everything else is secondary and anything that increases the potential for participants to drop out because the response burden on them is too high should be avoided at all costs.

Participant adherence. Adherence to or compliance with the protocol is another aspect of participant retention (Whitney and Dworkin, 1997). Adherence refers to the extent to which participants in clinical trials act in accordance with the protocol to which they have been randomized. Participants who do not adhere to a trial can introduce a level of variability in the data that can obscure or bias a treatment effect. Tracking adherence and reasons for nonadherence can also be very informative as it may reflect an aspect of the intervention that may adversely affect its acceptance in clinical practice.

There are a variety of ways to determine if participants are adhering to various protocol requirements. Robiner (2005), for example, refers to a number of strategies for assessing and enhancing adherence, including the use of biological markers to quantify exposure to pharmacological agents and microchip-based monitoring systems (embedded in medication dispensers) to identify drug compliance. Of course, simply opening a bottle or tube or counting pills at participant visits does not ensure that participants ingested the pills as prescribed. Corroborating information is necessary to ensure that pills, for example, have actually been ingested after having been removed from the bottle or that other aspects of the protocol have been followed.

A point raised by Milgrom et al. (1997) is important here. They note that, for treatment trials in particular, many of the participants are those individuals who have not been adherent to either prevention strategies or other treatment approaches. That is to say they are eligible for a treatment trial because their behavior was such that they did not adhere to preventive or other treatment regimens and now are seeking help with a health problem. Past behavior is often the best predictor of future behavior, particularly when health practices are concerned. While investigators may be tempted to enroll only individuals who are likely to adhere to the protocol, such an approach can result in a homogeneous sample, which may limit the generalizability of the findings and violate some of the underlying assumptions of the statistical tests employed in the analysis. Results from a homogeneous sample may overestimate the efficacy of the intervention. In general, it is preferable to have a heterogeneous sample, one that will include both adherent and nonadherent participants. In such situations, we come back to the intent-to-treat design that can adjust for nonadherence and drop out in a way that will more accurately reflect the overall impact of the experimental intervention patient populations.

12.7   Oversight of the phase III trial: shared responsibilities

The fact that most phase III clinical trials involve multiple centers not only increases the administrative complexity in conducting the trial but it also increases the complexity and difficulty of providing timely and sufficient oversight. Several independent groups may be responsible for overseeing parts or all of the trial. These include the trial's Steering Committee, Institutional Review Boards, Data and Safety Monitoring Board, the trial sponsor, and possibly regulatory agencies such as the FDA. Each of these groups plays a unique role. Together they complement each other in providing oversight of the trial. A general framework for a trial's oversight and operations is given in Figure 12.3.

Requirements of the various oversight groups or committees may vary. For example, while most oversight groups use similar definitions for adverse events, the required content

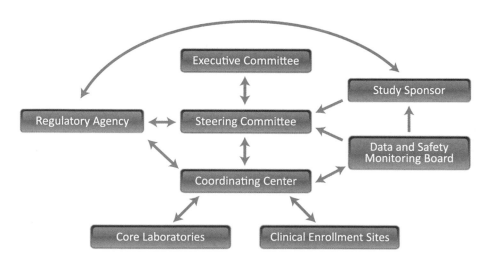

Figure 12.3   General oversight structure and relationships for phase III clinical trials. Adapted, with minor revisions, from Califf and DeMets (2002).

of event reports and the timing of their submission following discovery of an event may vary among the DSMB, regulatory bodies, and IRB. Meeting the needs and requirements of all relevant oversight bodies can be particularly challenging in multinational trials, where laws and policies concerning human subject research may vary by country and region. Study leaders must clarify any disparate requirements before the trial commences and establish a reporting protocol that meets the requirement of all the relevant oversight bodies. Investigators should not underestimate the amount of time and effort needed to oversee these aspects of phase III trial operations. Tasks and responsibilities should be delegated to specific study personnel or groups in the MOP and progress toward meeting these responsibilities should be monitored regularly throughout the trial.

12.7.1   Institutional review boards

The reader is referred to Chapter 3 for a more detailed discussion of Institutional Review Boards. In general, IRBs act to ensure that investigators and the trial meet the Belmont principles of respect (for persons), justice, and beneficence. This independent review board helps ensure that participants are not subject to undue or inappropriate risks and that their participation remains voluntary and based on a clear understanding of the trial, its risks, and alternatives.

In addition to providing preapproval for each phase III trial site, the IRB must be informed when a serious adverse event, particularly an unexpected one, occurs at any site. This enables the IRB to assess if the risk–benefit ratio for the trial has changed, regardless of where or when the event(s) occurred. Adverse event reports and any deidentified follow-up information may be sent by the study manager to the local site PI and the respective IRB. The Data and Safety Monitoring Board can also facilitate this process (see below).

12.7.2   Data and safety monitoring boards

The U.S. government requires that all government-sponsored, multicenter phase III trials establish a DSMB. DSMB serve in an advisory role to both the investigators and the funding agency and should include experts in biostatistics, clinical trial methodology, ethics, and the relevant medical or dental discipline. The DSMB can include ex officio members from the data coordinating center, the investigative team, and the funding agency. Generally, only independent members are allowed to vote on issues brought before the DSMB.

The major roles of the DSMB are to review and approve the study's plans to ensure patient safety, monitor compliance with or deviations from the study protocol, and evaluate the overall performance of the trial and the integrity of the data being collected. They are independent of the investigative group and sponsor and should have no vested interests in the trial's outcomes or conflicts of interests. It is advisable to ask each member of the DSMB to sign a prepared statement indicating that they have no real or perceived conflicts of interest in terms of affiliation with the study team or with regard to any products used in the study. These signed statements should be kept on file by the study team.

The size of the DSMB and the frequency of its meetings are dictated by the nature, complexity, and size of the trial. It should review the trial's progress on a regular basis, typically annually. Changes in the timing of DSMB meetings may be dictated by interim analyses or accumulated adverse events. During their review, using the trial timeline developed before the beginning of the trial, members of the DSMB typically evaluate the trial's progress with recruitment, enrollment, randomization, and follow-up. Individuals attending closed portions of DSMB meeting, particularly ex officio members, must be unmasked since the DSMB receives and discusses interim endpoint reports during this period.

The DSMB also monitors the well-being and safety of participants by reviewing the occurrence of sentinel health events, or side effects. While these events are not typically used as endpoints in clinical trials, they can be indicators that an intervention is harmful to health in general even though it may be effective in addressing a particular disease. Side effects may not only result directly from administration of the intervention being tested but, depending on the specific design of the trial, may also be the result of the type of control condition(s) used.

In the Children's Amalgam Trial (DeRouen et al., 2002; McKinlay et al., 2003), the two study groups monitored participants for any unexpected medical diagnoses or health events during the trial. Both groups developed systems for monitoring sentinel events. In one of the trials (DeRouen et al., 2002), a three-component monitoring system was used. The system involved an annual short health history questionnaire sent to parents of participants, a structured set of health history questions administered by a dental hygienist at the time of the annual exam, and consultation with teachers and school officials, including the school physician, to detect specific diagnoses and/or extended absences that might be related to illness. If any of these sources suggested a health problem, designated trial personnel sought consent to access to the medical records and confirm the event(s). Annual reporting to the DSMB included endpoint information and statistical analyses of sentinel health events.

The DSMB can facilitate the work of the IRB by providing regular feedback to them throughout the trial. Meeting summaries and recommendations are sent to the IRB following each meeting. Because the DSMB review study progress, interim data, and adverse events reports across clinical sites, they are often very well positioned to assess overall risk to participants and can use this information to inform individual the IRB. Because the DSMB review otherwise masked interim results, the IRB may defer to them and not require investigators to submit interim results from their site. Reports from the DSMB to the IRB, however, report adverse events or toxicity reports in aggregate.

12.7.3   Steering committees

In a multicenter phase III clinical trial, the SC designs, executes, and disseminates the study (Califf and DeMets, 2002). The SC generally consists of the overall principal investigator, the directors of the data coordinating center and laboratory cores, several enrollment site PI, and possibly an individual from the trial's sponsor. The specific roles and responsibilities of the SC vary from trial to trial. In general, however, it is responsible for the trial's overall operations. Most SCs are responsible for the distribution of resources to the various components of the trial. They may target additional resources to lagging or underperforming sites or, on occasion, redistribute resources by closing some sites and identifying new ones. For larger trials, an executive committee, made up as a subgroup of the SC, is charged with managing more time-sensitive or critical issues that arise during the trial.

Trial monitoring plans, which are developed by the SC with input from the data co-ordinating center, should consider the number of enrollment sites, study procedures, and amount of clinical and laboratory data collected. Study leaders should ensure that all phases of the trial are monitored in a meaningful, consistent, and regular manner. Problems with protocol violations and data quality can arise in phase III clinical trials when the SC assumes but does not verify that operations are being conducted as planned. Importantly, the SC must ensure that study site coordinators are aware of all protocol updates and reconsent participants using updated informed consent documents if necessary.

SCs may also review proposals for ancillary studies. Publications subcommittees, which review proposals for meeting abstracts, presentations, and manuscripts, are generally appointed by or are subsets of the SC. The SC should develop or adopt a detailed and clear publications policy when the MOP is written in order to minimize later confusion and potential conflict regarding authorship. SCs typically are responsible for final review and approval of trial manuscripts.

With few exceptions, the SC remains masked in the trial. It neither review interim results nor review adverse events or protocol violations that require the study to become unmasked. Only members of the DSMB and the study biostatistician are unmasked. The SC should, however, monitor enrollment progress, protocol violations, and data quality reports summarizing the timeliness and accuracy of data submissions. The SC can also provide advice and assistance to the underperforming enrollment sites. Specific parameters for improved performance should be communicated in writing to affected sites. The SC can assist underperforming sites by arranging face-to-face meetings or videoconferences between personnel from well- and underperforming centers. The focus of the SC's initial work in this regard should be to provide assistance and guidance to underperforming sites. However, as indicated earlier, when sufficient attention is paid to organizational and communication issues early in the trial planning process, problems involving underperforming sites can be minimized and identified quickly.

12.8   Concluding comment

Throughout this chapter, we have emphasized that phase III trials test the efficacy of new interventions under highly structured conditions. We have also emphasized that phase III trial results are generalizable to the extent that the trial's conditions and participants mirror the broader clinical and patient communities. Einstein is credited with saying that, in constructing experimental models, "everything should be made as simple as possible, but not simpler." While in some instances, this approach can help us understand complex phenomena such as those involved in testing the safety, effectiveness, and efficacy of an intervention, it may also contain an inherent danger of simplifying something that is inherently very complex. As clinical researcher/orthodontist, Sheldon Baumrind (1993) states:

> If the experimental model one studies underestimates or misrepresents the complexity of the system(s) in which one is really interested, the answer(s) one arrives at is (are) likely to be simplistic rather than simple.

The art of designing and carrying out phase III clinical trials lies in reaching an appropriate balance between developing the appropriate experimental model, one that represents the idealized clinical situation while not oversimplifying an otherwise highly complex system. With careful and broad-based planning, phase III trials can become experimental models of clinical practice in which decisions about what is best for our patients are dictated by reliable and valid data.

References

Angell M. 1997. The ethics of clinical research in the third world. *New England Journal of Medicine* 337:847–849.

Annas GJ, Grodin MA. 1998. Human rights and maternal-fetal HIV transmission prevention trials in Africa. *American Journal of Public Health* 88:560–563.

Atchison KA, Fagan L. 2003. Understanding health behavior and perceptions. *Dental Clinics of North America* 47 (Special Issue 1: Minority Oral Health): 21–39.

Barrow SL, Xionan X, LeGeros AR, Mijares DQ, Legeros RZ, Galvis DL, Snead M, Tavares M, Cruz GD. 2003. Dental caries prevalence among a sample of African American adults in New York city. *Dental Clinics of North America* 47 (Special Issue 1: Minority Oral Health): 57–65.

Baumrind S. 1993. The role of clinical research in orthodontics. *The Angle Orthodontist* 63:235–240.

Bayer R. 1998. The debate of maternal-fetal HIV transmission prevention trials in Africa, Asia and the Caribbean: racist exploitation or exploitation of racism? *American Journal of Public Health* 88:567–570.

Begg C, Cho M, Eastwood S, Horton R, Moher D, Olkin I, Pitkin R, Rennie K, Schultz F, Simel D, Stoup DF. 1996. Improving the quality of reporting of randomized controlled trials. *Journal of the American Medical Association* 276:637–639.

Braunholtz DA, Edwards SJ, Lilford RJ. 2001. Are randomized clinical trials good for us (in the short term)? Evidence for a "trial effect". *Journal of Clinical Epidemiology* 54:217–224.

Brownlee S. 2007. *Overtreated: Why Too Much Medicine Is Making Us Sicker and Poorer*. Bloomsbury: New America Foundation.

Burns DR, Elswick RK. 2001. Equivalence testing with dental clinical trials. *Journal of Dental Research* 80:1513–1517.

Califf RM, DeMets DL. 2002. Principles from clinical trials relevant to clinical practice: part II. *Circulation* 106:880–886.

Craig RG, Yip JK, Mijares DQ, Boyland RJ, Haffajee AD, Socransky S. 2003. Destructive periodontal diseases in minority populations. *Dental Clinics of North America* 47 (Special Issue 1: Minority Oral Health): 103–114.

Cruz GD, Galvis DL, Barrow SL, LeGeros AR, Xionan X, Taveres M, LeGeros RZ. 2003. Dental health status and indicators of treatment needs of four hispanic subgroups in New York city. *Dental Clinics of North America* 47 (Special Issue 1: Minority Oral Health): 41–55.

Dasanayake AP, Russell S Boyd D, Madianos PH, Foster T. 2003. Preterm low birth weight and periodontal disease in African Americans. *Dental Clinics of North America* 47 (Special Issue 1: Minority Oral Health): 115–125.

DeRouen TA, Leroux BG, Martin MD, Townes BD, Woods JS, Leitao J, Castro-Caldas A, Braveman N. 2002. Issues in design and analysis of a randomized clinical trial to assess the safety of dental amalgam restorations in children. *Controlled Clinical Trials* 23:301–320.

DiAmici D, Klersy C, Ramajoli F, Brustia L, Pierluigi P. 2000. Impact of the Hawthorne effect in a longitudinal clinical study: the case of anesthesia. *Controlled Clinical Trials* 21:103–114.

Fleming TR. 2005. Surrogate endpoints and FDA's accelerated approval process. *Health Affairs* 24:67–78.

Fleming TR, DeMets DL. 1996. Surrogate end points in clinical trials: are we being misled? *Annals of Internal Medicine* 125:605–613.

Formica M, Kabbara K, Clark R, McAlindon T. 2004. Can clinical trials requiring frequent participation contact be conducted over the internet? Results from an online randomized controlled trial evaluating a topical ointment for herpes labialis. *Journal of Medical Internet Research* 6 (1), e6. Available online at http://www.jmir.org/2004/1/e6/.

Friedman LM, Furberg CCD, DeMets DL. 1998. *Fundamentals of Clinical Trials, Third Edition.* New York: Springer.

Karim SS. 1998. Placebo controls in HIV perinatal transmission trials: a South African's viewpoint. *American Journal of Public Health* 88:564–566.

Katz RV, Kegeles SS, Green BL, Kressin NR, James SA, Claudio C. 2003. The Tuskegee legacy project: history, preliminary scientific findings, and unanticipated society benefits. *Dental Clinics of North America* 47 (Special Issue 1: Minority Oral Health): 1–19.

Katz RV, Kegeles SS, Kressin NR, Green L, James SA, Wang MQ, Russell SL, Caludio C. 2008. Awareness of the Tuskegee Syphilis study and the US presidential apology and their influence on minority participation in biomedical research. *American Journal of Public Health* 98:1137–1142.

Koch GG, Paquette DW. 1997. Design principles and statistical considerations in periodontal clinical trials. *Annals of Periodontology* 2:42–63.

Korn EL, Baumrind S. 1991. Randomized clinical trials with clinician-preferred treatment. *The Lancet* 337:149–152.

Leathers R, Le AD, Black E, McQuirer JL. 2003. Orofacial injury in underserved minority populations. *Dental Clinics of North America* 47 (Special Issue 1: Minority Oral Health): 127–139.

Levine RJ, Dennison DK. 1997. Randomized trials in periodontology: ethical considerations. *Annals of Periodontology* 2:83–94.

Linke HAB, Kuyinu EO, Ogundare B, Imam MM, Kahn SH, Olawoye OO, LeGeros RZ. 2003. Microbiological composition of whole saliva and caries experience in minority populations. *Dental Clinics of North America* 47 (Special Issue 1: Minority Oral Health): 67–86.

MacEntee, MI, Wyatt C, Kiyak HA, Jujoel PP, Persson RE, Persson GR, Powell LV. 2002. Response to direct and indirect recruitment for a randomized dental clinical trial in a multicultural population of elders. *Community Dental Oral Epidemiology* 30:377–381.

Marks RG. 2004. The future of web-based clinical research in dentistry. *Journal of Dental Research* 83 (Special Issue): C25–C28.

Marks R, Conlon M, Pepine CJ. 2001a. Enhancing clinical trials on the internet: lessons from INVEST. *Clinical Cardiology* 24:17–23.

Marks RG, Conlon M, Ruberg SJ. 2001b. Paradigm shifts in clinical trials enabled by information technology. *Statistics in Medicine* 20:2683–2696.

McKinlay S, Meurer EA, Assmann SF, Bellinger D, Taveres M, Daniel DB, Clarkson T, Cernichiari E, Barregard L, Braveman NS. 2003. The children's amalgam trial: design and methods. *Contemporary Clinical Trials* 24:795–814.

Meinert CL. 1986. *Clinical Trials: Design, Conduct and Analysis.* New York: Oxford University Press.

Michalowicz BS, Hodges JS, DiAngelix AJ, Lupo VR, Novak MJ, Ferguson JE, Buchanan W, Bofill J, Papapanou PN, Mitchell DA, Matseonane S, Tschida PA. 2006. Treatment of periodontal disease and risk of preterm birth. *The New England Journal of Medicine* 355:1885–1894.

Milgrom PM, Hujoel PP, Weinstein P, Holborow DW. 1997. Subject recruitment, retention and compliance in clinical trials in periodontics. *Annals of Periodontology* 2:64–74.

Moseley JB, O'Malley K, Petersen NJ, Menke TJ, Brody BA, Kuykendall DH, Hollingsworth JC, Ashton CM, Wray NP. 2002. A controlled trial of arthroscopic surgery for osteoarthritis of the knee. *The New England Journal of Medicine* 347:81–88.

Naydeck BL, Sutton-Tyrrell K, Burek K, Sopko GS. 1996. Organizational structure and communication strategies of the bypass angioplasty revascularization investigation: a multicenter clinical trial. *Controlled Clinical Trials* 17:226–234.

Piantodosi S. 2005. *Clinical Trials (Second Edition).* New York: Wiley. Available online at http://www3.interscience.wiley.com/cgi-bin/bookhome/109921043?CRETRY=1&SRETRY=0.

Polson AM. 1997. The research team, calibration and quality assurance in clinical trials in periodontics. *Annals of Periodontology* 2:75–82.

Proceedings of the ICW–CCT. 2004. Proceedings: International consensus workshop on caries clinical trials (ICW–CCT). *Journal of Dental Research* 83 (Special Issue): 125–129.

Robiner WN. 2005. Enhancing adherence in clinical research. *Contemporary Clinical Trials* 26:59–77.

The Cardiac Arrhythmia Suppression Trial (CAST) Investigators. 1989. Preliminary report: effect of encainide and flecainide on mortality in a randomized trial of arrhythmia suppression after myocardial infarction. *The New England Journal of Medicine* 321:406–412.

Wager TD, Nitschke JB. 2005. Placebo effects in the brain: linking mental and physiological processes. *Brain, Behavior and Immunity* 19:281–282.

Whitehead J. 2004. Stopping rules of clinical trials. *Controlled Clinical Trials* 25:69–70.

Whitney CW, Dworkin SF. 1997. Practical implications of noncompliance in randomized clinical trials for temporomandibular disorders. *Journal of Orofacial Pain* 11:130–138.

13

Postmarketing surveillance

Eugenio D. Beltrán-Aguilar, DMD, MPH, MS, DrPH, and Michael C. Manz, DDS, MPH, DrPH

13.1 Objective

This chapter will review the scientific and regulatory basis, importance, and process of monitoring side effects of drug products and medical devices in the United States and abroad, focusing on areas of interest to dental researchers and clinicians.

13.2 Definitions

13.2.1 Public health surveillance and postmarketing surveillance

The Centers for Disease Control and Prevention (CDC) has defined *public health surveillance* as (Thacker and Berkelman, 1988):

> The ongoing, systematic collection, analysis and interpretation of health data essential to the planning, implementation, and evaluation of public health practice, closely integrated with the timely dissemination of these data to those who need to know. The final link of the surveillance chain is the application of these data to prevention and control.

When this definition is applied to the monitoring of health events specifically caused by the use of drug products, we enter into the domain of what is known as pharmacosurveillance. This term, however, tends to limit the scope of this type of surveillance to drug products. Medical devices are also the subject of surveillance. Therefore, in this chapter, the term *"postmarketing surveillance"* will include the monitoring of adverse health events caused by drugs and devices.

13.3   Three examples of side effects

The February 2008 issue of the *Journal of the American Dental Association* includes three articles with one underlying common issue: reporting on adverse effects of drugs or dental materials. The paper by Lauterbach and associates (Lauterbach et al., 2008) compared neurological outcomes among two groups of children participating in a 7-year randomized clinical trial. One group of children received mercury-based dental amalgams while the other received composite resins. The trial was designed to compare neurological outcomes, not to test the clinical performance of the dental materials. The second paper by Mandel and Alfi (2008) reported on two cases of HIV patients receiving highly active antiretroviral therapy causing unusual deposition of fat in the subcutaneous area of the parotid, a manifestation of lipodystrophy syndrome. The third paper by McCoy and associates (McCoy et al., 2008) presented self-reported side effects of chlorhexidine used as an adjunctive therapeutic in a clinical trial measuring the effect of periodontal treatment on glycemic control among veterans with poorly controlled diabetes.

Neurological outcomes (allegedly caused by mercury exposure), clinical enlargement of the parotideal area (a head and neck side effect of the antiretroviral therapy), and change in taste sensation and staining of teeth (produced by chlorhexidine) are examples of *adverse effects* in the head and neck area associated with pharmaceutical products (HIV antiretrovirals, chlorhexidine) or devices (dental amalgam). These adverse effects are of direct interest to patients, who experience the effects; the researcher and manufacturer, who either developed or tested the therapeutic agent or device; and the clinician who, most of the time, is the first to recognize signs and symptoms of these adverse effects. We should also mention that although dental professionals may notice specific adverse effects as a direct consequence of practicing dentistry (Schedle et al., 2008), these are clinical practice and occupational exposure issues not within the scope of this chapter.

13.4   Burden

No pharmaceutical is completely safe. Approximately 100,000 deaths and over 1.5 million hospitalizations occur every year in the United States due to adverse drug reactions/experiences (ADR or ADE—see definitions) (Lazarou et al., 1998; Elixhauser and Owens, 2007), and over 350,000 ADE occur in nursing homes (Gurwitz et al., 2000). In the 1990s, it cost $30 billion annually to treat ADE (Johnson and Bartman, 1995). The Agency of Healthcare Research and Quality estimates that it costs up to $5.6 million per hospital to treat ADE (www.ahrq.gov/qual/aderia/aderia.htm). What makes these data more compelling is that 20–70% of these events are preventable (Strom, 2005). Furthermore, drugs and medical devices are used to prevent, cure, or alleviate disease and its *sequelae*; thus, there is an expectation that they prevent disease or improve health, not otherwise.

According to the Pharmaceutical Research and Manufacturers of America (PhRMA, www.phrma.org), an organization representing the major pharmaceutical companies in the United States, the amount invested in research and development industry-wide was $58.8 billion in 2007, an increase of $3 billion from the previous year.

13.4.1   Adverse drug reaction, adverse drug experience

Adverse drug reaction is an undesirable or toxic effect produced or contributed by a marketed drug, including the failure of the pharmacologic agent to produce the desired effect (Arrowsmith-Lowe, 2000). Other terms used in the literature include "adverse effects," "side effects," and "adverse events." The Food and Drug Administration (FDA) uses the term "Adverse Drug Experience," which is defined as (U.S. Department of Health and Human Services, Food and Drug Administration, 1885[1]):

> Any adverse event associated with the use of a drug in humans, whether or not considered drug related, including the following: an adverse event occurring in the course of the use of a drug product in professional practice; an adverse event occurring from drug overdose, whether accidental or intentional; an adverse event occurring from drug abuse; an adverse event occurring from drug withdrawal; and any significant failure of expected pharmacological action.

Additionally, the FDA defines "serious" ADE, as those resulting in death, threat to life, hospitalization or prolongation of existing hospitalization, persistent or significant disability/incapacity, congenital anomaly/birth defect, and cancer or overdosing/dependence. "Unexpected" means that the ADE is not listed in the current labeling[2] for the drug or is of greater severity or specificity than that described in the current labeling.

13.4.2   Therapeutic agents (drugs)

Drug product means a finished dosage form, for example, a tablet, capsule, or solution, that contains a drug substance independent or in association with other ingredients. *Drug substance* means an active ingredient that is intended to produce a pharmacological effect or any other direct effect in the diagnosis, cure, mitigation, treatment, or prevention of disease ((U.S. Department of Health and Human Services, Food and Drug Administration, 1885), p. 7493). *New molecular entities* (*NME*) are chemically unique pharmaceuticals that have never before been marketed in the United States in any form.

13.4.3   Medical device

(See also Chapter 4)

A medical device is an object or instrument that is used for diagnosis therapeutic purposes. Examples include medical thermometers, x-ray machines, and surgical instruments. The FDA regulates approximately 1,700 different generic types of medical devices and classifies them into 16 medical specialties known as panels. Dental devices are discussed in Part 872 of Volume 21 of the Code of Federal Regulations (21CFR872), and include diagnostic, prosthetic, surgical, therapeutic, and other miscellaneous devices. The interested

---

[1] This information is taken from 21CFR314.80, the current Code of Federal Regulations from the U.S. Food and Drug Administration (number 21). This document is available as a searchable document at http://www.accessdata.fda.gov/scripts/cdrh/cfdocs/cfcfr/CFRSearch.cfm (search for "314.80").

[2] The terms "label" or "labeling" refers to the information included in the drug's package insert, which is also the information included in the Physician's Desk Reference (PDR) and the one agreed by the FDA and the manufacturer in terms of dosage and route of administration. However, once a drug is approved for prescription use, the FDA does not interfere or regulate with the use of the drug; thus, the physician can make therapeutic decisions based on her or his best judgment. The practice of prescribing drugs outside those recommended on the label of the product is known as "off-label" use of the drug.

reader should check www.fda.gov/cdrh/devadvice/3131html for a full list and definition of each of these devices and their intended uses. In addition, all medical devices are assigned into three regulatory classes based on the level of control necessary to ensure their safety and effectiveness. Class I devices present minimum potential for harm, for example, medical gloves and handheld surgical instruments including dental burs, but are subject to medical device reporting requirements. Class II devices are those requiring special labeling requirements, mandatory performance standards, and postmarketing surveillance, for example, powered wheelchairs, infusion pumps, caries detection devices, and amalgam alloy. Class III devices are those that support or sustain human life, are important in preventing impairment of human health, or present unreasonable risk of illness and injury. These require premarketing approval and postmarketing surveillance and include heart valves, breast implants, bone grafting material containing drugs that are therapeutic, and some dental implants (blade-form)[3]. A complete list of dental devices monitored by the FDA is available at www.accessdata.fda.gov/scripts/cdrh/cfdocs/cfrsearch.cfm?cfrpart=872.

13.4.4   Pharmacoepidemiology and pharmacosurveillance

A well-known textbook *Pharmacoepidemiology* (Strom, 2005) defines the title term as "the study of the use of and the effects of drugs in a large number of people." As such, this discipline involves the application of the principles of pharmacology and the tools of epidemiology in the analysis of effects of drugs in populations. One important component of this discipline is the gathering, analysis, and interpretation of data (clearly, a related surveillance activity), which is used either in detecting whether an ADE occurred above expected levels (pharmacosurveillance or postmarketing surveillance) or in establishing causation between the drug and the ADE.

13.5   Need for pharmacoepidemiology and pharmacosurveillance: how a drug or class III medical device is approved for use (premarket)

Recent data suggest that a new drug may cost $800 million to develop, averaging 10–12 years from concept to commercial use (DiMassi et al., 2003). In the United States, the FDA regulates marketing of drugs following a three-phase process. The following is a brief description of each phase; the interested reader should review FDA documentation starting with the FDA's "Drug Review Process: Ensuring Drugs Are Safe and Effective" available at www.fda.gov/fdac/features/2002/402_drug.html (see also Chapter 11).

Phase 1 focuses on evaluating the pharmacokinetic properties of the drug in a reduced number of healthy volunteers, typically 20–80. Phase 2 focuses on assessment of efficacy using short exploratory clinical trials in selected groups of patients, usually numbering in the hundreds. In phase 3, the manufacturer conducts confirmatory therapeutic clinical trials performed in larger samples of subjects, usually around 3,000 persons (Arrowsmith-Lowe,

---

[3]Postmarket requirements for medical devices should be distinguished from "postapproval requirements" (see http://www.fda.gov/MedicalDevices/DeviceRegulationandGuidance/HowtoMarketYourDevice/PremarketSubmissions/PremarketApprovalPMA/ucm050422.htm for further details).

2000) (see also Chapter 12). Thus, rare events, such as those occurring in 1 in 10,000 exposed or lower, have very little or no chance of occurrence during phase 3.[4] Moreover, because subjects in premarketing trials are selected for their higher probability to respond positively to the drug being tested and chosen from homogenous groups to maximize the probability of success, phase 3 trials tend to exclude childbearing woman, children, the elderly, and subjects with concomitant conditions or using other drugs (Friedman et al., 1999). Therefore, approved drugs are generally tested under very controlled circumstances, on a reduced number of subjects, reducing the chance of detecting uncommon ADE, ADE occurring with simultaneous use of other drugs, or ADE in persons with other preexisting conditions or diseases. Thus, there is a need to monitor effects of a drug once it is on the market.

Despite these limitations, this approach is reasonable in trying to balance a need for new drugs against protecting the public, as it would be impossible to predict and account for the hundreds of potential combinations of drug effects, disease factors, and demographics in designing phase 3 clinical trials. Thus, it is impossible to know all potential ADE before release in populations. Also, there are economic and social issues impacting drug development: the need of the manufacturer to reduce the cost of development and the societal needs of having drugs that are effective at a reasonable cost from the laboratory to the pharmacy in a timely manner.

During a new drug application, the FDA reviews the proposed labeling and proposed drug promotion to ensure the information is communicated accurately and risks and benefits are presented with clear balance. In some cases, the FDA may request postmarketing trials to further define risks among subgroups of the population with long-term use. These are often referred to as phase 4 (Friedman et al., 1999) and, if requested, are an integral part of postmarketing surveillance. It is clear that drug safety and efficacy should continue to be monitored as long as the drug is on the market.

13.6   History

Little attention was given to monitoring drug reactions until the late 1950s, when chloramphenicol was found to produce fatal aplastic anemia (Wallerstein et al., 1969). In 1960, the FDA sponsored hospital-based drug monitoring systems to explore the short-term effects of drugs (Cluff et al., 1964). In 1961, an unusually high number of a rare birth defect, known as phocomelia, was observed in Europe, followed by an alleged association with use of thalidomide, a drug prescribed to reduce nausea in pregnant women.[5] William McBride, a clinician, made the first report of this association to *The Lancet* (McBride, 1961). Lenz estimated that 7,000 infants were affected (Lenz, 1966). The drug was withdrawn from the European market in November 1961. Thalidomide was not marketed in the United States; thus, no cases were reported in the United States. However, the event led to passing of the Kefauver–Harris Drug Amendments on October 10, 1962 (see copy of the FDA's Food and Drug Review, November 1962 issue), requiring extensive preclinical testing and substantial

[4]Penicillin produces anaphylaxis in 1 in every 10,000 persons exposed. In the hypothetical case that penicillin would be submitted for approval, the supporting data would likely not show anaphylaxis as an ADE.

[5]Thalidomide causes phocomelia ("seal-like" limbs), amelia (absence of limbs), or micromelia (abnormally short limbs). In addition, it may cause internal and external ear, cardiac, and gastrointestinal malformations.

evidence of efficacy in well-controlled studies, and later the passing of Title 21 of the Code of Federal Regulations (21CFR) in 1985 (Faich et al., 1985; Arrowsmith-Lowe, 2000). Incidentally, thalidomide has been subsequently shown to have therapeutic effects in leprosy, multiple myeloma, and AIDS, and has entered the U.S. market in 1998 for the treatment of erythema nodosum leprosum (see news published in *The Lancet* on July 25, 1998).

Classic epidemiological research has been used to determine causality of observed ADE. For example, in the early 1970s, Herbst and associates reported on the delayed effects of in utero exposure of diethylstilbestrol in causing clear cell adenocarcinoma in young woman (Herbst et al., 1971). In other cases, the causality between some ADE and the alleged drugs or device was never convincingly proven but the drug/product was removed from the market. That seems to be the case with silicone breast implants, removed from the market in 1992 despite a lack of scientific consensus. The interested reader can find additional information in the book by Marcia Angell, former editor of the *New England Journal of Medicine* (Angell, 1996).

Other known examples of studies that have used surveillance data for establishing ADE causality of marketed drugs include salicylate use in children with viral illness and the development of Reye's syndrome (Waldman et al., 1982), and the risk of breast cancer associated with long-term oral contraceptive use (Centers for Disease Control, 1983).

13.7   Legislation and regulations in the United States

13.7.1   Drug products

Under Title 21 of the U.S. Code of Federal Regulations (21CFR), the FDA is responsible for monitoring ADE (U.S. Department of Health and Human Services, Food and Drug Administration, 1885). These regulations are reviewed once a year. Chapter 1 of 21CFR concerns the Food and Drug Administration. Each chapter has parts and sections. For example, Part 314 is "Applications for FDA approval to market a new drug or an antibiotic drug" and has a section 80 entitled "postmarketing reporting of adverse drug experience." The latter is referred to as section "314.80." The FDA website has a searchable system for specific sections within 21CFR available at www.accessdata.fda.gov/scripts/cdrh/cfdocs/cfcfr/cfrsearch.cfm. The interested reader should also review FDA's "Postmarketing surveillance and epidemiology: human drugs" available at www.fda.gov/cder/aers/chapter53.htm that provides guidance to the FDA field staff for the enforcement of the 21CFR sections on "Postmarketing Adverse Drug Experience Reporting Regulations" (i.e., 310.305, 314.80, and 314.98).

The purpose of postmarketing ADE regulation is "to obtain information on rare, latent, or long-term drug effects not identified during premarket testing" (www.fda.gov/cder/aers.chapter53.htm). Briefly, under this regulation, "sponsors, manufacturers, packers, and distributors are required to report all serious, unexpected (not listed in the drug product's current labeling) ADE to the FDA within 15 working days." The FDA Center for Drug Evaluation and Research (CDER) is responsible for receiving, tracking, and evaluating these reports using the Adverse Event Report System (AERS). Drugs most likely to have unexpected ADE are those approved for marketing over the previous 3 years, new molecular entities, and those known or suspected of having bioavailability or bioequivalence problems. Other ADE are required to be reported at quarterly intervals during the first 3 years following approval and annually thereafter (U.S. Department of Health and Human

Services and Food and Drug Administration, 1885). Manufacturers are also responsible for reporting to the FDA (within 15 days) of any report of ADE appearing in the medical literature, case reports, or as part of clinical trials. Health care professionals, including dentists, are not required to report ADE, but are strongly encouraged to do so (Garvin, 2006). To facilitate voluntary reporting, the FDA developed the MedWatch program (see below).

In 1992, the U.S. Congress started passing a series of legislative acts known collectively as the Prescription Drug User Fee Acts (PDUFA), which sought to expedite the FDA drug-review process and improve efficiency by collecting fees from the manufacturers. These fees were used to hire additional drug reviewers and support staff and upgrade computer infrastructure at the FDA. The average time for reviewing a new drug was reduced to 1 year, down from 3 years a decade before (Friedman et al., 1999). The latest 5-year PDUFA reauthorization plan is available for review at www.fda.gov/cdedr/pdufa/pdufa_IV_5yr_plan_draft.pdf. The plan endorses a single internet portal for reporting ADE by initiating the MedWatch[Plus] project (see below) and the integration of the adverse event reporting of all FDA-regulated products, which is labeled FAERS (FDA Adverse Event Report System). Every year, the FDA published fee rates in the Federal Register. As per the Act, fees continue to be collected to upgrade the agency's drug safety program, increase resources for review of television drug advertising, and facilitate more efficient development of safe and effective new medications. The fees for fiscal year 2009 were published on August 1, 2008.

There has been some concern among members of the U.S. Congress and the public in general that the FDA's approval process is too fast, and that there may be a need for an independent drug safety board (Kleinke and Gottlieb, 1998; Wood et al., 1998), but an FDA review concluded that there is no association between time for approval and later removal from the market (Friedman et al., 1999). It appears that this issue will continue to be debated as the need for new drugs is balanced against ensurance of efficacy and safety, emphasizing the importance of postmarketing surveillance.

Absence of ADE, however, does not mean that the drug product is safe, because the efficacy of the postmarketing systems depends on the thoroughness of the reporting systems, how widespread the drug is used, and the number of years the drug has been on the market.

Regulations on drugs and devices need to be constantly modified as new technologies and new methods are developed. The interested reader should check the FDA website (www.fda.gov) frequently for links to current and past FDA regulations and guidelines, as well as for information regarding recent withdrawals, recalls, field corrections, and notifications (www.fda.gov/cber/recalls.htm). These notifications also include medical devices and can be delivered to the interested person via e-mail if requested.

13.7.2 Medical devices

Under 21CFR822.1 (www.accessdata.fda.gov/scripts/cdrh/cfdocs/cfcfr/cfrsearch.cfm?cfrpart=822.1), the "FDA has the authority to order postmarket surveillance on any class II or class III device that meets the following criteria: (a) failure of the device would be reasonably likely to have serious adverse health consequences; (b) the device is intended to be implanted in the human body for more than 1 year; or (c) the device is intended to be used to support or sustain life and to be used outside the user facility" (www.fda.gov/cdrh/devadvice/352.html). Manufacturers are notified by letter and have 30 days to submit a postmarketing surveillance plan. The FDA will review the plan within

60 days of receipt to determine whether it will result in the collection of useful data, and whether the designated person (researcher) has the appropriate qualifications and experience to implement the surveillance plan or not. Manufacturers of class II and class III devices meeting these criteria should carefully review the definitions, exceptions, and requirements as required by 21CFR822.

Mandatory reporting for medical devices adverse events is required of user facilities, manufacturers, and importers. User facilities include hospitals, nursing homes, ambulatory surgical facilities, and outpatient diagnostic and treatment facilities, but do not include physicians or other health care providers outside of these facilities. Facilities are required to report device-related deaths and serious injuries (similar to serious events). Death reports should be submitted to the FDA and the manufacturer within 10 days of knowledge of the event. Serious injury reports are sent to the manufacturer within the same 10-day time frame. Manufacturers must submit reports to the FDA within 30 days of knowledge of the event as well as report on events necessitating a remedial action, which may include recalls, replacements, relabeling, notifications, within 5 days (Gross and Kessler, 1996).

Other federal legislations and regulations, for example, the Safe Medical Devices Act of 1990 (SMDA), and the Medical Device Amendments of 1992 (Public Law 102-300) and its final rule in 1995 affect postmarketing regulations of medical devices. The interested reader should visit www.fda.gov/chrh/mdr for additional information.

13.8   Monitoring ADE after drug approval

The core of the FDA process to monitoring ADE is the AERS, which gathers, tabulates, and analyzes mandatory reports from manufacturers or researchers and voluntary reporting from health care professionals and consumers through the MedWatch program (www.fda.gov/medwatch). The FDA recommends the use of MedWatch forms 3500 (by physicians, dentists, and other health care professionals) or 3500A (by manufacturers, user facilities), available in paper and computer-generated data entry (http://www.fda.gov/medwatch/getforms.htm) (see copy on page 255).

The structure of the AERS database is in compliance with guidelines issued by the International Conference on Harmonization (ICH) and clinically validated international medical terminology through the Medical Dictionary for Regulatory Activities (MedDRA). Data entered into AERS are evaluated by clinical reviewers of the FDA CDER and the Center for Biologics Evaluation and Research (CBER) to detect safety signals (Figures 13.1 and 13.2).

If the drug is found to produce serious ADE, then the FDA can require manufacturers to inform health care professionals through a "Dear Health Care Professional" letter and make changes in the labeling of the product such as the inclusion of "black box warning"—a boxed warning in the package insert. Black box warnings are the strongest warning the FDA can issue. For example, a recent "black box" warning placed on all antidepressant medications describing the increased risk for suicidal ideation in children and adolescents was followed, in one study, by up to 37% of practitioners modifying their prescription practices (Bhatia et al., 2008). On July 8, 2008, the FDA required a black box warning for fluoroquinolone antibiotics (e.g., Cipro) to alert about the increased risk of tendonitis and tendon rupture, especially among those above 60 years of age; among kidney, heart, and lung transplant

U.S. Department of Health and Human Services

MED WATCH

The FDA Safely Information and
Adverse Event Reporting Program

For VOLUNTARY reporting of
adverse events, product problems and
product use errors

Page ____ of ____   Page ____ of ____

Form Approved: OMB No. 0910-0291, Expires;10/31/08
See OMB statement on reverse

FDA USE ONLY

Triage unit
Sequence #

A. PATIENT INFORMATION

1. Patient Identifier	2. Age at Time of Event, or Date of Birth	3. Sex	4. Weight
In confidence		☐ Female ☐ Male	_____ lb or _____ kg

B. ADVERSE EVENT, PRODUCT PROBLEM OR ERROR

Check all that apply:

1. ☐ Adverse Event   ☐ Product Problem (e.g. defects/malfunctions)
☐ Product Use Error ☐ Problem with Dfferent Manufacturer of Same Medicine

2. Outcomes Attributed to Adverse Event
(Check all that apply)

☐ Death _____
(mm/dd/yyyy)
☐ Life-threatening
☐ Hospitalization - initial or prolonged
☐ Required interventior to Prevent Permanant Impairment/Damage (Devices)

☐ Disability or Permanent Damage
☐ Congenital Anomaly/Birth Defect
☐ Other Serious (Important Medical Events)

3. Date of Events (mm/dd/yyyy)	4. Date of this Report (mm/dd/yyyy) 01/15/2009

5. Describe Event, Problem or Product Use Error

6. Relevant Tests/Laboratory Data, Including Dates

7. Other Relevant History, Including Preexisting Medical Conditions (e.g. allergies, race, pregnancy, smoking and alcohol use, liver/kidney problems, etc.)

C. PRODUCT AVAILABILITY

Product Availabe for Evaluation? (Do not sent product to FDA)

☐ Yes ☐ No ☐ Returned to Manufacturer on:_____
(mm/dd/yyyy)

D. SUSPECT PRODUCT (S)

1. Name, Strength, Manufacturer (from product lable)

#1 _____

#2

2. Dose or Amount	Frequency	Route
#1		
#2		

3. Dates of Use (If unknown, give duration) from/to for best estimate)	5. Event Abated After Use Stopped or Dose Reduced?
#1	#1 ☐ Yes ☐ No ☐ Doesn't Apply
#2	#2 ☐ Yes ☐ No ☐ Doesn't Apply

4. Diagnosis or Reason for Use (Indication)	8. Event Reappeared After Reintroduction?
#1	#1 ☐ Yes ☐ No ☐ Doesn't Apply
#2	#2 ☐ Yes ☐ No ☐ Doesn't Apply

6. Lot#	7. Expiration Date	9. NDC # or Unique ID
#1	#1	
#2	#2	

E. SUSPECT MEDICAL DEVICE

1. Brand Name

2. Common Device Name

3. Manufacturer Name, City and State

4. Model #	Lot #	5. Operator of Device
Catalog #	Expiration Date (mm/dd/yyyy)	☐ Health Professional ☐ Lay User/Patient
Serial #	Other #	☐ Other

6. If Implanted, Give Date (mm/dd/yyyy)	7. If Explanted, Give Date (mm/dd/yyyy)

8. If this a Single-use Device that was Reprocessed and Reused on a Patient?
☐ Yes ☐ No

9. If Yes to Item No. 8 Enter Name and Address of Reproceesor

F. OTHER (CONCOMITANT) MEDICAL PRODUCTS

Product names and therapy dates (exclude treatment of event)

F. REPORTER (See confidentiality section on back)

1. Name and Address

Phone #	E-mail

2. Health Professional?	3. Occupation	4. Also Reported to:
☐ Yes ☐ No		☐ Manufacturer ☐ User Facility ☐ Distributor/Importer
5. If you do NOT want your identity disclosed to the manufacturer, place an "X" In this box: ☐		

FORM FDA 3500 (10/05) Submission of a report does not constitute an admission that medical perssonel or the product caused or contributed to the event.

(side text) PLEASE TYPE OR USE BLACK INK

Figure 13.1 FDA MedWatch form (FDA 3500) for voluntary reporting of adverse events or product problems. Downloadable printable form (accessed June 30, 2009) available on-line at http://www.fda.gov/downloads/Safety/MedWatch/HowToReport/DownloadForms/ ucm082725.pdf.

Form Approved: OMB No. 0910-0291, Expires;10/31/08
See OMB statement on reverse

U.S. Department of Health and Human Services
Food and Drug Administration

For use by user-facilities,
importers, distributors and manufacturers
for MANDATORY reporting

Mfr Report #
UF/Importer Report #

MEDWATCH

FORM FDA 3500A (10/05)   Page ____ of ____

FDA Use Only

A. PATIENT INFORMATION			
1. Patient Identifier	2. Age at Time of Event: or ———— Date of Birth:	3. Sex ☐ Female ☐ Male	4. Weight ———— lbs or ———— kgs
In confidence			

B. ADVERSE EVENT OR PRODUCT PROBLEM

1. ☐ **Adverse Event** and/or ☐ **Product Problem** (e.g. defects/malfunctions)

2. **Outcomes Attributed to Adverse Event** (Check all that apply)
☐ Death _____ (mm/dd/yyyy)   ☐ Disability or Permanent Damage
☐ Life-threatening   ☐ Congenital Anomaly/Birth Defect
☐ Hospitalization - initial or prolonged   ☐ Other Serious (Important Medical Events)
☐ Required interventio to Prevent Permanant Impairment/Damage (Devices)

3. **Date of Event** (mm/dd/yyyy)	4. **Date of This Report** (mm/dd/yyyy)

5. **Describe Event or Problem**

6. **Relevant Tests/Laboratory Data, Including Dates**

7. **Other Relevant History, Including Preexisting Medical Conditions** (e.g. allergies, race, pregnancy, smoking and alcohol use, hepatic/renal dysfunction, etc.)

C. SUSPECT PRODUCT(S)

1. **Name** (Give labeled strength & mfr/labeler)
#1
#2

2. **Dose or Amount & Route Used** #1 #2	3. **Therapy Dates** (if unknown, give duration) frin/to (or best estimate) #1 #2

4. **Diagnosis for Use** (Indication) #1 #2	5. **Event Abated After Use Stopped or Dose Reduced?** #1 ☐ Yes ☐ No ☐ Doesn't Apply #2 ☐ Yes ☐ No ☐ Doesn't Apply

6. **Lot #** #1 #2	7. **Exp. Date** #1 #2	8. **Event Reappeared After Reintroduction?** #1 ☐ Yes ☐ No ☐ Doesn't Apply

9. **NDC# or Unique ID**	#2 ☐ Yes ☐ No ☐ Doesn't Apply

10. **Concomitant Medical Products and Therapy Dates** (Exclude treatment of event)

D. SUSPECT MEDICAL DEVICE

1. **Brand Name**

2. **Common Device Name**

3. **Manufacturer Name, City and State**

4. **Model #** Catalog # Serial #	**Lot #** **Expiration Date** (mm/dd/yyyy) **Other #**	5. Operator of Device ☐ Health Professional ☐ Lay User/Patient ☐ Other

6. **If Implanted, Give Date** (mm/dd/yyyy)	7. **If Explanted, Give Date** (mm/dd/yyyy)

8. **If this a Single-use Device thaat was Reprocessed and Reused on a Patient?**
☐ Yes ☐ No

9. **If Yes to Item No. 8, Enter Name and Address of Reproceesor**

10. **Device Available for Evaluation?** (Do not send to FDA)
☐ Yes ☐ No ☐ Returned to Manufacturer on:_____ (mm/dd/yyyy)

11. **Concomitant Medical Products and Therapy Dates** (Exclude treatment of event)

E. INITIAL REPORTER

1. **Name and Address**	**Phone #**

4. Also Reported to:
☐ Manufacturer

2. **Health Professional?** ☐ Yes ☐ No	3. **Occupation**	4. **Initial Reporter Also Sent Report to FDA** ☐ Yes ☐ No ☐ Unk.

Submission of a report does not constitute an admission that medical perssonnel, user facility, importer, distributor, manufacturer or product caused or contributed to the event.

PLEASE TYPE OR USE BLACK INK

Figure 13.2 FDA MedWatch form (3500A) for mandatory report of adverse events or product problems by user facilities, importers, distributors, and manufacturers. Downloadable printable form (accessed June 30, 2009) available online at http://www.fda.gov/downloads/Safety/MedWatch/HowToReport/DownloadForms/ucm082728.pdf.

MEDWATCH

FORM FDA 3500A (10/05) *(continued)* Page ___ of ___

FDA Use Only

F. FOR USE BY USER FACILITY/IMPORTER *(Devices Only)*

1. **Check One**
☐ User Facility ☐ Importer

2. **UF/Importer Report Number**

3. **User Facility or Importer Name/Address**

4. **Contact Person**

5. **Phone Number**

6. **Date User Facility or Importer Became Aware of Event** *(mm/dd/yyyy)*

7. **Type of Report**
☐ Initial
☐ Follow-up # ______

8. **Date of This Report** *(mm/dd/yyyy)*

9. **Approximate Age of Device**

10. **Event Problem Codes** *(Refer to coding manual)*
Patient Code ☐ - ☐ - ☐
Device Code ☐ - ☐ - ☐

11. **Report Sent to FDA?**
☐ Yes ______ *(mm/dd/yyyy)*
☐ No

12. Location Where Event Occurred
☐ Hospital
☐ Home
☐ Nursing Home
☐ Outpatient Treatment Facility
☐ Other: ______ *(Specify)*
☐ Outpatient Diagnostic Facility
☐ Ambulatory Surgical Facility

13. **Report Sent to Manufacturer?**
☐ Yes ______ *(mm/dd/yyyy)*
☐ No

14. **Manufacturer Name/Address**

G. ALL MANUFACTURERS

1. **Cotact Office - Name/Address *(and Manufacturing site for Devices)***

2. **Phone Number**

3. **Report Source** *(Check all that apply)*
☐ Foreign
☐ Study
☐ Literature
☐ Consumer
☐ Health Professional
☐ User Facility
☐ Company Representative
☐ Distributor
☐ Other:

4. **Date Received by Manufacturer** *(mm/dd/yyyy)*

5.
(A)NDA # ______
IND # ______
STN # ______
PMA/ 510(k) # ______
Combination Product ☐ Yes
Pre-1938 ☐ Yes
OTC Product ☐ Yes

6. **If IND, Give Protocol #**

7. **Type of Report** *(Check all that apply)*
☐ 5-day ☐ 30-day
☐ 7-day ☐ Periodic
☐ 10-day ☐ Initial
☐ 15-day ☐ Follow-up # ___

8. **Adverse Event Terms(s)**

9. **Manufacturer Report Number**

H. DEVICE MANUFACTURERS ONLY

1. **Type of Reportable Event**
☐ Death
☐ Serious Injury
☐ Malfunction
☐ Other: ______

2. **If Follow-up, What Type?**
☐ Correction
☐ Additional Information
☐ Response to FDA Request
☐ Device Evaluation

3. **Device Evaluated by Manufacturer?**
☐ Not Returned to Manufacturer
☐ Yes ☐ Evaluation Summary Attached
☐ No *(Attach page to explain why not)* or provide code: ______

4. **Device Manufacture Date** *(mm/yyyy)*

5. **Labeled for single Use?**
☐ Yes ☐ No

6. **Evaluation Codes** *(Refer to coding manual)*
Method ☐ - ☐ - ☐ - ☐
Results ☐ - ☐ - ☐ - ☐
Conclusions ☐ - ☐ - ☐ - ☐

7. **If Remedial Action Initiated, Check Type**
☐ Recall ☐ Notification
☐ Repair ☐ Inspection
☐ Replace ☐ Patient Monitoring
☐ Relabeling ☐ Modification/ Adjustment
☐ Other: ______

8. **Usage of Device**
☐ Initial Use of Device
☐ Reuse
☐ Unknown

9. **If action reported to FDA under 21 USC 360i(f), list correction/ removal reporting number:**

10. ☐ **Additional Manufacturer Narrative** **and / or** 11. ☐ **Corrected Data**

The public reporting burden for this collection of information has been estimated ot average 66 Minutes per response, including the time for reviewing instructions, searching existing data sources, gathering and maintaining the data needed, and completing and reviewing the collection of information. Send comments regarding this burden estimate or any or any other aspect of this collection of information, including suggestions for reducing this burden to:

Department of Health and Human Services
Food and Drug Administration - MedWatch
10903 New Hampshire Avenue
Building 22, Mail Stop 4447
Silver Spring, MD 20993-0002
Please DO NOT RETURN this form to this address.

OMB Statement:
"An agency may not conduct or sponsor, and a person is not required to respond to, a collection of information unless it displays a currently valid OMB control number."

Figure 13.2 (*Continued*)

recipients; and among those taking steroids. Black box warnings can be controversial. For example, in July 2008, the FDA proposed a black box warning for epileptic drugs because they were associated with suicidal ideation. An outside panel convened by the FDA voted against such warning on the basis that it might prevent some patients from receiving the benefits of the drugs when the benefits outweight the risks.

If the risks associated with the drug use surpass the benefits, the drug can be withdrawn from the market. Most withdrawals from the U.S. market occur within a couple of years of approval—this is especially critical for new molecular entities.

Of interest to researchers, AERS data stripped of personal identifiers are available to the public for download and analysis at www.fda.gov/cder/aers/default.htm. The interested researcher should check a description of the databases available at CDER at www.fda.gov/cder/cder_db_description.htm. For example, Wysowski and Swartz reviewed 33 years of AERS data and summarized about 2.3 million case reports on approximately 6,000 marketed drugs. These researchers reported that 75 drugs/drug products were removed from the market due to safety problems and 11 drugs had special requirements for prescription or restricted distribution imposed (Wysowski and Swartz, 2005).

13.9   Monitoring medical devices

As described above, adverse events of medical devices are reported to the FDA using the same MedWatch form 3500A used to report adverse drug events. Once received, AE are evaluated by the FDA clinical staff to determine if the AE poses a real or potential risk to the public health (Gross and Kessler, 1996). After review and initial evaluation, the FDA may do one of the following: (1) issue a report with no further action; (2) request additional information from the manufacturer or reporter; (3) request a physical inspection of the manufacturing plant; or (4) initiate an internal FDA decision-making process to consider additional communication activities, risk communication, and compliance options by the manufacturer (Gross and Kessler, 1996).

The FDA uses public health notifications to disseminate the results of postmarketing surveillance to the public. A public health notification is a message from the FDA's Center for Devices and Radiological Health (CDRH) describing a risk associated with the use of a medical device and providing recommendations to avoid or reduce the risk. A preliminary public health notification is similar to a public health notification, but it is issued when the information is still evolving and the FDA determines that the information needs to be released to allow for informed clinical decisions. The notifications are listed by date at www.fda.gov/cdrh/safety.html and are automatically delivered to subscribers by e-mail. Interestingly, two of the five public health notifications since December 2007 relate to dental issues: on December 12, the FDA reported serious patient injuries, including third-degree burns, associated with the use of poorly maintained electrical dental handpieces (www.fda.gov/cdrh/safety/121207-dental.html). On February 2008, a notification was posted on serious allergic reactions caused by denture cleansers (www.fda.gov/cdrh/medicaldevicesafety/atp/022508-denturecleansers.html).

Data reported to the FDA's CDRH are entered into the Manufacturer and User Facility Device Experience (MAUDE) database. The Device Experience Network (originally DEN, now MDR) database is a legacy database for reports prior to 1996 and is no longer being updated. The MAUDE database includes reports from manufacturers, importers, and user facilities. MDR files are available for downloading at www.fda.gov/cdrh/mdrfile.html. An online query system allows searching the database for reports of death or serious injuries from 1984 to 1996. MAUDE contains voluntary reports since June 1993, user facility reports since 1991, distributor reports since 1993, and manufacturer reports since August 1996 (www.fda.gov/cdrh/maude.html). Compressed (zipped) files are available for downloading at the same website.

13.10   Monitoring AE of interest to oral health researchers and clinicians

As described in the beginning of this chapter with the three examples from JADA, oral health researchers may be involved in developing new drugs or devices for the diagnosis and treatment of oral diseases and dental clinicians use devices and prescribe drugs to their patients. Furthermore, some dental materials (devices) have been associated with adverse events in patients, for example, mercury in dental amalgam. In this section, we provide additional examples of studies related to AE.

Biphosphonates are drugs used in a variety of clinical situations to reduce osteoporosis, bone pain, hypercalcemia, and skeletal complications associated with multiple myeloma, Paget's disease, and breast, lung, and other cancers. Since 2003, reports in the medical literature have proposed links and showed evidence of biphosphonate-associated osteonecrosis (BON) in the jaws. The majority of these cases have been diagnosed after a dental procedure, such as tooth extraction, but some cases have been reported as occurring spontaneously (Ruggiero et al., 2004). Furthermore, there appears to be a different outcome whether the drugs are administered through an intravenous or oral route. Because BON is rare, it is expected that continued postmarketing surveillance would identify additional cases that, in turn, may provide more statistical power to conduct further analysis. An expert panel convened by the American Dental Association Council on Scientific Affairs has reminded and encouraged dentists to report cases of BON to the FDA MedWatch program (American Dental Association and Council on Scientific Affairs, 2006).

The recent trend to propose, develop, and validate diagnostic procedures for systemic diseases using oral tissues and fluid will benefit from postmarketing surveillance. For example, a CDC team used postmarketing surveillance to assess the validity of rapid HIV-1 antibody test (OraQuick) and compared validity (sensitivity, specificity) when applied to whole blood and oral fluid (Wesolowski et al., 2006).

Dental materials may be associated with adverse events. Most information currently available in the literature on these AE, however, is not directly focused on the specific events, and do not use a standardized data collection process (Schedle et al., 2008). Furthermore, reports are based on spontaneous reporting of subjective symptoms followed by amelioration after the alleged material is removed (Lygre et al., 2003). Thus, a causation link cannot be established. The main methodological limitation is that most AE symptoms associated with dental materials are subjective and could be attributed to other physiological or pathological simultaneous conditions.

13.11   International issues

Postmarketing surveillance of drug products, dental and medical devices, and vaccines varies across countries. There are different levels of enforcement, protocols for reporting, and databases that have changed over time within and across countries. Common characteristics in all these systems are the presence of some level of underreporting and the lack of comparison groups to assess causality (Heeley et al., 2001). These limitations make international comparisons difficult.

The European Union (EU) has established the EudraVigilance project to have standardized electronic reporting of all human adverse reactions between EU and national health authorities, marketing authorization agencies, and pharmaceutical companies. The project has been run since December 2001 by the European Medicines Agency (EMEA). For further information about the EudraVigilance system, visit www.eudravigilance.emea.eu/human/index.asp.

There are current efforts to reduce the duplication of efforts in the research and development of new medicines by standardization of guidelines and processes for new pharmaceuticals. One such effort is the International Conference on Harmonization of Technical Requirements for Registration of Pharmaceuticals for Human Use (ICH) (www.ich.org). The primary objective of this project is to bring together regulatory authorities of Europe, Japan, and the United States, and pharmaceutical companies to discuss scientific and technical aspects of pharmaceutical product development and registration. Established in 1990, the ICH focuses on issues of quality, safety, and efficacy of products providing guidelines, including those in pharmacovigilance. One interesting set of ICH guidelines is the (MedDRA), which provides standard terminology for information throughout the medical product life cycle (www.ich.org/cache/compo/276-254-1.html). ICH guidelines have been endorsed by the WHO Advisory Committee on safety of medical products. Other efforts include those of the EMEA (www.emea.europa.eu), an agency of the European Union with responsibility on protection of public and animal health through the evaluation and supervision of medical products (www.emea.europa.eu/htms/aboutus/emeaoverview.htm), and the World Health Organization (WHO) program for International Drug Monitoring, established in 1971 and residing at the WHO Collaborating Center for International Drug Monitoring Uppsala Monitoring Center in Sweden. The database contains over three million reports of suspected adverse drug reactions (www.who.int/medicines/areas/quality-safety/safety_efficacy/advdrugreactions/en/index.html). WHO releases *Drug Alerts* when a serious problem with any medical product is detected. The website www.who.int/medicines/publications/drugalerts/drugalertindex/en/index.html includes the most recent *Drug Alerts* released. As mentioned earlier in the chapter, the CDER's AERS is in compliance with ICH international safety reporting guidance, and events are coded following MedDRA terms.

13.12   Future challenges

The number of prescription drug products available in the U.S. market has increased over the past two decades and Americans are using a greater number of pharmaceuticals than they were using a decade ago. It is expected that these numbers will continue to increase in the future. Thus, there is a potential for larger number of ADE to be detected and reported. Currently, the FDA receives more than 250,000 potential ADE a year from all sources. At the same time, these databases are growing in size and complexity; the evolution of informatics systems allows constant access to this information almost in real time. As mentioned earlier, the 2008 PDUFA IV 5-year plan proposes a MedWatch[Plus] program that will take advantage of information technology and a single internet portal to encourage timeliness and accuracy of spontaneous reporting and user-friendly access to consumers of product safety information from the FDA. Also, the plan proposes integration of all FDA-regulated products.

With increased globalization, manufacturers will initiate simultaneous approval in different countries or use the process initiated in one country to apply for marketing in another. This will require from each country harmonization of criteria and language but, at the same time, consideration for each country's rules and regulations.

Also with globalization and increased communication capabilities, researchers, including dental scientists, will cooperate more closely on new drugs and devices that will require more detailed postmarketing surveillance plans. Thus, researchers must stay aware of new legal and regulatory requirements for application and postmarketing surveillance of their products. Some of these requirements will include postmarketing investigations (phase 4 studies) to clarify rare but serious events. At the same time, a greater contribution of the dental practitioner in monitoring drugs and devices and reporting suspect AE is expected and needed. The NIDCR Dental Practice-Based Research Network initiative may be a good starting point to promote postmarketing surveillance of drugs and dental devices (www.nidcr.nih.gov/research/DER/clinicalresearch/DentalPracticeBasedResearch Networks.htm).

Acknowledgments

The authors would like to thank Amy Collins, William Kohn, and Stephen Sykes for their editorial review and comments.

References

American Dental Association, Council on Scientific Affairs. 2006. Dental management of patients receiving oral biphosphonate therapy. Expert panel recommendations. *Journal of the American Dental Association* 137:1144–1150.

Angell M. 1996. *The Clash of Medical Evidence and the Law in the Breast Implant Case*. Hardcover edn. New York: W. W. Norton & Company.

Arrowsmith-Lowe J. 2000. Post-market safety surveillance for pharmaceuticals. In: Teutsch SM, Churchill RE (eds). New York: Oxford University Press, pp. 343–363.

Bhatia SK, Rezac AJ, Vitiello B, Sitorius MA, Buehler BA, Kratochvil CJ. 2008. Antidepressant prescribing practices for the treatment of children and adolescents. *Journal of Child and Adolescent Psychopharmacology* 18:70–80.

Centers for Disease Control. 1983. Cancer and steroid hormone study: long-term oral contraceptive use and the risk of breast cancer. *The Journal of The American Medical Association* 249:1591–1595.

Cluff LE, Thornton GF, Seidl LG. 1964. Studies on the epidemiology of adverse drug reactions. I. Methods of surveillance. *The Journal of The American Medical Association* 188:976–983.

DiMassi JA, Hansen RW, Grabowski HG. 2003. The price of innovation: new estimates of drug development costs. *Journal of Health Economics* 22:151–185.

Elixhauser, Owens. 2007. Adverse drug events in U.S. hospitals, 2004. United States Agency for Health Research and Quality (AHRQ). Available online at www.hcup-us.ahrq.gov/reports/statbriefs/sb29.pdf.

Faich GA, Knapp D, Dreis M, Turner W. 1985. National adverse drug reaction surveillance: 1985. *The Journal of The American Medical Association* 257:2068–2070.

Friedman MA, Woodcock J, Lumpkin MM, Shuren JE, Hass AE, Thompson LJ. 1999. The safety of newly approved medicines. Do recent market removals mean there is a problem? *The Journal of The American Medical Association* 281:1728–1734.

Garvin J. 2006. FDA urges dentists to report adverse events to MedWatch. *ADA News*. 2006-01-09. p. 6.

Gross TP, Kessler LG. 1996. Medical device vigilance at the FDA. *Studies in Health Technology and Informatics* 28:17–24.

Gurwitz JH, Field TS, Avorn J. 2000. Incidence and preventability of adverse drug events in nursing homes. *American Journal of Medicine* 109:87–94.

Heeley E, Riley J, Layton D, Wilton LV, Shakir SAW. 2001. Prescription-event monitoring and reporting of adverse drug reactions. *The Lancet* 358:1872–1873.

Herbst AL, Ulfelder H, Poskanzer DC. 1971. Adenocarcinoma of the vagina: association of maternal stilbestrol therapy with tumor appearance in young woman. *New England Journal of Medicine* 284:878–881.

Johnson HA, Bartman JL. 1995. Drug related morbidity and mortality. *Archives of Internal Medicine* 155:1949–1956.

Kleinke JD, Gottlieb S. 1998. Is the FDA approving drugs too fast? Probably not—but drug recalls have sparket debate. *British Medical Journal* 317:899.

Lauterbach M, Martins IP, Castro-Caldas A, Bernardo M, Luis H, Amaral H, Leitão J, Martin MD, Townes B, Rosenbaum G, Woods JS, DeRouen T. 2008. Neurological outcomes in children with and without amalgam-related mercury exposure. *Journal of the American Dental Association* 139(2):138–145.

Lazarou J, Pomeranz BH, Corey PN. 1998. Incidence of adverse drug reactions in hospitalized patients: a meta-analysis of prospective studies. *The Journal of The American Medical Association* 279:1200–1205.

Lenz W. 1966. Malformations caused by drugs in pregnancy. *American Journal of Diseases of Children* 112:99–106.

Lygre GB, Gjerdet NR, Grønningsaeter AG, Björkman L. 2003. Reporting on adverse reaction to dental materials—intraoral observations at a clinical follow-up. *Community Dentistry and Oral Epidemiology* 31:200–206.

Mandel L, Alfi D. 2008. Drug-induced paraparotid fat deposition in patients with HIV. Case reports. *Journal of the American Dental Association* 139(2):152–157.

McBride WG. 1961. Thalidomide and congenital abnormalities. *The Lancet* 2:1358.

McCoy LC, Wheler CJ, Rich SE, Garcia RI, Miller DR, Jones JA. 2008. Adverse events associated with chlorhexidine use. Results from the Department of Veterans Affairs Dental Diabetes Study. *Journal of the American Dental Association* 139(2):178–183.

Ruggiero SL, Mehrotra B, Rosenberg TJ, Engroff SL. 2004. Osteonecrosis of the jaws associated with the use of bisphosphonates: a review of 63 cases. *Journal of Oral and Maxillofacial Surgery* 62:527–534.

Schedle A, Örtengren U, Eidler N, Ensten A. 2008. Do adverse effects of dental materials exist? What are the consequences, and how can they be diagnosed and treated? *Clinical Oral Implants Research* 18(Suppl. 3):232–256.

Strom BL. 2005. What is pharmacoepidemiology? *Pharmacoepidemiology*. West Sussex: John Wiley & Sons, Ltd, pp. 3–15.

Thacker SB, Berkelman RL. 1988. Public health surveillance in the United States. *Epidemiology Reviews* 10:164–190.

U.S. Department of Health and Human Services, Food and Drug Administration. 1885. *New Drug and Antibiotic Regulations.* pp. 7451–7519.

Waldman RJ, Hall WN, McGee H, Van Amburg G. 1982. Aspirine as a risk factor in Reye syndrome. *The Journal of The American Medical Association* 247:3089–3094.

Wallerstein RO, Condit PK, Kasper CK, Brown JW, Morrison FR. 1969. Statewide study of chloramphenicol therapy and fatal aplastic anemia. *The Journal of The American Medical Association* 208:2045–2050.

Wesolowski LG, MacKellar DA, Facente SN, Dowling T, Ethridge SF, Zhu JH, Sullivan PS. 2006. Post-marketing surveillance of OraQuick whole blood and oral fluid rapid HIV testing. *AIDS* 20:1661–1666.

Wood AJJ, Stein CM, Woosley R. 1998. Making medicines safer—the need for an independent drug safety board. *New England Journal of Medicine* 339:1851–1854.

Wysowski DK, Swartz L. 2005. Adverse drug event surveillance and drug withdrawals in the United States, 1969–2002: the importance of reporting suspect reactions. *Archives of Internal Medicine* 165:1363–1369.

14

Dental practice-based research networks

Donald J. DeNucci, DDS, MS, and the CONDOR Dental
Practice-Based Research Networks

14.1 Introduction to dental practice-based research networks (PBRN)

Dental practice-based research is a form of research conducted in clinical practices by practitioners and their staff and is designed to answer questions that dentists face in the routine care of their patients. Practice-based research (PBR) holds great potential for answering these clinical questions and for expediting the translation of research findings into clinical practice. A group of practitioners engaged in coordinated practice-based research constitutes a PBRN.

Practice-based research began when small groups of European medical practitioners began sharing information pertinent to patient care and clinical outcomes. The early precursors to today's practice-based research networks can be traced back to the European sentinel networks of the 1970s. This sentinel model soon took hold in the United States as the Ambulatory Sentinel Practice Network (ASPN) which was followed closely by the establishment of the Pediatric Research in Office Settings (PROS) in 1984 (Green and Hickner, 2006). Currently, there are over 120 primary care PBRN known to be active in the United States, which include about 20,000 practices of pediatrics, family medicine, and general internal medicine located in all 50 states. These practices provide care for more than 20 million Americans (Agency for Healthcare Research and Quality, 2008). The dental profession has only recently recognized the value of practice-based research with the establishment of the Community Research for Oral Health Wellness Network (CROWN) in 2001 (Case Western Reserve University, 2008) and finally the three National Institute of Dental and Craniofacial Research (NIDCR) funded practice-based research networks in 2005 (National Institute of Dental and Craniofacial Research, 2008).

This chapter will focus on the important aspects of the conduct of oral health research in general dental practices. It will include sections on practice-based research network infrastructure requirements, practitioner recruitment and retention, study development, study deployment, data acquisition and analysis, the protection of human research subjects, and the translation of the acquired scientific evidence into clinical practice.

14.2   Network infrastructure development and governance including fiscal issues

Jonathan A. Ship, DMD, **and Anne S. Lindblad,** PhD for the PEARL Dental Practice-Based Research Network

14.2.1   Infrastructure of the PBRN

The creation of a successful PBRN requires a comprehensive infrastructure that must include representation from a variety of individuals from different backgrounds and groups of experts responsible for key goals of the network (Lindbloom et al., 2004) (an example of PBRN infrastructure is provided in Figure 14.1). The most important component is the practitioner-investigators (P-I) themselves, who ideally are qualified, interested, and dedicated clinical scientists who are willing to participate in clinical investigations supported

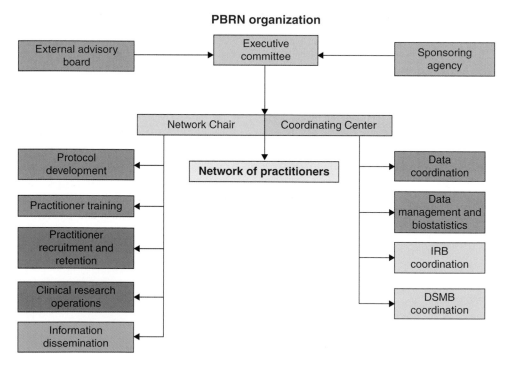

Figure 14.1 Organizational outline for a practice-based research network, consisting of a Network Chair, coordinating center, practitioner-investigators, and advisory groups.

by the PBRN. The practitioner-investigators can come from a variety of settings, depending upon the needs of the network and individual study requirements (Rust and Cooper, 2007). Clinicians from private practices, public clinics, academic institutions, hospitals, nursing homes, and other settings can all be considered part of a network infrastructure and its governance. Their practices should represent a wide variety of patient profiles with respect to race, ethnicity, and socioeconomic status. Diversity among the practitioner-investigators including professional training is also important. Heterogeneity among patient populations and practitioner-investigators promotes a richer input into setting a research agenda and specific study planning with the goal of speeding the translation of research results into practice. Specifically, it is necessary to conduct studies in populations as representative as possible of patients in the communities where the study is being conducted, and that the study design reflects current practices (Green et al., 1994).

The governance of a PBRN should involve primarily practitioners, as the PBRN is a network designed to answer common questions encountered in clinical practice that perhaps cannot be addressed by more traditional industry/government/foundation grants (Culpepper and Froom, 1998). It is this constituency that will support the research from idea inception to implementation. The governance of a PBRN requires a small team, or executive committee (EC), to oversee the scientific agenda, set policies, and monitor the progress of the network in achieving its goals. Membership includes practitioners from the network, often on a rotating basis via election or appointment, representatives from the Network Chair (NC), or clinical operational component, representatives of the coordinating center (CC), which provides the data collection and analysis infrastructure, and a representative from the sponsoring agency (see Figure 14.1). This executive committee receives input from an external advisory committee, consisting of experts in clinical research and PBRN, not otherwise connected with the network, as well as a patient advocate. They can advise and guide the network, provide scientific critiques, and help the network avoid common problems encountered by earlier funded PBRN. The executive committee works with the sponsoring agency (private, government, foundation) so that their needs and demands are satisfied early on in the design and implementation process and throughout the life cycle of the network.

An efficient PBRN is a collaboration between the organizing scientists/clinicians (typically based at an academic or medical institution; frequently referred to as the Network Chair) and a coordinating center (this can be part of an academic or medical institution or could be a private organization such as a Clinical Research Organization (CRO)). Together they form the switchboard that connects practitioner-investigators and their patients with research. The Network Chair and the coordinating center provide the network with expertise in scientific method, study design, administration, quality control and assurance, regulatory adherence, and information dissemination.

14.2.2   Financial support for the PBRN

Substantial financial support is required for a large gamut of network duties that include the following: organization of the network; recruitment, retention, and training of the practitioner-investigators; development of clinical research protocols from idea inception through the Institutional Review Board (IRB) approval process; support from advisory committees and experts; clinical research operations; data coordination, management, quality control, and biostatistics; and finally, dissemination of the research findings. The financial resources to run the network should be the responsibility of the Network Chair and the coordinating center with input from the executive committee. Finances are needed not only to maintain the structure of the PBRN, but also for conducting the clinical research studies supported by the network.

Serious financial consideration must be given for critical areas of the clinical research enterprise such as hiring of clinical research coordinators (CRC) or associates to serve as a liaison with each practitioner to assist with training and assessment of data quality; organizing an electronic database for on-site, web-based data entry with subsequent data management and biostatistician analysis; reimbursement to consultants, committee members, and other advisory experts; reimbursement to practitioners and their patients for participating in clinical investigations; support for presentation of findings at regional, national, international meetings; preparation of network newsletters and other periodic communication formats; and publication of findings in peer-reviewed journals. Reimbursement to practitioner-investigators must take into consideration the cost to perform the study in the practice. For most practitioner-investigators, it is important that participation in clinical research does not result in loss of practice revenue.

Consideration of including compensation to patients for their participation must take into account ethical issues. If compensation is allocated, it is included within the practitioner agreement. Compensation to patients must not be seen as an enticement that may interfere with the patient's free choice of participation. An Institutional Review Board will typically review this aspect of the trial with respect to its ethical acceptability.

Close scrutiny of finances will help determine the size and scope of studies that can be supported by the network. Furthermore, the PBRN leaders must consider fiduciary issues well into the future, so as to plan grant applications and fund raising initiatives. A stable source of financing will ensure the survival and hopefully the growth of the network for many years of productive clinical research that will help advance the practice of health care.

14.3   Practice-based research in large group dental practices

D. Brad Rindal and Dan Pihlstrom for the Dental Practice-Based Research (DPBRN) Collaborative Group

Large group practices share characteristics that facilitate implementation of PBR and provide unique opportunities to conduct studies that may not be possible in other delivery models. Examples of large group practices are independent or corporately owned group practices as well as government managed health care systems to include the Department of Veterans Affairs, the Department of Defense, and the Public Health Service.

As a class, large group practices are quite diverse in the way they are organized and operate; however, many similarities exist that differentiate them from solo and small group practices. Large group practices typically provide dental services to a diverse and large number of patients through a network of regional offices or clinics. They may be integrated with medical services through a clinical information system that uses a common patient identifier for dental and medical information. Compensation for dentists is often different from a solo or small group practice and may be comprised of a salary and include incentives designed to promote a common set of evidence-based care guidelines. This treatment philosophy often plays an important role in operational and clinical aspects of a large group practice. One example is the use of a standardized dental chart that incorporates disease risk assessment tools and diagnosis codes. In addition, large group practices have a centralized administrative structure that actively supports dentists and facilitates communication between offices.

Large group practices provide certain efficiencies when deploying a PBRN study. Staff meetings provide a vehicle to discuss studies and encourage participation. The organic communications infrastructure provides economical and timely ways to communicate and coordinate with participating dentists. Quality control is more efficient because of access to patient charts and electronic data.

Large group practices often utilize an electronic dental record (EDR). The EDR screens can be created or altered to allow collection of the research data elements for a study. This avoids the need for a separate form to collect data, saving a significant amount of charting time for the dentist. The EDR also allows for remote viewing by the regional coordinator following the initial training of the clinician. Early evaluation of deviation from the protocol and incomplete data allow for early follow-up communications that improve data quality.

Large group practices provide ready access to robust dental, medical, and pharmacy data. These data allow for studies that examine the relationships between oral health and other medical conditions. Studies of this type can be carried out if the organizations are connected with researchers, statisticians, and programmers. Prior collaborative projects utilizing this type of data include examinations of the impact of xerostomic medications on caries-related restorations (Rindal et al., 2005; Maupomé et al., 2006) and of the caries risk assessment tools being used by the two groups (Bader et al., 2005; Rindal et al., 2006; Bader et al., 2008). In addition, access to large populations with reasonable levels of stability provides an opportunity to conduct studies that require longer observation periods. Longitudinal studies and registries are well suited for these types of large group practices.

14.4   Recruitment and retention strategies for practice-based research network investigators

Frederick A. Curro, Van Thompson, Ron Craig, and Don Vena for the PEARL Dental Practice-Based Research Network

14.4.1   Determinants of the size of a practice-based research network

A PBRN is defined as a group of practitioners who conduct research in their practices and are centrally linked to a governance and coordinating organization. These central organizations can take the form of academic centers or other contract research entities. These governance and coordinating organizations are responsible for practitioner recruitment and retention.

The ability to sustain an existing PBRN is dependent upon both the number and the intensity of the clinical studies being conducted and the retention of the practitioner-investigators within the network. The type of study conducted also affects the optimal size of a PBRN. A general research design principle for studies being conducted by a PBRN is to have a large number of practitioner-investigators recruit a relatively small number of subjects from each of their clinical practices into a given study. Conversely, for certain study designs, such as the randomized controlled clinical trial (RCT), it is preferable to have a smaller number of practitioner-investigators that recruit a relatively larger number of subjects from their practices into the study.

The PBRN design permits creativity and innovation in conducting clinical research and also allows the assessment of more inclusive populations, such as those necessary for drug effectiveness and safety studies (Mold and Peterson, 2005). The PRBN also has the ability to capture data not otherwise available in selected populations, such as that which is observed in a typical clinical practice (Lanier, 2005). If a research protocol can be easily incorporated into the work flow of a dental or medical practice, a relatively large PBRN can undertake a study and only be limited by the practice support staff's time to qualify the data collection, that is, the availability and motivation of CRC at the practice site as well as the clinical research associates (CRA) representing the PBRN (Nutting et al., 1998). Therefore, study design is very important to ensure both success of the PBRN protocol and the economic necessities of the participating practice (Genel and Dobs, 2003). The ability to design studies that fit within a time frame consistent with the practice's daily dynamics is vital to ensure that practices do not lose interest, reduces investigator turnover, keeps the office staff motivated, and reduces overhead costs of the PBRN.

In general, the more intensive studies such as randomized controlled trials demand a large cadre of well-trained and highly motivated practitioners. As a consequence, the business of conducting studies has to be balanced with the networks ability to recruit, retain, and train practitioners. Long periods of inactivation will increase practitioner turnover and thus cost. The PBRN must establish mechanisms to maintain contact with its practitioner-investigators during periods of relative inactivity to sustain practitioner-investigator interest.

It is generally accepted that recruitment and retention are best accomplished by establishing a personal relationship between practitioners and PBRN central organizations. Because the training of relatively research naïve practitioners to conduct sound clinical research is extremely expensive, the establishment of a personal relationship with practitioners by the PBRN is considered to be of great importance in reducing practitioner turnover and avoiding the high costs of training new practitioners. Strategies that maximize the potential for establishment of a personal relationship with practitioners must strive to engender a sense of ownership that ultimately makes each PBRN member a key recruitment asset for the organization.

14.4.2   Mechanisms for recruitment and retention of practitioner-investigators

Enrollment criteria must be established to select potential practitioner-investigators that will be successful in the network. One of the most important selection criteria is the willingness on the part of prospective members to enroll patients in network studies. For example, in the PEARL Dental Practice-based Research Network, practitioners interested in participating in the PBRN are generally mid-career, are involved with financially secure, well-established practices, and have a desire to contribute to the evidence base of their profession. However, even in financially successful practices, the level of practice disruption demanded by research is of paramount importance to practitioners.

Mass recruitment efforts have generally not met with significant success. However, the effect of network name branding as a result of these strategies is important and ultimately may enhance recruitment. Examples of mass recruitment strategies include network visibility at professional meetings, alumni functions, and in professional periodicals, newsletters, and advertisements.

It is generally agreed that the most successful recruitment strategies incorporate personalized contact with practitioners. This can be accomplished by designating for each PBRN member a recruitment emissary for the organization. In addition, the PBRN should strongly consider initiating personal contact with prospective members and even offering to visit practices that have indicated an initial willingness to join the network.

14.4.3 Stratification of practitioner-investigators in a practice-based research network

It is important that PBRN attempt to stratify their practitioner members based on their willingness and ability to complete network studies. The criteria for this stratification into tiers can be based on the willingness to enroll subjects, level of training and expertise, distance from the academic hub, and motivation to complete studies in a timely fashion. For example, organizing practitioners into three tiers has proven successful in some PBRN. Tier-one practitioners are the most motivated, most highly trained, and experienced investigators. These practitioners are generally selected to conduct more complex studies including randomized clinical trials. Conversely, tier-three practitioners have basic research training and skills, may be distant from the PBRN hub, and may only be interested in completing relatively simple studies involving survey and observational data. A critically important component of any PBRN is the ability to ensure the integrity of the data generated by the network. By organizing practitioners into tiers with at least one of the criteria being distance from the PBRN hub, the issues associated with ensuring data integrity can be addressed more effectively (see Figure 14.2).

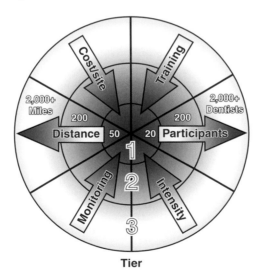

Figure 14.2 Three-tier system of participation of practitioner-investigators (P-I) in a practice-based research network. Tiers are defined by level of P-I participation, intensity of the research study, level of monitoring required, distance from the Network Chair (see Figure 14.1), cost/site for participating in the study, and level of required training for the study.

14.4.4   Recruitment of scientific content experts in support of the PBRN

PBRN must make a concerted effort to recruit and attract scientific content experts and engage them in the study development process. Recruitment incentives include an opportunity to engage in the PBRN research process that many investigators find attractive. The PBRN must recruit content experts in various fields, both scientists and those with clinical practice experience, to serve as consultants early in the study design phase. These individuals work closely with PBRN staff and certain key practitioner-investigators to discuss study design, funding, and feasibility issues. This assures the design of scientifically sound studies that address important clinical questions and are feasible in practitioner offices.

14.5   Study idea acquisition, prioritization, and development

Jack Ferracane, PhD, **and Tom Hilton,** DMD, MS, for the Northwest PRECEDENT (NWP) Dental Practice-Based Research Network

One of the essential themes of any PBRN is that it be practitioner centric. This may be achieved by encouraging practitioner involvement in as many activities as possible. Practitioner "buy-in" to research is necessarily predicated on their level of interest in its outcomes. Therefore, it is critical that the practitioners assume a significant role in identifying study ideas if the network is to be successful. Furthermore, it is important to engage the practitioner members early on in studies that they consider most relevant to their daily activities. Thus, the practitioner members should be involved in the process of prioritizing the studies to be pursued by the network. Finally, practitioner interest will most likely be maintained at a high level when they are somehow involved in the development of the study ideas and protocols, and not solely in their conduct.

This section of the chapter will address these important considerations. While reference may be made to the NIDCR-funded NWP dental practice-based research network, the systematic process is likely applicable to any dental practice-based research network (see Figure 14.3).

14.5.1   Research idea acquisition

Members initially enroll in the network by registering on the network website and completing a survey about their practice characteristics. In the course of responding, they may be asked to provide ideas for studies that interest them and that they would like to see conducted in the network. Study ideas are also solicited at various professional meetings from practitioners interested in joining the PBRN. These study questions range from the very general such as "What protocol works best to eliminate tooth decay?" to the more specific such as "Do dental implant supported prosthetics, that is, crowns and fixed partial dentures, have a shorter life expectancy in patients that have been chronic bruxers as compared to

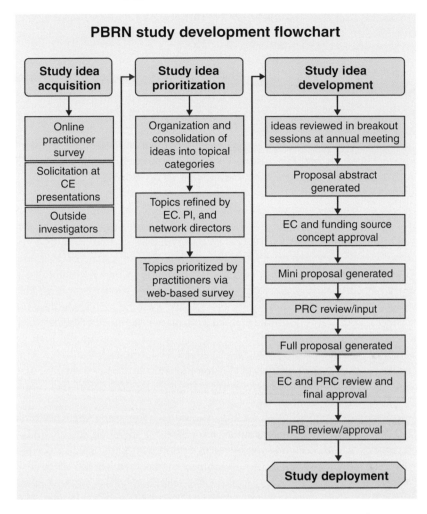

PBRN study development flowchart

Study idea acquisition	Study idea prioritization	Study idea development
Online practitioner survey	Organization and consolidation of ideas into topical categories	ideas reviewed in breakout sessions at annual meeting
Solicitation at CE presentations		Proposal abstract generated
Outside investigators	Topics refined by EC. PI, and network directors	EC and funding source concept approval
	Topics prioritized by practitioners via web-based survey	Mini proposal generated
		PRC review/input
		Full proposal generated
		EC and PRC review and final approval
		IRB review/approval
		Study deployment

Figure 14.3 From idea to reality: how a practitioner-generated proposal becomes a PBRN study.

nonbruxers?" Finally, additional study ideas may be submitted by nonmember practitioners and other investigators at the affiliated academic centers and other institutions who view the PBRN as an attractive research venue.

A multifaceted approach for eliciting study ideas has been shown to be popular in medical PBRN, where both practitioner members and outside investigators are active in identifying study questions. The process has been described as "bottom-up" when study ideas are elicited directly from the members, or from a steering committee composed of members, and has been reported in the literature by both dental and medical practice-based research networks (Wotman et al., 2001; Graham et al., 2007). In a recent national survey of 86 primary care research networks conducting practice-based studies, only 14% relied on their leaders or members to generate study ideas. Similarly, only 25% solicited research ideas from outside sources. Conversely, 61% of PBRN used a combination of their members and outside investigators to generate study ideas (Tierney et al., 2007).

14.5.2   Research idea prioritization

The study ideas received from the network members are compiled into topic categories by the office of the Network Chair that includes the network director, codirector, and the coinvestigators of the network. Study ideas are grouped together by theme and topic. Some of the topic areas that are suggested by one or two members only are combined with other studies to which they are broadly related. This consolidation is accomplished to assign the study topics into a diverse but manageable number of categories. A list of 10–20 topical categories provides sufficient variety without becoming too burdensome.

Consideration is also given to the available expertise for addressing all of the potential study ideas. From the refined list of study topics, PICO-type questions can be written by the network principal investigators. PICO is an acronym that serves as a guide to generating well-designed clinical research questions, where P refers to the patient or problem, I to the intervention, C to the comparison or control group, and O to the outcome to be assessed (Schlosser et al., 2007). PICO was originally introduced by Richardson et al. (1995) and has since been promoted for use in many disciplines, including evidence-based dentistry (Faggion and Tu, 2007). It is desirable that the practitioner members of the network receive instruction in the development of PICO questions as a part of the required PBRN training program (DeRouen et al., 2008).

When the study list is complete, it is submitted to the PBRN executive committee for approval. The EC consists of the network leadership, the study principal investigators, a funding agency representative, and a group of network practitioner-investigators, the latter comprising the majority vote on the committee. The study ideas are considered individually by the EC. Recommendations are made for maintaining the study idea as submitted, modifying, and refining the concept, or eliminating the study from the PBRN research agenda. This final list is then submitted to the membership at large for their consideration.

Most PBRN members have a strong interest in restorative dentistry. In order to diversify the PBRN research portfolio, modifications may be made to the priority list before studies are submitted for development. For example, all three of the NIDCR-funded dental networks were asked to develop and participate in a large, trans-network, case–control study on risk factors associated with osteonecrosis of the jaw (ONJ). Although an ONJ study had been ranked of moderate interest to the member practitioners, the EC voted to participate in the study because of the potential public health implications.

14.5.3   Research idea development

Once the research topics of greatest interest have been selected and research portfolio finalized, the top research ideas are submitted for development. Studies are usually developed by a team composed of academic professionals and practitioners. Issues considered in this process include feasibility, study design, and the probability that the study will serve to fill an existing knowledge gap in clinical practice. Once the study has been developed, it may be presented to the practitioners in conceptual form at the PBRN annual meeting. It is reasonable to efficiently present and discuss several study ideas in this way. A brief oral presentation is made to the entire assembly of practitioner members, and then the members are given the opportunity to select the specific studies they want to review further in small group breakout sessions.

Study discussions and breakout sessions are of enormous benefit to the study designers. Perhaps more importantly, they serve to energize the practitioner members by enabling them to participate in the study development process and raising their level of anticipation about the coming studies. These breakout sessions also provide an opportunity for practitioner members to identify themselves as part of a future "working group" assembled by the study developers to respond to specific questions arising during the development of the complete protocol.

Once the final study idea is formulated, an abstract is generated and submitted to the EC for approval. Once all of the approvals have been acquired, a more comprehensive study abstract or "mini-proposal" is prepared and submitted to the network CC. The CC provides the data analysis plan and sample size calculations. It is at this stage that the practitioner working group is engaged via e-mail communication and internet surveys to further refine the study protocol and provide additional input that will aid further in developing and refining the protocol.

The "mini-proposal" typically consists of a 4–6 page protocol describing the background, objectives, specific aims, hypotheses, significance, research design, and data analysis. It is reviewed and refined by the PBRN. It is then resubmitted to the EC for final approval. This then signals that the protocol is ready to undergo preliminary scrutiny by an external protocol review committee (PRC).

The PRC is a scientific review body ideally composed of individuals with expertise in biostatistics, general dentistry, PBRN administration, and clinical investigation with nonvoting membership by the funding agency. For the sake of objectivity, the members of the PRC are selected and appointed by an entity not related to the PBRN. The role of the PRC is to assess the scientific merit of the study and to evaluate study design and feasibility. Three outcomes are possible. These are as follows:

1. Approval
2. Disapproval with recommendation for resubmission
3. Disapproval and not recommended for resubmission

If the protocol is approved, it is then submitted to an IRB to assure that human subjects are protected during the conduct of the study. If the protocol is disapproved with recommendations for resubmission, study proponents revise the protocol incorporating the critiques provided by the PRC. The study is then resubmitted to the PRC for a second formal review.

Once the IRB approval is obtained, the study is ready for deployment to practitioner-investigators in a pilot study group, typically about five practices, in order to determine compensation and to identify any final changes in the protocol before the deployment of the full study. Because each practice is compensated for their participation time in each study, an estimate of the time required to complete the protocol is obtained and an acceptable compensation rate plan is determined based on the distribution of practitioner and staff effort. Feasibility issues are again assessed in the pilot deployments and the study is further refined based on the recommendation of the practitioners. Many criteria are used to determine whether or not a particular practice is to be included in a study. These include the number of studies previously completed, practice configuration, staff motivation, patient demographics, and other criteria specific to each study.

In summary, one of the main attractions for doing research in practice-based networks is the "real-world" nature of the outcomes. But the inherent variability of the proposition requires tremendous attention to study protocol details in order to obtain results of high quality, and in a way that is acceptable and exciting to the variety of practitioner-investigators involved.

14.6   Study deployment, implementation, and coordination

Anita H. Sung, Brooke Latzke, and Andrea Mathews
for the CONDOR Dental Practice-Based Research Group

14.6.1   Identifying interested practitioners and office staff members

Once a study protocol is approved by the IRB but before it is deployed, a survey is prepared to assess the interest of the network's P-I and their staff in participating in the study. The new study protocol and the corresponding interest survey are announced to the network via e-mail and posted on the network's website. These are typically followed by a reminder e-mail and faxes to the practitioners. If a practice initially fails to respond, a follow-up phone call is made to determine whether or not a practice is interested in participating in a particular study.

This interest survey includes a one-page summary of the protocol with study procedures, projected timeline, and responsibilities of the P-I and their staff. The survey also includes a list of the inclusion/exclusion criteria for patient eligibility to aid the practitioners and office staffs in considering whether their patient population is appropriate for the study. On the basis of this information, the practitioners are asked to decide whether their offices have the resources to commit to the study as well as to estimate the number of study patients they anticipate enrolling in the study.

Clinical study monitors (CSM) and/or pharmaceutical industry clinical research associates are typically employed in the conduct of PBRN interest surveys. CSM and CRA are staff specially trained in the principles of conducting a clinical study under good clinical practice (GCP) and knowledgeable in the aspects of clinical study auditing. Their primary responsibility is to assure that office personnel are properly trained and that the studies are conducted in accordance with the prescribed protocols. They typically attempt to recruit practices that are a good fit for a particular study.

The dialogue stimulated by the preliminary surveys gives practices a headstart in preparing for an upcoming study while providing the network clinical study monitors an opportunity to select sites for participation and to prepare study materials, and other resources for training, certification, and approval.

14.6.2   Study pilot testing

Before full network deployment of a study, it is pilot tested in a representative sample of practices to assess feasibility and the operational aspects of data collection. This process also provides an opportunity to test educational materials and the strategies that will eventually be used to train personnel. In general, pilot testing is an extremely effective means of assessing the operational aspects of a study. It provides a significant opportunity to identify and resolve potential problems and to refine the study design to assure compatibility with the office environment.

14.6.3   Practitioner and office staff training

Incorporating clinical research into a dental practice is a rather new concept. Typically, the vast majority of dental offices are naïve to the principles involved in clinical research. For many of the practitioners, this will be their first exposure to the conduct of clinical research. This presents particular challenges to the PBRN that require a unique approach to research training. Fortunately, office staff are often receptive to research training because of their enthusiasm for the novel concept of practice-based research. Practitioners and office staff will be required to rapidly become familiar and facile with research terminology. Although practice-based research strives for minimal office disruption, some modification of daily office routines will be required to conduct clinical research.

Perhaps of greatest importance to a practice considering involvement with a particular study is to assess the level of disruption that the study-related processes will cause. Seamlessly integrating clinical research into daily practice differs for each office. Training materials, tutorials, and other study resources can be provided in a variety of formats to accommodate these practice differences. Communication between clinical study monitors and practices may be accomplished by e-mail, fax, and telephone based on the office preference.

While clinical study monitors and clinical research associates seek to provide support and helpful suggestions for incorporating research into clinical practice, the participating dental offices are also encouraged to communicate with one another. The latter provides opportunities to share experiences and strategies for incorporating clinical research into daily office operations. Collaboratively, this provides a forum for the exchange of ideas and experiences while engendering a sense of camaraderie.

Research involving human subjects is subject to stringent government regulations designed to protect research participants. Training is required in human subject research, good clinical practices, and the Health Insurance Portability and Accountability Act (HIPAA). Training in human subjects protection is offered by the National Institutes of Health (NIH) and the Collaborative IRB Training Initiative. Recertification in good clinical practice, HIPAA, and human subjects protection is generally required on an annual basis.

In addition, training specific to each study is provided to the office staff. This training may be in the form of tutorials or other educational materials. While training is frequently offered in a classroom setting, web- or DVD-based tutorials may be substituted or used to augment the other venues. Practitioners and other office staff are frequently awarded continuing dental education credits by the PBRN-affiliated academic center upon completion of this training. Annual meetings offer an additional training opportunity.

Before study deployment at individual sites, clinical study monitors conduct training sessions during which they provide the prospective participating practices with a study binder containing the study protocol, informed consent documents, IRB approval documents, and a Manual of Procedures (MOP). The MOP, one the most important training documents, may include a training manual, study forms, study logs, and source document worksheets. Office staff and practitioners are also provided training in data collection and submission procedures. Although electronic data capture (EDC) over a secure website is the preferred mode for data acquisition, offices not equipped to use EDC have the option to use paper forms that are then transmitted to data coordinating centers.

Once didactic training is completed, clinical study monitors and clinical research associates may spend additional time in offices to provide additional training and to assure adherence to the study protocol procedures. For the remainder of the study, the clinical study monitor is always available by telephone or e-mail to answer questions, resolve problems, and, if necessary, return to the office to provide additional assistance when required.

Training in the protection of human subjects and the informed consent process is extremely important. This training can be conducted using a variety of venues and media. Each provides a detailed explanation of the informed consent process as it pertains to the study procedures. It also includes a section on risks and benefits, HIPAA considerations, and other important issues related to the protection of human research participants.

In addition to detailed study protocol instructions, each site is provided with a condensed version of the protocol suitable for quick reference in the treatment room. These are usually laminated one- or two-page documents that contain essential information on subject eligibility criteria, protocol flowcharts, and the steps involved in the informed consent process.

Study sites are required to keep all study-related documents in a study binder. This binder is periodically reviewed by the clinical study monitor and clinical research associate to verify adherence to the protocol, to assure the timely and appropriate entry and submission of data, and compliance with other regulations pertaining to good clinical research practices. This assists PBRN clinical study monitors and clinical research associates in assuring that studies are conducted in accordance with all applicable guidelines and regulations.

14.6.4   Role of the Practice Research Coordinator

Practice Research Coordinators are members of the practitioner office staff who will be actively engaged in the conduct of research. At least one Practice Research Coordinator is appointed at each study site. When multiple Practice Research Coordinators are appointed, one of these is designated the lead Practice Research Coordinator in that office. These personnel work closely with the clinical study monitors to assure that studies are conducted in accordance with the protocol and that there is adherence to all pertinent regulatory requirements.

Practice Research Coordinators may include office managers, hygienists, dental assistants, and sometimes receptionists. The enthusiastic participation and cooperation of office staff are important if the study is to be conducted with minimal interruption to the daily operations of the practice. When multiple office staff members are involved, each is encouraged to take responsibility for a specific study task or tasks and to work as a team to prevent overburdening any one member of the team.

Practice Research Coordinators typically assist with the identification of potential research participants, participate in the informed consent process, administer survey instruments, enter and submit research data, conduct study participant follow-up, and distribute participation incentives. Although the practitioner-investigator is ultimately responsible for study implementation and conduct, the Practice Research Coordinators perform the majority of the day-to-day operations associated with the conduct of research in the office.

One of the most important functions of the Practice Research Coordinator is to serve as a liaison with the PBRN Director and the coordinating center. The Practice Research Coordinator serves as a conduit for information and frequently participates on network conference calls designed to assess study progress, participant recruitment, and to provide feedback to the PBRN on the entire research experience.

14.6.5   Memoranda of understanding and other legal documents

Practitioner-investigators and their respective practice research coordinators are required to execute memoranda of understanding and other documents that legally bind them to conduct the study in accordance with the protocol and comply with all related training requirements. In addition, they agree to submit to periodic site monitoring inspections.

All documents pertaining to this participation in the PBRN are maintained in a regulatory document file. Required documentation may include curriculum vitae, dental license, cardiopulmonary resuscitation certification, Drug Enforcement Agency certificate, Controlled Substance Registration certificate, and other clinical research training certificates. All PBRN retain copies of IRB approvals, executed agreements, and study site visit reports for each practitioner-investigator. When practice or research participant remuneration is involved, PBRN maintain clinical trial collaborative agreements, individual investigator agreements, a memorandum of agreements, and scope of work documents.

14.6.6   Research quality assurance procedures

To assure research quality and data integrity, PBRN clinical study monitors conduct standardized procedures for monitoring studies. Clinical study monitors based at the PBRN academic centers are assigned to a specified number of offices and are a source of training, guidance, and assistance throughout the period of implementation and the subsequent life span of each study. Clinical study monitors contact the offices on a regular basis, monitor data entry, and are available for support via phone and e-mail. It is important that office staff view clinical study monitors as a valuable resource for assistance during the study. Clinical study monitors strive to build a positive, supportive relationship with each practice. Overall, the PBRN attempt to engender a collaborative environment aimed at building a community of researchers. Clinical study monitors perform a pivotal role in this process.

Specific duties of the clinical study monitor include review of informed consent documentation, confirmation of study patient eligibility, and verification of the accuracy of data transfer from source documents to case report forms. Clinical study monitors conduct study initiation visits and study closeout visits as appropriate. Periodic study monitor visits are scheduled with a frequency sufficient for the enrollment and the expected volume of study data generated by the sites. Clinical study monitors are authorized to file IRB reports related to adverse events, protocol deviations, and violations. They also facilitate communication among the various study sites, the PBRN academic centers, coordinating centers, and certain other regulatory entities.

14.6.7   Encouraging practitioner and patient participation

It is critical to maintain the interest of both the practitioners and office staff both during and after the conduct of a study. In the course of a given study, clinical study monitors play a critical role in maintaining practice interest by scheduling meetings and conference calls. After the conclusion of a study, clinical study monitors provide sites with periodic updates on study results. This serves to provide feedback to the participating practices and reinforces in each practice the importance of their participation in network research.

A well-trained and highly motivated office staff is key to study patient recruitment and ultimately study success. To this end, PBRN studies are specifically designed to minimize the burden on both the patient and the office staff. Conducting practice-based research is nevertheless different from daily clinical practice. However, the greatest success is achieved when studies can be designed that will have minimal impact on the daily clinical practice.

PBRN studies are typically designed so that the research process can be accomplished during the patient's regularly scheduled dental appointment. This requires expert coordination by the office staff so that the research component is seamlessly integrated into the regular dental appointment without unduly disrupting clinical operations. If a study requires follow-up appointments, the Practice Research Coordinator reminds the patient that additional appointments will be required to complete their participation in the study. The Practice Research Coordinator may also be responsible for arranging follow-up appointments and subsequently contacting patients to remind them of their obligations under the terms of the research protocol should compliance become an issue.

14.6.8   Data capture and management

Data from the majority of PBRN studies are recorded on paper at the office site and submitted electronically via an EDC system to the coordinating center. Most electronic data capture systems are designed to detect spurious data entries and to generate a query requesting that the data be entered in accordance with the design of the study. Electronic data capture is clearly the most efficient means of data capture but requires that each research site has a broadband internet connection.

Once data are submitted to the coordinating center, it is reviewed by clinical study monitors for any irregularities. These are flagged in the data entry system and the research site is notified and provided instructions for correcting the entry. Again, clinical study monitors have a critical role in assuring the integrity of study data.

14.6.9   Study design and variances from the standard of care

Clinical studies appropriate for the PBRN model may include surveys as well as retrospective and prospective observational studies. These protocols are typical standard-of-care studies in which the practitioner provides the care that would normally be accomplished at the patient's dental appointment. These studies tend to be low risk and involve less complexity than prospective cohort studies, retrospective case–controls studies, interventional studies, and randomized controlled trials.

Interventional studies that vary from the standard of care may require discussions with dental insurance carriers to resolve reimbursement issues, particularly when a practitioner receives compensation from the PBRN for study participation.

Finally, it is important that the length of time from initial site recruitment to study initiation be minimized to assure compliance with all aspects of the study protocol by leveraging the impact of training closely approximated to study initiation.

In summary, study deployment, implementation, and coordination are critical phases of practice-based research. Most practices are naïve to the concept of clinical research. The process requires collaboration between PBRN personnel and practitioner-investigators to assure that appropriate practices are recruited and then rigorously trained in clinical research. PBRN must strive to conduct studies that minimize the impact on the daily routines of dental offices while assuring adherence to study protocols, maintenance of data integrity, and compliance with applicable regulations.

14.7   Data acquisition and analysis

O. Dale Williams, PhD, **Anne S. Lindblad,** PhD, **Brian G. Leroux,** PhD for the CONDOR Dental Practice-Based Research Group

Subsequent to the critical decisions as to study design and participant eligibility, selection, and recruitment, perhaps the next most important components of any research endeavor are those associated with data acquisition, data management, and analyses. These are perhaps best considered as processes and they tend to be more complex, demanding, and time consuming than is often recognized. Thus, they may either take longer to complete than planned or they may not receive attention commensurate with their importance and data quality may suffer unnecessarily. Six broad categories for these components include the following:

1. Decisions as to which data are to be collected.
2. How the data are to be collected in terms of measurements, questionnaires, and procedures.
3. How the data are to be transmitted and processed through the various steps that are required to get results from their initial source all the way into reports and publications.
4. Quality assurance and quality control for data collection and processing activities.
5. Utilization of appropriate statistical analysis procedures.
6. Review of data and results for appropriateness and correctness.

Dental practice-based research networks must approach these issues in a somewhat different context than is often the case for other types of research. Research done in a practice setting collecting data from or about patients involved in care delivery encounters cannot be overly disruptive. Specifically, it must not impact negatively on care delivery. Typically, this means that the volume of data obtained during patient encounters needs to be quite limited. For example, in one network, the target is the equivalent of two pages of questionnaires or less per patient encounter. Further, the mechanism for data acquisition itself should not distract the dentist or other care providers from their delivery of care responsibilities.

In this context, developing and implementing data collection instruments require careful attention. These activities can be guided by the considerable experience of previous research endeavors (Knatterud et al., 1983; DePauw, 1989; Christiansen et al., 1990; Spilker and Schoenfelder, 1991; Hosking et al., 1995; McFadden, 1998). An essential step for study development is piloting the procedures and data collection instruments prior to their full implementation, a step especially important for a practice-based research setting. Ensuring that practices are aware of the expected workload of study participation can help maximize the chance of successful implementation. Piloting can identify areas where the flow of questions does not conform to typical practice procedures, questions are unclear, or response categories are incomplete.

Also important is the quality and standardization of data collection procedures (Williams, 1979; Whitney et al., 1998), especially for practice-based settings since the primary data collection typically is undertaken by dental care providers and their staff, in contrast to research conducted in university settings that employs personnel specifically trained in research methodology. For some projects, the local dental office may collect limited data on, say, 50 consecutive patients so that there is a need only for a one-time training session, with special emphasis on the importance of a truly consecutive sample.

In other cases, the study may involve several patient encounters over an extended period. This situation creates special problems in that the encounters may be relatively infrequent and thus data collection staff may not utilize the procedures sufficiently frequently to become skilled and adept at the process. Or they may not be equipped with tools to manage patient adherence to a follow-up visit schedule with the rigor required by a research study.

Dental practice-based research networks tend to collect three broad categories of data:

1. Data from surveys of practitioners across their networks about practitioner or practice characteristics that does not require information from specific patient encounters

2. Data from the practitioner relating to issues during specific patient encounters

3. Data from measurements or questionnaires directly from patients

Each of these three basic data types require somewhat different approaches to data acquisition for reasonable efficiency and also to statistical analyses so that the analytical approaches properly reflect data structure. Also, the three types may be used for collecting data for a variety of study designs, ranging from surveys to clinical trials. All types require competent and efficient data management and processing procedures for effective study operations. General discussions of these procedures are readily available and can be most helpful in setting up systems for new studies (DuChene et al., 1986; DePauw, 1989; Hosking et al., 1995; McFadden et al., 1995; McFadden, 1998; Society for Clinical Data Management, 2003; Association for Clinical Data Management, 2005).

14.7.1   Quality assurance

Training in human subjects protection and good clinical practices for research prior to initiating research helps set the groundwork for study-specific training. A good training program is just the beginning. Ongoing monitoring and close contact with investigators are essential to reinforce good research practices and provide additional training as needed. A roving coordinator approach can help in this process as well as scheduled study calls to discuss problems encountered and potential solutions. Using an experienced study coordinator who regularly contacts sites both via telephone and in person provides an important personal connection and resource to practice-based research sites. Ongoing data monitoring for completeness and consistency and prompt reporting to the practice of deficiencies with follow-up for resolution can help prevent small problems from growing and impacting study quality.

14.7.2   Patient selection and statistical analysis considerations

An essential ingredient for all statistical analyses is that the analytical approach and tools used need to match the structures of the population selected and the data being analyzed. Study design and analysis must take into account how patients will be enrolled in the study. For surveys and case series, selection bias and nonresponse bias can severely limit the value of a study. For example, if consecutive patients will be selected as the population, ensuring scheduling practices do not introduce bias is an important consideration (Lilienfeld and Lilienfeld, 1980).

For dental practice-based research, the data structures can be especially complex because of the varying levels of dependencies, or lack of complete independence of data elements in the data set. For example, *within practices*, dentists are likely to approach some issues in a common fashion so that they tend to be somewhat more alike each other than like dentists in other practices; *within dentists*, patients are likely to be treated in a rather consistent manner and this may be somewhat different than it is for patients of other dentists; *within patients,* different teeth are subjected to a vast array of issues common to that patient; *within teeth*, different surfaces or tooth components are likely to be subjected to some common issues that may be somewhat different from those of surfaces on other teeth within the same person.

Statistical analyses that take these factors into account can be quite challenging because of their multilevel structure. Statistical methods that can accommodate multilevel dental data are available. However, the application of these methods is not straightforward because it involves careful choice of an appropriate model on which to base the analysis. The interested reader can refer to the book by Lesaffre et al. (2009) for details.

14.7.3   Data sharing

Comparability across networks, across studies within networks, and over time within studies is an important consideration as the above issues are implemented. For example, the PBRN funded by NIDCR that make up CONDOR have established procedures to develop common data elements in the context of the caBIG program (https://cabig.nci.nih.gov/) for studies undertaken within the networks. This approach will allow researchers to combine data across studies in various networks with some confidence in the comparability of the data.

14.8   Participant protection and scientific peer review in dental PBRN

Gregg H. Gilbert, DDS, MBA, **O. Dale Williams,** PhD, **Sheila D. Moore,** CIP, for the DPBRN Collaborative Group

14.8.1   Aspects of the PBRN context that make it different with regard to human participants protections

The PBRN research context presents unique challenges to designing and implementing research studies (Genel and Dobs, 2003; Lindbloom et al., 2004; Mold and Peterson, 2005;

Graham et al., 2007; Westfall et al., 2007; Gilbert et al., 2008). Unlike studies conducted in academic health centers, PBRN studies are conducted by clinicians in community-based settings, whose main job is still to provide clinical care even while they are participating in a clinical research study. Furthermore, these persons may be doing their first research study and therefore have no experience in doing research.

Unique to the PBRN context, a healthy tension exists between the need to conduct research directly relevant to clinical practice, to protect the rights of participants (including the confidentiality and privacy of all personnel such as patients, practitioner-investigators, and the practice's staff), to provide and document informed consent, yet also to minimize burden on practices and their patients. This all must be accomplished within a single study design that often includes different geographic regions and very different types of clinical settings. Because all of their potential research participants are also patients for whom they will continue to provide clinical care, practitioner-investigators and their staff must also be sensitized to the need to avoid any sense of pressure, intimidation, or appearance of a conflict of interest during the informed consent process.

IRB need to have written, contractual assurance that potentially inexperienced PBRN personnel understand all applicable procedures and regulations so that they can be compliant with them. Federal regulations governing these assurances have changed or evolved at times. Indeed, a key aspect of these requirements, the individual investigator agreement mechanism (discussed later), is itself only from 2005 (OHRP, 2005).

Many PBRN studies are observational in design and only record information about treatment from the chart or treatment record—treatment that will be done regardless of whether the patient agrees to become a participant in the research study about that treatment. Consequently, there may be an opportunity to propose to Institutional Review Boards an informed consent process that includes a waiver of documentation of consent and thereby is streamlined and less burdensome to the flow of busy clinical practices.

IRB can make three conclusions about PBRN studies. IRB can conclude for an individual study that the (1) practitioner-investigators are the only subjects in the study; (2) patients are the only subjects of the study; or (3) that both patients and practitioner-investigators are subjects in the study. With conclusions #1 and #3, practitioner-investigators will need to provide informed consent. With conclusion #2, only patients need to provide informed consent.

14.8.2   Procedures required to participate in clinical studies

Common to requirements for clinical studies done in academic settings, certifications for PBRN research also require that key personnel who are employed by the academic institution also obtain training and certification in human participants research. These faculty and staff are named in the IRB applications and receive approval to conduct the PBRN research as employees, much as if the research were to be conducted in an academic setting instead of the PBRN context.

Community-based practitioner-investigators and other personnel who are not employees of the academic institution but are key personnel are also required to complete training in human participants research. Some PBRN provide this training during a face-to-face meeting with practitioner-investigators (such as an annual meeting of all practitioner-investigators in which results from the PBRN's studies are discussed), while other PBRN may allow an online training and certification option. One option used in some PBRN is a course provided by the National Institutes of Health (National Cancer Institute, 2008). Practitioner-investigators may review a printed version supplied by the PBRN, log onto the website, take a test to document competency, print and save electronically a certificate, and then e-mail that certificate to their PBRN staff coordinator.

The administrative home base for the PBRN, which is typically a university, may obtain IRB approval for general network operations separately. These general operations may include recruitment of practitioner-investigators, communications with them and their staff, collection of questionnaire data about characteristics of the practitioner-investigators and their practices, and related activities. Specific research studies are then approved via separate, study-specific IRB protocols.

Practitioner-investigators can participate in studies only after an IRB has approved their participation for a specific study. Thus, each practitioner-investigator is included at the time of submission or added to each study separately, on a study-by-study basis. To be added to a particular study, practitioner-investigators must complete requirements in addition to their human participants training, such as other IRB documents or contracts. These requirements can vary substantially from one IRB to the next.

Practitioner-investigators may need to sign a study-specific amendment to a study already approved by their host IRB. This is done to document that they have read and understood the protocol, that their human participants certification is up-to-date. They may also need to sign an informed consent form if they themselves are subjects of the study. The consent form would be maintained by the principal investigator.

Community-based practitioner-investigators are typically attached to their IRB via a written agreement, such as a memorandum of understanding developed by the IRB's institutions or an individual investigator agreement, a mechanism allowed by the agency responsible for oversight of U.S. federally funded studies (OHRP, 2005). A sample agreement is provided at the agency's website.

PBRN that involve more than one IRB create a circumstance where the IRB for the PBRN's administrative site will need to accept the review done by the IRB in another region. For studies funded by U.S. agencies, the IRB for the administrative site will require that the other IRB be registered with the U.S. Office for Human Research Protections (OHRP, 2008a, 2008b). In addition to accepting the review by the other IRB, the administrative site IRB will need documentation from the other IRB that particular practitioner-investigators have been approved to do that particular study. Only then can the PBRN's administrative site and the PBRN's coordinating center accept data from that practitioner-investigator.

In addition to human participant assurances, a mechanism is necessary to remunerate practitioner-investigators, to contractually obligate them to follow federal and local regulations, and to assure no conflict of interest. This mechanism can be handled by a contract such as a memorandum of agreement that each practitioner-investigator or participating clinic authority signs. This agreement may subsequently be amended for each of the PBRN's studies.

Requirements differ depending on whether practitioner-investigators are community based or whether they are employees of an organization. Practitioner-investigators who are employees will have already been named as investigators when an IRB application for a specific study is submitted to their IRB. Consequently, they do not have to sign study-specific amendments, individual investigator agreements, or memoranda of agreement. The same circumstance applies to faculty investigators and staff who are employees of affiliated research foundations or universities.

14.8.3   Variations among IRB

The literature provides evidence of substantial variation in IRB reviews for multicenter studies (Gold and Dewa, 2005; Wolf et al., 2005; AAMC, 2006; Blustein et al., 2007). See Chapter 3 for institutional requirements of IRB. Different conclusions made by IRB can not only cause prolonged delays in network-wide implementation of studies, but may also force PBRN to choose between (1) changing the study design to reach a consensus among the network's IRB and (2) not being able to implement the study in all the network's regions.

With the first clinical study in one dental PBRN (Gilbert et al., 2009), substantial streamlining of protocols did result from engaging IRB in a series of discussions. This study required practitioner-investigators to collect data about the reasons for placing the first restoration on a previously unrestored tooth surface. The study did not alter treatment. Instead, it recorded information about routine dental treatment that was going to be done anyway. One dental PBRN IRB approved a waiver of documentation of informed consent. In another dental PBRN region, a protocol was submitted using an informed consent form that was standard for most projects approved by that IRB. Early feedback from practitioner-investigators and patients using these forms was that this process was cumbersome, inconsistent with the notion that this was a minimal-risk study of routine treatment, and raised suspicion among patients instead of decreasing it. Following additional discussions with that IRB, a revised protocol was submitted and approved. In the revised protocol, participants were provided a one-page information sheet, the study was discussed with them, informed consent was obtained verbally, and documentation of consent was noted in the patient's chart and a study log of enrolled participants. Comparable reductions in the length of the consent process were subsequently obtained with two other IRB in that PBRN.

This same dental PBRN also has a Scandinavian region, which involves IRB in three different countries (Gilbert et al., 2008). Different arrangements were necessary between the IRB at the administrative site (University of Alabama at Birmingham, UAB) and each of these countries. For one country, the UAB IRB serves as the IRB of record. In another country, the UAB IRB required a formal agreement with the host IRB because although that IRB was registered with the U.S. federal system, its FWA was not active. For the third Scandinavian country, the UAB IRB interacts with that host country's IRB in a manner very similar to the IRB in the U.S. DPBRN regions.

Instead of viewing IRB as potentially adversarial, customized solutions for minimal risk, observational studies can be identified by engaging IRB in collegial discussions that identify common ground within regulatory bounds. These solutions can improve acceptability of PBRN research to patients, practitioners, and university researchers.

14.8.4   Data and Safety Monitoring Boards in PBRN

Data and Safety Monitoring Boards (DSMB) are committees of independent experts with overview responsibilities for the conduct of clinical trials. The value and importance of creating an outside, independent group of experts, expected to be free of conflicts of interests for the trial in question, to monitor the ongoing activities of clinical trials, has been recognized for some time. In fact, the need for such boards was first articulated in 1967 in what is known as the Greenberg Report (1967). Since that initial recommendation, the need for and functioning of such boards have received considerable attention (Friedman et al., 1998; Ellenberg et al., 2002; DeMets et al., 2006; NIH, 2008). At this point, the funding agencies for most clinical trials require monitoring by an independent board including members with appropriate expertise. In general, this process puts the primary responsibility for assessing the status of an ongoing trial in the hands of a group that would not benefit financially or otherwise from the consequences of board recommendations.

These boards tend to have variable names, including DSMB, data monitoring committees, and Safety and Data Monitoring Boards. Their overarching purpose is to protect the safety of the participants in the trials and to assess scientific appropriateness, efficacy, study quality, and study performance. Their role reflects the fact that clinical trials tend to be conducted on the interface between science and society, and the boards functioning reflects this interface in the sense that good science is conducted in a manner that does not cause harm to participants and that is to the public good. The role of DSMB for non-PBRNs is described in Chapter 12 on phase 3 clinical trials.

14.8.5   Charge and topics addressed

The charge to DSMB reflects their overarching purpose of protecting the safety of trial participants so that adverse events and endpoint frequency are always critical issues to be assessed. Beyond this, the boards also address scientific appropriateness and quality. Specifically, this includes the status of participant recruitment, allocation to treatment groups, data quality and timeliness, and the ever so critical issue of possible early termination.

14.8.6   The peer review process in PBRN

A key operating principle for most PBRN is that the research questions originate from practitioner-investigators, and that the answers to these questions have the potential to improve the practice of dentistry. This situation creates a healthy tension between the needs of a sound research project and the need not to be overly disruptive of daily clinical practice. In this sense, the process requires neither the researchers to become practitioners nor the practitioners to become full-time researchers.

PBRN will commonly obtain input on the design of each study from research staff who will most directly interact with practitioner-investigators during data collection. This input may lead to changes in the study design to make the study more feasible to conduct in clinical practice. Either before or after (or both) receiving input from research staff, a PBRN will typically have an executive committee that serves as its main decision-making body. Ideally, this committee would have its majority voting authority reside with practitioner-investigators, not with academic faculty. In this manner, review occurs among practitioners' peers very early in the process. It is not uncommon for studies to be rejected at this point because they are judged not to be of broad interest to practitioners or because they are not feasible to conduct in a busy clinical practice.

Most PBRN end the formal peer review process at this point. The three dental PBRN funded by NIDCR have an additional step in peer review. Once study applications have been approved by the executive committee, they are sent for final scientific review to the protocol review committee. This committee comprises dental clinical scientists, a biostatistician, a medical PBRN director, a practicing dentist, and an NIDCR representative. This committee, constituted by NIDCR, not the PBRN, has the mandate to approve, disapprove, or recommend changes to all studies. All committee members are unaffiliated with the dental PBRN so as to provide an objective and independent scientific review.

If the protocol review committee approves the study, the PBRN then submits IRB applications from each of its regions. Data collection forms and study processes are typically pilot tested with an initial group of practitioner-investigators across the network. Pilot testing may lead to substantial changes in the forms and in that sense serves as a last step in the peer review process for study implementation.

14.9   Translation of research into practice

Ruth McBride, PhD for the CONDOR Dental Practice-Based Research Group

The translation of research findings into clinical practice is important but challenging aspect of research conducted in any venue. Balas and Boren (2000) estimated that it requires an average of 17 years from the first report of research results to implementation in a clinical practice. Various explanations have been provided for this apparently excessive time to translation including the inability of practitioners to adequately review the literature (Williamson et al., 1989) and conflicting results from several studies that confuse practitioners and patients alike (Haynes and Haines, 1998) (see also Chapter 1).

In an effort to improve the quality of health care delivered in the United States and elsewhere, there has been a move to implement "evidence-based medicine" or "evidence-based health care." Evidence-based medicine has been defined as "the conscientious and judicious use of current best evidence from clinical care research in the management of individual patients" (Sacket et al., 1996). In 2003, the American Dental Associations defined evidence-based dentistry as "an approach to oral health care that requires the judicious integration of systematic assessments of clinically relevant scientific evidence related to the patients oral and medical condition and history, with the dentist's clinical expertise and the patient's treatment needs and preferences" (ADA Policy Statement, 2003).

Although much work remains to be done to determine how best to facilitate the translational process, one review suggests that interactive educational experiences were more likely to facilitate the translational process than were educational materials or lectures (Bero et al., 1998). In addition, it has been suggested that patients have become more influential in determining treatment decisions due to the proliferation of direct-to-consumer advertising and marketing (McGlone et al., 2001).

The infrastructure and organization of practice-based research networks appear to be designed to support a more expeditious translation of research findings into practice. It is possible that practice-based research findings may be translated more rapidly in the PBRN setting because the practitioner-investigators and their staff are directly engaged in data collection. This research model may engender a sense of ownership and involvement that may enhance the early adoption of new techniques and strategies into clinical practice when the evidence to support this change is the result of research in which the dental team participated. Also, the collaborative nature of practice-based research may lend itself to improved communication among practices and between practices and academic centers. Practice-based research networks are engaged in a self-assessment process to determine whether this model for clinical research can truly enhance and expedite the process of translating clinical evidence into improvements in clinical practice.

Dedication

This chapter is dedicated to the memory of Jonathan Ship whose boundless energy and unwavering support for dental practice-based research served as an inspiration to all.

References

Section 14.1: Introduction to dental practice-based research networks (PBRN)

Agency for Healthcare Research and Quality. 2008. *Primary Care Practice-Based Research Networks.* Available online at http://www.ahrq.gov/about/highlt07b.htm. Accessed on November 23, 2008.

Case Western Reserve University. 2008. *CROWN Dental Practice-Based Research Network.* Available online at http://www.case.edu/dental/dentalpractice/about/. Accessed on November 23, 2008.

Green L, Hickner J. 2006. A short history of practice-based research networks: from concept to essential research laboratories. *Journal of the American Board of Family Medicine* 19(1):1–10.

National Institute of Dental and Craniofacial Research. 2008. *Dental Practice-Based Research Networks.* Available online at http://www.nidcr.nih.gov/Research/DER/ClinicalResearch/DentalPracticeBasedResearchNetworks.htm. Accessed on November 23, 2008.

Section 14.2: Network infrastructure development and governance including fiscal issues

Culpepper L, Froom J. 1998. The International Primary Care Network: purpose, methods, and policies. *Family Medicine* 20(3):197–201.

Green LA, Hames CG, Sr., Nutting PA. 1994. Potential of practice-based research networks: experiences from ASPN. Ambulatory Sentinel Practice Network. *Journal of Family Practice* 38(4):400–406.

Lindbloom EJ, Ewigman BG, Hickner JM. 2004. Practice-based research networks: the laboratories of primary care research. *Medical Care* 42(Suppl. 4):III45–III49.

Rust G, Cooper LA. 2007. How can practice-based research contribute to the elimination of health disparities? *Journal of the American Board of Family Medicine* 20(2):105–114.

Section 14.3: Practice-based research in large group dental practices

Bader JD, Perrin NA, Maupomé G, Rindal DB, Rush WA. 2005. Validation of simple approach to caries risk assessment. *Journal of Public Health Dentistry* 65:76–81.

Bader JD, Perrin NA, Maupomé G, Rush WA, Rindal DB. 2008. Exploring the contributions of components of caries risk assessment guidelines. *Community Dentistry and Oral Epidemiology* 36(4):357–362.

Maupomé G, Peters D, Rush WA, Rindal DB, White BA. 2006. The relationship between cardiovascular xerogenic medication intake and the incidence of crown/root restorations. *Journal of Public Health Dentistry* 66(1):49–56.

Rindal DB, Rush WA, Perrin NA, Maupomé G, Bader JD. 2006. Outcomes associated with dentists' risk assessment. *Community Dentistry and Oral Epidemiology* 34:1–6.

Rindal DB, Rush WA, Peters D, Maupomé G. 2005. Antidepressant xerogenic medications and restoration rates. *Community Dentistry and Oral Epidemiology* 33(1):74–80.

Section 14.4: Recruitment and retention strategies for practice-based research network investigators

Genel M, Dobs A. 2003. Translating clinical research into practice: practice based research networks—a promising solution. *Journal of Investigative Medicine* 51(2):64–71.

Lanier D. 2005. Primary care practice based research comes of age in the United States. *Annals of Family Medicine* 3(Suppl.):S2–S4.

Mold JW, Peterson KA. 2005. Primary care practice-based research networks: working at the interface between research and quality improvement. *Annals of Family Medicine* 3(Suppl. 1): S12–S20.

Nutting PA, Beasley JW, Werner JJ. 1998. Practice-based research networks answer primary care questions. *Journal of the American Medical Association* 281(8):686–688.

Section 14.5: Study idea acquisition, prioritization, and development

DeRouen TA, Hujoel P, Leroux B, Mancl L, Sherman J, Hilton T, Berg J, Ferracane J; Northwest Practice-Based Research Collaborative in Evidence-Based Dentistry (PRECEDENT). 2008. Preparing practicing dentists to engage in practice-based research. *Journal of the American Dental Association* 139:339–345.

Faggion DM, Tu Y-K. 2007. Evidence-based dentistry: a model for clinical practice. *Journal of Dental Education* 71(6):825–831.

Graham DG, Spano MS, Stewart TV, Staton EW, Meers A, Pace WD. 2007. Strategies for planning and launching PBRN research studies: a project of the Academy of Family Physicians National Research Network (AAFP NRN). *Journal of the American Board of Family Medicine* 20(2):220–228.

Richardson W, Wilson M, Nishikawa J, Hayward R. 1995. The well-built clinical question: a key to evidence-based decisions. *ACP Journal Club* 123:A12–A13.

Schlosser RW, Koul R, Costello J. 2007. Asking well-built questions for evidence-based practice in augmentative and alternative communication. *Journal of Communication Disorders* 40:225–238.

Tierney WM, Oppenheimer CC, Hudson BL, Benz J, Finn A, Hickner JM, Lanier D, Gaylin DS. 2007. A national survey of primary care practice-based research networks. *Annals of Family Medicine* 5(3):242–250.

Wotman S, Lalumandier J, Nelson S, Stange K. 2001. Implications for dental education of a dental school-initiated practice research network. *Journal of Dental Education* 65(8):751–759.

Section 14.6: Study deployment, implementation, and coordination

No references

Section 14.7: Data acquisition and analysis

Association for Clinical Data Management. 2005. *ACDM Guidelines to Facilitate Production of a Data Handling Protocol*. St. Albans (United Kingdom): Association for Clinical Data Management. Available online at www.acdm.org.uk/files/pubs/DHP%20Guidelines.doc. Accessed on September 26, 2009.

Christiansen DH, Hosking JD, Dannenberg, AN, Williams OD. 1990. Computer-assisted data collection in epidemiologic research. *Controlled Clinical Trials* 11:101–115.

DePauw M. 1989. Forms: design and content. In: Rotmensz N, Vantongelen K, Renard J (eds). *Data Management and Clinical Trials*. New York: Elsevier.

DuChene AG, Hultgren DH, Neaton JD, Grambsch PV, Broste SK, Aus BM, Rasmussen WL. 1986. Forms control and error detection procedures used at the coordinating center of the multiple risk factor intervention trial (MRFIT). *Controlled Clinical Trials* 7S:34–45.

Hosking JD, Newhouse M, Bagniewska A, Hawkins BS. 1995. Data collection and transcription. *Controlled Clinical Trials* 16:66S–103S.

Knatterud GL, Forman SA, Canner PL. 1983. Design of data forms. *Controlled Clinical Trials* 4:429–440.

Lesaffre E, Feine J, Leroux B, Declerck D (eds). 2009. *Statistical and Methodological Aspects of Oral Health Research*. Oxford: Wiley.

Lilienfeld AM, Lilienfeld DE. 1980. *Foundations of Epidemiology*, 2nd edn. New York: Oxford University Press, pp. 199–209, 267.

McFadden ET. 1998. *Management of Data in Clinical Trials*. New York: John Wiley & Sons, Inc.

McFadden ET, LoPresti F, Bailey LR, Clarke E, Wilkins PC. 1995. Approaches to data management. *Controlled Clinical Trials* 16:30S-65S.

Society for Clinical Data Management. 2003. *Good Clinical Data Management Practices*. Milwaukee (Wisconsin): Society for Clinical Data Management. Available online at www.scdm.org/GCDMP. Accessed on September 26, 2009.

Spilker G, Schoenfelder J. 1991. *Data Collection Forms in Clinical Trials*. New York: Raven Press.

Whitney CW, Lind BK, Wahl PW. 1998. Quality assurance and quality control in longitudinal studies. *Epidemiologic Reviews* 20:71–80.

Williams OD. 1979. A framework for the quality assurance of clinical data. National Conference on Clinical Trials Methodology, Bethesda, MD (October 2–4, 1977). *Clinical Pharmacology and Therapeutics* 25(No. 5, Part 2):700–702.

Section 14.8: Participant protection and scientific peer review in dental PBRN

American Association of Medical Colleges. 2006. *Alternative IRB Models. 2006. National Conference on Alternative IRB Models: Optimizing Human Subjects Protection*. Proceedings available online at http://www.aamc.org/research/irbreview/irbconf06rpt.pdf. Accessed on September 26, 2009.

Blustein J, Regenstein M, Siegel B, Billings J. 2007. Notes from the field: jumpstarting the IRB approval process in multicenter studies. *Health Services Research* 42(4):1773–1782.

DeMets D, Furberg C, Friedman L. 2006. *Data Monitoring in Clinical Trials. A Case Studies Approach*. New York: Springer.

Ellenberg SS, Fleming TR, DeMets D. 2002. *Data Monitoring Committees in Clinical Trials. A Practical Perspective*. West Sussex: John Wiley & Sons.

Friedman L, Furberg C, DeMets D. 1998. *Fundamentals of Clinical Trials*, 3rd edn. New York: Springer.

Genel M, Dobs A. 2003. Translating clinical research into practice: practice-based research networks, a promising solution. *Journal of Investigative Medicine* 51(2):64–71.

Gilbert GH, Qvist V, Moore SD, Rindal DB, Fellows JL, Gordan VV, Williams OD; DPBRN Collaborative Group. 2009. Institutional review board and regulatory solutions in the dental PBRN. *Journal of Public Health Dentistry*; [Epub 2009 Aug 20].

Gilbert GH, Williams OD, Rindal DB, Pihlstrom DJ, Benjamin PL, Wallace MA; DPBRN Collaborative Group. 2008. The creation and development of the dental practice-based research network. *Journal of the American Dental Association* 139(1):74–81.

Gold JL, Dewa CS. 2005. Institutional review boards and multisite studies in health services research: is there a better way? *Health Services Research* 40(1):291–307.

Graham DG, Spano MS, Manning B. 2007. The IRB challenge for practice-based research: strategies of the American Academy of Family Physicians National Research Network (AAFP NRN). *Journal of the American Board of Family Medicine* 20(2):181–187.

Greenberg Report. 1967. Organization, review, and administration of cooperative studies (Greenberg report: a report from Heart Special Project Committee to the National Advisory Heart Council by the Heart Special Project Committee). *Control Clinical Trials* 9:137–148.

Guidelines for NIH Intramural Investigators and Institutional Review Boards on Data and Safety Monitoring. 2008. Available online at http://ohsr.od.nih.gov/info/pdf/InfoSheet18.pdf. Accessed on September 25, 2009.

Lindbloom EJ, Ewigman BG, Hickner JM. 2004. Practice-based research networks: the laboratories of primary care research. *Medical Care* 42(Suppl. 4):III45–III49.

Mold JW, Peterson KA. 2005. Primary care practice-based research networks: working at the interface between research and quality improvement. *Annals of Family Medicine* 3(Suppl. 1):S12–S20.

National Cancer Institute, U.S. National Institutes of Health, U.S. Department of Health Human Services. 2008. *Human Participant Protections Educations for Research Teams*. Available online at http://cme.cancer.gov/clinicaltrials/learning/humanparticipant-protections.asp. Accessed on January 10, 2008.

Office for Human Research Protections, U.S. Department of Health Human Services. 2005. *Guidance on Extension of an FWA to Cover Collaborating Individual Investigators and Introduction to the Individual Investigator Agreement, January 31, 2005*. Available online at www.hhs.gov/ohrp/humansubjects/assurance/guidanceonalternativetofwa.htm. Accessed on January 10, 2008.

Office for Human Research Protections, U.S. Department of Health Human Services. 2008a. *Code of Federal Regulations, Title 45, Public Welfare*. Available online at http://www.hhs.gov/ohrp/humansubjects/guidance/45cfr46.htm#46.101. Accessed on January 10, 2008.

Office for Human Research Protections, U.S. Department of Health Human Services. 2008b. *Home Page*. Available online at http://www.hhs.gov/ohrp/. Accessed on January 10, 2008.

Westfall JM, Mold J, Fagnan L. 2007. Practice-based research—'blue highways' on the NIH roadmap. *Journal of the American Medical Association* 297(4):403–406.

Wolf LE, Walden JF, Lo B. 2005. Human subjects issues and IRB review in practice-based research. *Annals of Family Medicine* 3(Suppl. 1):S30–S37.

Section 14.9: Translation of research into practice

ADA Policy Statement on Evidenced-based Dentistry. 2003. Available online at www.ADA.org. Page updated on February 28, 2008; last accessed on September 22, 2009 (RMcB).

Balas EA, Boren SA. 2000. Managing clinical knowledge for health care improvement. *Yearbook of Medical Informatics*. 2000:65–70.

Bero LA, Grilli R, Grimshaw JM, Harvey E, Oxman AD, Thomson MA. 1998. Getting research findings into practice: closing the gap between research and practice: an overview of systematic reviews of interventions to promote implementation of research. *British Medical Journal* 317:465–468.

Haynes B, Haines A. 1998. Getting research findings into practice. *British Medical Journal* 317:273–276.

McGlone P, Watt R, Sheiham A. 2001. Evidenced-based dentistry: an overview of the challenges in changing professional practice. *British Dental Journal* 190(12):636–639.

Sacket DL, Rosenberg WMC, Gray JA, Haynes RB, Richardson WS. 1996. *British Medicine Journal* 312(7023):71–72.

Williamson JW, German PS, Weiss R, Skinner EA, Bowes F. 1989. Health service information management and continuing education of physicians. A survey of U.S. primary care practitioners and their opinion leaders. *Annals of Internal Medicine* 110(2):151.

15

The technology transfer process for life science innovations in academic institutions

Robert J. Genco, DDS, PhD

15.1   Introduction

Bringing a discovery from the laboratory or clinic to development as a useful product or service is a very necessary part of research. This process, called technology transfer, is often the ultimate goal of research and involves bringing scientific findings to benefit humanity through products that save lives, contribute to quality of life, provide energy, communications, and other entities that contribute to progress in the standard of living. It is the end game resulting in bringing the fruits of scientific discovery to benefit the public. It occurs in industry as well as in academic institutions. The process in academic institutions will be the focus of this chapter, as industry practices vary from company to company and are usually set by company policy. University policies are generally similar to each other, and involve academic researchers interacting with those from the legal, financial, and accounting professions, as well as business people. It is those who will hopefully benefit from this chapter.

The technology transfer process often leads to economic development since it involves the participation of university researchers and educators interacting with the business community to start new businesses, and to provide innovation for existing companies. This alliance among the academic and external communities is not often easy or natural and must be carefully developed to ensure timely and effective transfer of research innovations to benefit society.

The process of transferring scientific findings from academia for the purpose of development and commercialization typically includes the following:

1. Identifying new technologies from research done at the academic institution through inventor disclosures, called new technology disclosures (NTD).

2. Protecting the intellectual property in these technologies through patents, copyrights, trademarks, and trade secrets.

3. Developing commercialization strategies by either licensing technologies to existing companies or creating new start-up companies.

4. Facilitating the early development of these start-up companies through assistance with facilities (incubators), legal, financial, and business plan assistance.

A reference that provides detail on these processes can be obtained from the Association of University Technology Managers (AUTM) (2006).

Academic and research institutions are increasingly engaging in technology transfer as it offers considerable benefit to the institution and also fulfills an obligation they have to society. The reasons for engaging in technology transfer by an academic institution include the following:

1. Improving the health, well-being, and standard of living of society.

2. Compliance with federal regulations, namely, the Bayh–Dole Act (to be discussed later and Chapters 2 and 3).

3. Attraction and retention of talented faculty and students.

4. Recognition of discoveries made by the faculty and students at the institution.

5. Attraction of corporate support.

6. Licensing and equity revenues that further support research and education.

7. Local economic development, mainly through start-up business activity.

The ultimate beneficiary of technology transfer is the public who benefits from the products and services that result from university research. The regional economy is often enriched by the jobs and wealth created from the development and sale of new products and services.

15.1.1   U.S. national effort in innovation from academia

The activities of research and intellectual property protection and commercialization are pursued in over 4,000 universities throughout the United States, without disrupting the core mission of research, teaching, and service provided by the university. In fact, technology transfer serves the service and research missions, and sometimes the educational mission of academic institutions. For example, a service to the community is provided by creating jobs and wealth and, if properly managed, does not impede sharing of major findings of research programs.

Transferring the intellectual property from research institutions is critical in transition from a manufacturing-based economy to a technology-based economy. Academic institutions are becoming focal points for economic development and many governments are developing programs to enhance economic development through technology transfer from local academic institutions. For example, the U.S. federal government participates heavily through the Small Business Innovation Research (SBIR) and Small Business Technology Transfer (STTR) programs for small businesses, as well as through specific, targeted research grants and other support given to university and academic institutions to develop technologies of interest to government agencies such as the Departments of Defense, Transportation, Health, Agriculture, and Commerce.

15.2   The technology transfer premise

The technology transfer premise operating in U.S. academic institutions is based on the following:

1. Federal agencies fund university research.

2. Discoveries made from the funded research may benefit the public good.

3. Industry investment is often required to complete development and to commercialize discoveries.

4. Patents and other forms of protection of intellectual property often provide the exclusivity industry needs to protect their investment in bringing the invention to the market.

A paradigm shift was brought about by the Bayh–Dole Act of 1980, which allows universities and companies to own inventions they make with federal funding. The universities can use these discoveries royalty-free for their own purposes. Universities, however, have a mandate to partner with industry to translate research results into products benefiting the public. The resulting university licensing income is invested in further research as well as in rewarding scientist-inventors and supporting technology transfer offices.

Universities that accept federal funding for research are required to carry out their best efforts to protect intellectual property resulting from the research and to commercialize the inventions and discoveries. The impact of the Bayh–Dole Act was put into perspective by the *Economist Technology Quarterly,* December 14, 2002, with the following statement:

> Possibly the most inspired piece of legislation to be enacted in America over the past half century was the Bayh–Dole Act of 1980 ... More than anything, this single policy measure helped reverse America's precipitous slide into industrial irrelevance.

American academic centers performed more than $40 billion worth of research in 2005, and this is increasing each year. Most of this basic research is where cutting-edge discoveries with long-term potential effects occur. Many industries recently have reduced funding for long-term discovery and basic research projects, focusing on shorter range applied research. These two complementary research and development efforts, that is, short-term applied industrial research and development with long-term basic research from American academic centers, provide a key competitive advantage to the twenty-first century economy and competitiveness.

Since the Bay–Dole Act was enacted in 1980, more than 5,000 new companies had been formed based on university research results. Nationally, 85% of these new start-ups are located in close proximity to the university, and most of these stay in the communities where they were founded with regional economic impact. University patenting has exploded from 495 issued patents in 1980, prior to Bayh–Dole Act, to 3,278 in 2005. In 2005 alone, U.S. universities helped introduce 527 new patents to the marketplace. Between 1998 and 2005, 3,641 new products were created from university and academic center research.

Academic center technology transfer operation creates billions of dollars of direct benefits to the U.S. economy every year. A former president of the NASDAQ stock market estimated that 30% of its value is rooted in university-based, federally funded research results that may have never commercialized had it not been for the Bayh–Dole Act.

The public also benefits from the Bayh–Dole Act. Significant innovations and drug technologies were developed under the Bayh–Dole Act. These include the following:

- Synthetic penicillin

- Citracal, a calcium supplement

- Cysplatin and carboplatin, cancer therapies

- Human growth hormone

- Treatment for Crohn's disease

- Avian flu vaccine

- Clean water technologies

Many of these drugs and technologies improve the health and quality of life of people globally.

On December 6, 2006, the Sense of Congress resolution was passed by the U.S. House of Representatives, and this statement was made:

> The Bayh–Dole Act (Public Law 96-517) has made substantial contributions to the advancement of scientific and technological knowledge, fostered dramatic improvements in public health and safety, strengthened the higher education system in the United States, served as a catalyst for the development of new domestic industry that has created tens of thousands of new jobs for American citizens, strengthened States and local communities across the country, and benefitted the economic and trade policies of the United States.

It is clear that academic research and technology transfer play an important part in our economy, and benefits the public. The innovations and discoveries are the end result and often the culmination of long-term basic research projects is commercialization of these discoveries, which fits well within the context of the mission of universities and other academic institutions (see also Chapter 3 on Institutional Responsibilities).

> Academic research has remained strong and has not been compromised by increased technology transfer activities. U.S. based authors were listed one-third of all scientific articles worldwide in 2001. Researchers in the United States lead the world in the volume of articles published and the frequency in which these authors are cited by others. (Rising Above the Gathering Storm, 2007)

15.3   The technology transfer process in academic institutions

The process is illustrated in Figure 15.1. Scientific research discoveries are identified and the inventions are formally presented usually to the technology transfer office or some other administrative unit in the university or academic institution. This is a new technology disclosure and is a formal, legal document that sets precedence for the discovery. This disclosure is reviewed by the technology transfer officers or other administrators and a decision is made that (a) the technology is not appropriate for intellectual property protection since it is already patented, the technology is not well thought out, or there is little or no need for the technology; (b) the technology requires further research; and (c) the technology is worthy of intellectual property protection.

Once a decision is made to proceed to protect the intellectual property, there are several possibilities. In general, for new and innovative, unique discoveries or inventions, these can be patented. This can include composition of matter, new devices, new processes, and even unique software algorithms. Other discoveries can be copyrighted or trademarked if commercialization would benefit from such designation. Finally, the technology may be best kept as a trade secret if it involves, for example, a process that is difficult to reproduce, except in experienced laboratories.

Once the intellectual is protected, the technology transfer office proceeds to license the technology. The licensing can be exclusive or nonexclusive and it can be done to an existing company or to a new start-up company. If licensed to an existing company, a detailed license with terms may be drawn up dealing with issues including royalties and equity, milestone

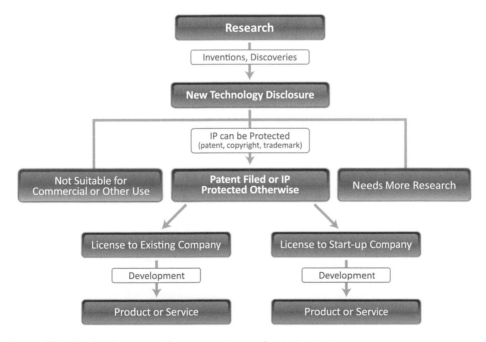

Figure 15.1 Technology transfer process in academic institutions.

payments to the university, performance milestones, liability, indemnity, and sublicensing. If licensed to a start-up company, similar terms are developed, but more often, equity might be taken in a start-up company.

The existing or start-up company then carries out research and development to bring the product to market. Often, the existing company can do this on its own, or may form a liaison with another company for marketing or manufacturing. The start-up company often can proceed through to marketing, but, for example, in the case of drugs, often joins forces and alliances with major drug companies to finance the very expensive regulatory clinical trials, formulation and toxicity studies needed, as well as manufacturing and marketing.

15.4   What is the role of the scientist in the process of technology transfer?

Scientists engaged in federally funded or other research are encouraged to develop a critical attitude toward application of the knowledge. Basic research is fundamentally driven by a quest for knowledge, how things work, and understanding nature; however, often clues to practical application come from results. These then should be discussed with technology transfer officers to determine if there is a potential use to benefit mankind. If so, they should be disclosed (as an NTD) before publication. It is very important not to compromise patent rights by prepublishing before filing for patents. The rules are different for the United States and foreign patents.

It is of critical importance for the scientist to understand that once protection is obtained, information can be published, just as any other scientific finding, without compromising the patentability. Efficient technology transfer offices can make the decision and file provisional patents, for example, in the United States, within 2–3 months of receiving a technology disclosure. Many universities give technology transfer offices 6 months to make this decision, after which the invention may be turned back to the scientist to proceed to patent or protect the technology if he or she wishes. Most technology transfer offices take less than 6 months in most cases, and the investigator can be working on a publication if appropriate, and the publication can be submitted within days of the filing of the provisional patent. Most often, there is very little delay in publication.

15.4.1   Licensing the technology

The inventor may participate in assisting the technology transfer office in identifying possible licensees among existing companies. Often, the inventor knows the scientists or vice president for research who can be champions for the technology within their company and this interaction often leads to licensing. The Association of University Technology Managers has surveyed the source of contact for licenses and found that over 60% are the inventors.

15.4.2   Start-up companies

Inventors also may have a strong desire to form a company around the technology, especially if it is an appropriate technology such as a platform technology with a wide variety of potential products. In this case, the technology transfer office often has legal, financial, and management consultation resources, as well as business plan expertise, to assist the inventor in developing a start-up company. Once a start-up company is formed and initial financing is obtained, most university faculties feel they want to be associated with a company as a scientific advisor or the chief technical officer and not as the business person running the company, in which case the small company would hire a CEO with scientific and business background. However, some scientists have the talent to do both and make arrangements with their department chair and/or dean to take time off, work part-time, or leave the university to run the company. A clear memorandum of understanding and management of conflicts of interest should be in place before a company is formed to avoid misunderstandings between the academic inventor, who is an officer of the company, and the university.

Many universities and communities have workshops and courses that researchers can take to determine the extent to which they want to participate in the formation of the company. These are extremely valuable, since starting a company is a major endeavor and should not be entered into lightly.

15.5   The role of the technology transfer officer at academic institutions

Technology transfer officers are charged with protection of intellectual property and commercialization of the inventions and discoveries made by the researchers at their academic institution. If the academic institution has accepted federal funds for research, they have a mandate to apply best practices to commercialize the inventions and discoveries made through federally funded research. Usually, the mandate is given by the university to the technology transfer office to protect and commercialize all research done at the university, regardless of funding.

15.5.1   Initial evaluation of technology

Technology transfer officers will perform outreach to assist faculty, especially new faculty, in understanding the disclosure, patenting, and commercialization pathway processes at their university. After receiving a technology disclosure, they will carry out an initial market analysis including the need and size of the market, percent of the market the product may fill, and also competitors in the market. In addition, the technology transfer office will assess the patentability of the technology by carrying out initial patent searches to reveal any major existing patents, which may preclude or alter patenting strategies.

15.5.2   Protection of the intellectual property

Once this is done, a decision is made, usually along with the investigator, to proceed to protect the intellectual property, or that further research is needed, or that this is an avenue that probably should not be pursued. Most often, universities will invest their own funds in the patent; other universities have arrangements where funding for the patent is covered by the investigator or another source. Most universities fund promising inventions for patenting, at least for provisional patenting. Often, licensees are sought before national and foreign patent filings, who may be asked to share in these expenses.

15.5.3   The commercialization pathway

Next, the commercialization pathway is usually assessed. Are there leads for licensing to existing companies? Technology transfer officers will market the technology to companies and, as mentioned above, often the investigator has contacts at various candidate companies that are critical in licensing. If a start-up business is the commercialization pathway of choice, the technology transfer office will generally help with the legal and other aspects of business formation including business plan development and initial funding.

15.5.4   Research parks and incubators

Many universities have research parks and incubators where companies can use the facilities and services offered. Incubation of start-up companies is generally thought to be successful, and studies show that the success rate of companies that are incubated is five to six times greater than companies that do not have the benefit of spending their early years in a nurturing incubator environment. Incubators can provide not only space, sometimes subsidized, but also advice, opportunity to network, services of the university, and other benefits that help in the early stages of the company.

15.6   University start-up companies

It is often appropriate to form a start-up company to develop a technology, especially an early technology with a broad technology platform and multitude of products that can be developed from this platform. Often, single-product technologies are best licensed to existing companies, for example, a single drug or diagnostic test. For example, if there is a chemical drug synthesis process that can lead to production of a series of drugs, this may be a platform for a start-up business.

15.6.1   Role of the faculty inventor in the start-up company

The role of the faculty inventor has to be clear in this start-up company. Often, they are the major person behind the company in the first year or so.

However, once seed or initial funding is available, the inventor may become the chief technical or scientific officer, and a CEO with business and scientific expertise is brought in to run the company. In any event, conflict of interest of the inventor should be formally worked out by the department chair and dean, as appropriate, to eliminate any potential misunderstanding as to the role of the inventor in the company versus the role of the inventor as an academic faculty member.

One of the early activities in a start-up company will be to develop a business plan or commercialization plan and this is a major effort necessary to obtain funding. Funding can be obtained through private venture firms, seed capital firms, governmental seed capital, or governmental funding.

15.6.2   Government funding for start-up of businesses

Federal government funding for start-up businesses is often obtained through the SBIR and STTR programs. Approximately 2.5% of the funds in the major divisions of government, such as the Departments of Health, Transportation, Defense, Energy, Commerce, and Agriculture, are set-aside for SBIR and STTR grants. These are competitive grants, and information can be found at http://grants.nih.gov/grants/funding/sbir.htm.

These applications fund in the range of $150,000 for phase I studies to $1 million for phase II studies, and in some instances, a fast-track phase I and II can be applied for. The funds are granted to start-up businesses, but approximately, one-third of the research can be subcontracted back to the university. Funding requires that the principal investigator of the SBIR grant be at least 51% employed by the business; hence, full-time faculties do not qualify as principal investigators. The SBIR grants require rigorous justification of use of the funds for technological development, as well as business plan. STTR grants allow a larger portion of the funds to be used by the university, and the university faculty member can be the principal investigator even if full-time.

Many states as well as non-U.S. governments have funds for start-up companies, which help bridge the gap between research funding and private venture funding.

15.6.3   Legal structure and management

The legal structure of university companies can be of different sorts. It can be an LLC or an S or C corporation, and usually the technology transfer officers have had experience with these various structures and can recommend legal help for structuring these companies.

Management. It is important for the university investigators to consider obtaining management assistance in the first few years of the company since the activities of the company soon get to be overwhelming and are often inconsistent with a full-time academic career. Some investigators decide to go part-time or full-time with the company, and others prefer to retain their full-time academic position and hire management.

Facilities. Often, universities offer some type of facilities-use agreement to use university facilities at a discounted rate, or are associated with incubators that often have subsidized rent. These arrangements usually come with critical services that are useful to a company, such as access to the internet, library services, university laboratories, computers, mail and copy services, and conference room services. The more effective incubators, for example, offer help in finding management and financing for the start-up companies.

15.7   Licensing to existing companies

Over three-quarters of technologies from academic institutions in the United States are licensed to existing companies. This offers the advantage that the existing company usually has adequate funds and personnel to do the necessary research and development to take products to the market. This is particularly important with products in the life sciences, such as drugs that require many years and tens of millions of dollars to bring the drug through the toxicity, preclinical, and clinical studies required by the FDA for approval.

It is important for the university scientist and technology transfer officers to make sure that licenses are well crafted, dealing with a myriad of subjects including performance, subcontracts, royalties, indemnity, and other issues. It is probably best for faculty to consider working with experts in the technology transfer office in crafting and negotiating these licenses, which often take several months to a year to negotiate. Faculty should not feel pressured or frustrated with the time that it takes to negotiate a truly comprehensive license that will be in the best interest of the inventor, the university, and the company.

15.8   Innovations in dentistry

Innovations developed in dentistry and transferred to existing companies or start-up companies for development often enter the profession through dental practice as well as through dental schools. This is probably true for many innovations in medicine also. The important thing is that innovations take time to gain acceptance in the community and this should be a realism accepted by the inventor. Often, even though the innovation has been fully developed, approved by the government regulatory agencies, and marketed, it may take time to be accepted by the profession and/or the public. Considerable education and effort may have to be expended by the licensing company often aided or guided by the inventor in making sure the innovation is accepted by the profession and used in the appropriate manner.

Examples of innovations that have emanated from academic research to real-world application are tabulated by the AUTM and can be found at www.betterworldproject.net. Innovations from 2008 have recently been posted and include innovations in agriculture, biotechnology, computer science, construction, education, electronics, energy, environment, food, health services, information services, manufacturing, medical, pharmaceutical, safety, and software technology.

References

AUTM Technology Transfer Practice Manual. 2006. *Association of University Technology Managers.* 3rd edn. Available online at http://www.autm.net/about/ dsp.pubDetail2.cfm?pid=35.
Rising Above the Gathering Storm. 2007. *Energizing and Employing America for a Brighter Economic Future.* Washington, D.C.: The National Academies Press.

16

Adoption of new technologies for clinical practice

Maxwell H. Anderson, DDS, MS, MEd

16.1   The problem?

A new scientific truth does not triumph by convincing its opponents and making them see the light but rather because its opponents eventually die, and a new generation grows up that is familiar with it. (Rogers, 2003)
   (Max Planck (1858–1947); winner of Nobel Prize in Physics in 1918)

Max Planck was a theoretical physicist engaged in the study of thermodynamics and blackbody radiation and is viewed by many as the father of quantum physics. Others argue that Einstein, using Planck's quantized energy formula (wherein lies Planck's constant), fathered quantum physics. In either case, these theories were the topic of much debate at the time they were put forth and not well accepted by the scientific community for a number of years. In fact, Planck initially rejected Einstein's special theory of relativity because he clung to Maxwell's theory of electrodynamics, the then prevailing belief.

His statement reflects, albeit pessimistically, how the community of science adopted new knowledge.

For a more medically and dentally relevant adoption sequence, we can study the term "Limey," which is an American and Canadian slang term used to describe British sailors. The story behind the term is a study of adoption of new methods in health care. The following is an attenuated history of the adoption of lime juice as a method of defeating scurvy by the British seagoing community.

16.2   The scurvy problem

Scurvy is a deficiency disease resulting from inadequate intake of vitamin C that is required for appropriate collagen synthesis. Most vitamins must be derived from exogenous sources since the body does not synthesize these nutrients in sufficient quantities. Scurvy is manifest orally as "spongy gums" and bleeding from the mucus membranes. In advanced cases, tooth loss is common. The systemic manifestations are far worse with ulcers on the lower extremities, opening of old wounds, depression, hallucinations, blindness, bones that break easily, and eventually death. The natural sources of vitamin C are fruits and vegetables.

When the British Navy and merchant marine began to explore the world's oceans and established trade routes with sea voyages that outlasted their supply of fruits and vegetables, scurvy became a major problem. It is estimated to have killed more sailors than all other seagoing hazards of that day. Scurvy was also an equal opportunity deficiency. It affected Navy men, merchant sailors, and the pirates that preyed on the merchant marine fleet equally.

While today we know that this malady is a vitamin deficiency, historically we did not have either an association or a known cause and effect. The problem was so severe that many seagoing units experimented with different solutions. There were many opinion camps about what worked and what did not.

In 1601, Captain James Lancaster, later of the East Indian Company, conducted an experiment during a voyage to India, Ceylon, and Sumatra (Wikipedia, 2008). He had four ships under his command. On one ship, he gave each sailor three teaspoons of lemon juice each day in addition to their normal diet. The other three ships received the normal diet, sans lemon juice. By the half-way point of the voyage, 110 of the 278 men on the three non-lemon-juice ships had died while those on Lancaster's ship remained healthy (Rogers, 2003). Given the clear results, a concise recommendation by Captain Lancaster, and the magnitude of the problem for the multiple constituencies, adoption of the practice of feeding lemon juice to crews on long voyages should logically have happened very quickly. It did not.

In 1747, after an intervening 146 years, a British Naval physician, James Lind (1716–1794), was researching hygiene and scurvy on British ships when he read and resurrected Lancaster's work. He was enamored with Lancaster's formula because it was his belief that acidic foods and liquids prevented scurvy. Based on his belief and Lancaster's previous work, he conducted another lemon-juice experiment in what was one of the first recorded "clinical trials." The experiment involved 12 sailors in six test groups. One group received two oranges and one lemon per day and the other five groups got other popular acidic interventions such as vinegar. The remainders of all diets were controlled and identical. These interventions were given to only those with overt clinical signs of scurvy. Only the fruit had substantial effects. It provided a "cure" in the 6-day trial for one sailor and great improvement in the other. While the sample size and testing period was far too small to have scientific merit, logic would again dictate that the results should have stimulated even further research on greater numbers of scurvy victims. Not so! It was not until 1795, 48 years later, that the British Navy adopted the policy directing the eating of citrus fruits, effectively wiping out scurvy in the British Navy. It took another 70 years for the British merchant marine to adopt the same policy.

The actual practice adopted was to provide lime juice or limes to sailors not the originally tested lemon juice. This practice was adopted because the British colonies in the Caribbean were rich in lime fruit rather than lemons.

In total, almost 200 years passed between the first demonstration of an effective cure for scurvy and the British Navy's adoption of the practice. Hundreds and probably thousands of deaths and disabilities from scurvy occurred during this period while many popular but unsuccessful remedies came and went.

These are but two examples of the diffusion of innovation into the world of science. They are representative of how innovation actually diffuses in scientific cultures such as physics and health care. The time frame for adoption of the scurvy cure is extreme but the factors that led to this slow adoption are instructive and are still in play today.

A rationale question concerning either of these examples is as follows: "Since the "systems" in which these discoveries occurred were made up of smart (arguably brilliant) individuals, what kept them from adopting the scientific advances?"

16.3   Why the failure to adopt?

The adoption of scientific knowledge or inventions within a field of sciences such as medicine and dentistry involves a myriad of influences affecting those who might adopt the new science or invention. The adoption of new policies or practices is referred to as "*diffusion*" in the current literature, and *diffusion of innovation* is the tagline for clinical practice(s) adoption. Researchers in the social and communications sciences have parsed out a number of factors that influence why practices are adopted or abandoned/ignored. These include but are not limited to the following:

- The character of the innovation that is being examined for potential adoption.

- The asymmetry of information—how different is the innovation from the current practice/belief?

- How and by whom the innovation is communicated?

- The social system in which the innovation occurs and in which it is communicated. In the case of this chapter, the social system is a pseudonym for the health care community.

- The time for adoption.

Each of these general categories has a milieu of nuances and studying the combinations of these variables is the stuff of academic careers. There are, however, within these data, good principles on which we can base the understanding of how diffusion of new science occurs in health care without examining every permutation (see also Chapter 1 on Clincal Translation).

In the case study of scurvy above, Rogers (2002) draws the conclusions that this discovery and rediscovery took 200 years to be adopted by the British Navy because there were competing belief systems about the causes of and cures for scurvy. These competing beliefs were being pervaded by pundits who were better connected to the then-current communications channels. Those pundits had higher status in the professional/social system.

In essence, those that proclaimed "the Earth is flat" had the ear of those who might have changed the current practices. Those with the actual "truth" did not. In today's "evidence-based" parlance, the "expert opinion" of the day was wrong.

16.4   Evidence-based X

Whether the "X" represents medicine, dentistry, nursing, pharmacy, or some other health profession, the goals of evidence-based evaluations and studies are the same. Evidence-based evaluations reduce the likelihood of making errors when deciding on health care actions. At its essence, this is an activity that targets reducing uncertainty in clinical practice and health care policy making.

There are a number of groups that provide "evidence-based" reviews and all their missions are virtually identical. As an example, the Cochrane Collaboration (http://www.cochrane.org/) lists as its primary mission, "Improving healthcare decision-making globally, through systematic reviews of the effects of healthcare interventions..." Their work is not limited to dentistry, but they have a dental component that has done a number of reviews on dental topics (see also Chapter 18).

The utility of the work they and others do in this arena is to provide an assessment of the validity of specific interventions and, because of control groups in many studies, noninterventions.

This "objectivity" would likely have tempered the advice of the pundits who advocated for scurvy therapies that were ineffective. At a minimum, the reviewers of the day would have noted that the studies of the day were poorly done and further research was needed to determine whether an intervention was successful. The review of their opinions would have been listed as "expert opinion," the lowest level of evidence in a hierarchy of evidence. However, trusted experts remain quite powerful in their opinions as we can see with an example of the adoption of the practice of placing bone at implant sites.

16.5   A current example

A current example of an expert opinion dilemma is that of providing bone augmentation for dental implant therapy. Depending on the practitioner, academic center, or institution, they may or may not believe that there is an advantage to placing bone grafts at the sight of a future or immediate implants. The Cochrane Collaboration has published their research into this topic initially in 2003 and then performed a substantive updated in 2006.

The reviewers tested the null hypothesis that there are no differences in the success, function, morbidity, and patient satisfaction between different bone augmentation techniques for dental implant treatment with the special objectives of testing whether and when augmentation procedures are necessary. The conclusions are that there is no clear evidence of benefit and that the trials conducted to date include few patients, with sometimes short follow-up periods and often being judged to be at risk of bias (http://www.cochrane.org/reviews/en/ab003607.html).

In the face of these and other objective reports (Block and Jackson, 2006), a number of opinion leaders advocate for placing bone or bone substitutes at extraction sites in preparation for implants and adjacent to immediately placed implants. When challenged for the evidence, the most commonly articulated defense for their support of the practice is that "this works effectively in my office" and that "lack of evidence does not equate to lack of efficacy." Both statements are in all probability true. However, there is no evidence that outcomes are improved by the practices and the unstated counter is also true. "Lack of evidence does not suggest efficacy."

Opinion leaders are just that. In spite of a lack of evidence, they can sway those who trust their counsel to reduce uncertainty in their adoption practices. In fairness, as noted above, they may be right. We do know that there is an increased frequency of infection where the grafting material is autogenous bone. Several authors use the surrogate measure of "bone height" to address the initial question regarding successful implant retention stating that when bone height improves, there is a greater probability of implant success. These same authors do not report on the quality of the bone deposited. This area of implant research is still evolving. Well-conducted studies over time will allow evidence seeking reviewers to evaluate new studies to reduce the current levels of uncertainty.

16.6   Why do we change?

Health professionals change practices for a limited number of reasons. Most adoption of new practices, techniques, materials, or equipment is undertaken as solutions to perceived problems or the inadequacies of the current state of the art/science.

The same can be said for those who develop innovations, particularly those with a financial incentive. It is not a good business practice to develop solutions to problems that have no viable markets.

Professionals adopt changes with specific patterns of behavior. First, a professional becomes aware of a problem. This may be a finding in specific practice issues or the awareness may come from an external source. Once the policy maker or practitioner is aware of a problem, they generally investigate potential solutions and can be persuaded to adopt solutions that have a perceived advantage over the current practice; is compatible with their belief system and values; lacks complexity; is trialable; and is observable. This is all part of deciding to switch to a new policy or practice.

16.7   Awareness of a problem

If a problem is serious enough to rise to the level of either a clinician's or policy maker's attention, they begin seeking knowledge about potential solutions. The problem may also be called out by others having influence with the individual or group who will actually implement the change(s). The knowledge quest takes many forms and ranges from significant research into the reviewed literature, seeking "evidence-based" materials where some other entity has done the research or simply seeking the advice of a friend or expert.

16.8   Persuasion to adopt

Depending on what is discovered in researching the problem and its solutions, a clinician or policy maker forms an opinion about the potential solutions. Some may be favorable and others may be unfavorable. The strength of belief in the findings relies in large part on the perceived reliability of the information. If from a trusted or authoritative source, the research knowledge is more likely to be accepted.

If the information about a solution to the problem is favorable, then a series of steps ensue. The decision to adopt the solution(s) is a process. If the solution to the problem has specific attributes that make adoption easier, it is more likely that the solution will be incorporated into routines.

16.9   Deciding

16.9.1   Perceived relative advantage

Health professionals change their practices and policies over the current way of addressing an issue, when they believe the change will have an advantage over the current practice. The use of "evidence-based" materials is a method of reducing uncertainty while adopting a new strategy, material, or practice where an expressed outcome has a recognizable advantage. This is an external validation of the probability that a solution will provide the perceived advantage. This "advantage" can be based on numerous drivers such as economic returns, increased efficiency, social prestige, convenience, or personal satisfaction. These can be subjective or objective measures. We seek added information to increase the probability that we will achieve a relative advantage.

16.9.2   Compatibility

Any new practice, material, or technique has a better chance of adoption when it is consistent with our existing beliefs, values, perceived needs, and past experiences. The lemon-juice application in an "acidic" remedy belief system is a historic example of matching an existing belief system. Some of the great historical intellectual battles in periodontics were waged between those wanting to preserve a belief system and those trying to change that belief. The prolonged debates on surgical interventions with bone recontouring and more conservative therapies are examples of existing and emerging techniques competing for practice and policy adoption.

16.9.3   Lack of complexity

Practitioners recognize the difficulty of changing clinical routines. Even minor changes to a routine affect the health care delivery team. Established patterns are initially hard to break and there is a cost in productivity and on the delivery system's social system. The simpler the change, the easier it is to make. Said differently, if the innovation is "dirt simple," it has a higher probability of being adopted. This is one of the major driving forces behind dental products manufacturers seeking effective "one-step" bonding agents for restorative systems. With experience, practitioners recognize that the fewer the steps in a procedure or process, the fewer opportunities there are to introduce errors that can influence the success of the practice or procedure.

16.9.4   Trialability

When an innovation is "trialable," the probability of adoption is increased. Dental conventions, trade shows, and manufacturer's representatives are a common vehicle for providing "trialability." Practitioners obtain samples or actually practice with a device or material to evaluate how it "feels" and its utility for their practice.

Most new techniques or practices require experience to become proficient at practicing the new technology. This may be achieved through "hands-on" training courses or through the application directly to practice. The risks of failure and abandonment of adoption are diminished as the practitioner gains experience. Using an early example for implants, the Brånemark group intensively trained both the early surgeons and restorative dentists in the placement and restoration of dental implants. They restricted sales to those who had completed their training programs. In essence, they created a "privileging" system for their implants. While there are good and sufficient product safety and liability reasons for doing this, there was an equal "adoption" rationale for "trialability."

16.9.5   Observability

Observability is the degree to which the results of innovation that is a candidate for adoption can be seen. The more immediate the results, the more likely an innovation to be adopted. Conversely, the longer it takes to realize the "advantage" of the innovation, the slower the adoption.

This is part of the reason that the practice of using dental sealants to "seal in" *incipient* caries has been slow to be adopted. Excising the demineralized tooth structure and replacing it with one of the current restorative materials provides an immediate "observable" result. Covering the incipiency has less surety for many practitioners.

16.10   Implementing

After deciding to adopt a change, policy makers or practitioners then begin using the adopted policy or practice. With the exception of the "trial" of the new policy or practice, the work to this point has been primarily a mental evaluative process. "Implementing" is an action phase wherein the policy or practice requires a defined behavior change. There may be more information gathering at this stage but it is now focused on how best to practice the mentally adopted change.

While changes are difficult in all settings, those in academic and other larger institutions face more significant challenges than those in smaller office settings. In general, the larger the organization, the more difficult the change process even though the reasons for change may still be compelling.

Once employed, the more frequently a new policy or practice is performed, the more rapidly it is adopted. If a practitioner changes their bonding agent in a restorative dominated practice, the frequency of use will likely be high and the change adopted more rapidly than the same change in a periodontal practice where fewer adhesive restorations are placed. Once the policy or practice is familiar, the concept of being "new" submerges and it becomes routine.

16.11   Reinvention

If a device, practice, or material has the potential for postadoption alteration, the use of an innovation is more likely to be attempted.

Within "reinvention" lies an area that is not well addressed in the current diffusion literature. In many situations in health care, adoption of an innovation is a purchasing decision. That is, the newly adopted practice requires an investment in new materials or piece of equipment with which to practice the innovation. In a buying decision, one of the considerations besides the direct and indirect cost of the innovation is whether the materials or instruments of the innovation can be redeployed or have other uses. If the purchase equipment or materials have other uses, it limits financial exposure. Many of those who were very early adopters of laser technologies found alternative uses for the lasers. Some as office plant holders but many others innovated different uses, sometimes outside dentistry, for these early devices.

The category of "reinvention" also embraces follow-on innovation. The use of dental implants as anchorage devices for orthodontic movement is a reinvention innovation that grew from the broader work in dental implants. Reinvention increases the probability that an innovation will be adopted. In essence, it gives alternative uses to an innovation and an outlet for the inventiveness of the adopters.

16.12   Confirmation

Individuals or systems that adopt a change to affect better outcomes continually reevaluate the new practice through their own experience and through other channels of communication. If the new practice delivers on the promise of a relative advantage over a previous practice, adoption is strengthened. If it does not, the decision is weakened and if the outcomes are unfavorable enough in either degree or frequency, the adopted practice may be abandoned. Unfavorable influences may also come from other trusted sources of information. A review by a trusted practitioner that is unfavorable may be sufficient to cause a marginal improvement to be abandoned. A favorable review by that same practitioner further strengthens the adoption behavior.

16.13   Adoption and current practices

The social, behavioral, and communications sciences have learned many things about the diffusion of innovation and adoption of new practices in health systems.

In spite of this body of work, today, there remains a significant gap between the discovery, revelation, and validation of an innovation that solves real problems and its adoption by practitioners.

This issue of the lack of adoption of new practices is not limited to health care. The U.S. Department of Energy hosts a division titled "Office of Scientific & Technical Information." One of their primary goals is to "accelerate the diffusion of knowledge to advance science" (Office of Science, 2008). Many other government divisions have equivalent organizations.

Congress established the Agency for Health Care Policy and Research (AHCPR), a division of HHS, in 1989, partially to accelerate the transfer of health care innovation to practice. The agency is now called AHRQ—Agency for Healthcare Research and Quality—with the express mission "to improve the quality, safety, efficiency, and effectiveness of health care for all Americans." To the extent that this agency fulfills its mission, it can help satisfy the needs of health care practitioners for external validation of emerging policies and practices (Quality, 2008).

AHRQ has a number of mandates including examining the outcomes and effectiveness of care, reducing medical errors, and disseminating the results to the professional communities. One of the mechanisms they are using to fulfill their mission is through the use of evidence-based studies.

16.14   Adoption examples from dentistry

In dentistry's past, a number of adoption patterns can be observed. The introduction of the Borden air rotor and acid etching to facilitate retention of restorative materials are two clear examples.

In more contemporary cases, dental sealants, posterior resins, periodontal maintenance, and surgical periodontal practices and dental implants offer good examples of the profession's adoption practices.

16.15   Dental sealants

Sealants offer a unique look at a technology innovation that has had a very slow adoption in the United States and other countries (Horowitz and Frazier, 1982; Bohannan et al., 1984; Frazier, 1984; Eklund, 1986; Cohen et al., 1988; Nakata et al., 1989; Chapko, 1991). Virtually, all papers on the adoption of sealants in either private or public health practices note that adoption has been slow (Figure 16.1).

Dr. Michael Buonocore, a truly innovative dental scientist at the Eastman Dental Center, published his research on acid etching enamel with a weak acid to enhance the mechanical retention of polymeric sealants in 1973 (Buonocore, 1973). His work was targeted at a significant need in the dental community, pit, and fissure caries. After repeated successful trials showing an average reduction in caries incidence of approximately 70% (Ahovuo-Saloranta et al., 2004), changes in state practice acts to allow sealant placement by hygienists and in some states dental assistants, evidence that intentionally or inadvertently sealing demineralized areas does not lead to progression (Griffin, 2008) and changes to remuneration practices by both public and private payers, there is still a significant gap in adoption.

There are a number of reasons cited for this lack of adoption. One of the major hurdles that any new technology must face is the "compatibility" issue. Until very recently, dentistry has been primarily a surgical reparative science. When pathology occurred, it was surgically repaired. Surgeons generally dislike waiting to see the outcome of a conservative, nonsurgical intervention such as sealants. This practice was reinforced by those who initially practiced dentistry from the 1920s through to the 1960s. Dental caries was pandemic in the United States and most of the world and the rate of progression of detected dental lesions made early restoration a practical and well-accepted imperative. With the advent of fluorides, the concomitant decline in caries rates, and the decreased speed of progression, the practice of "watchful waiting" was incompatible with a practitioner's experience.

Policy makers, both public and private, also hindered the adoption of sealants. Their payment policies lagged behind the science whereas payment for the repair/restoration of the tooth remained intact as an incentive to operate.

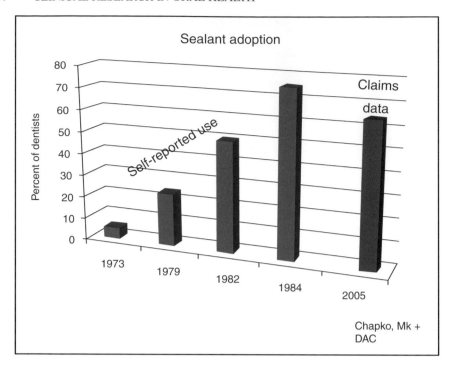

Figure 16.1 Use of dental sealants. Self-reported use versus insurance claims data regarding the percent of dentists using sealants in their practices. Chapko (1991) and Delta Data Analysis Center (2005).

Today, large data sets of insured individuals show that approximately 64% of general practitioners (GP) use sealants (Delta Dental Data Analysis Center, 1998). Some of this lack of adoption is a reflection of the pronouncements of current "experts" who cite hidden decay found in their laboratories when they section teeth. This observation is reinforced by the occasional clinical discovery that a pit or fissure area perceived as being minimally demineralized has far greater destruction than anticipated. Both the pronouncement and clinical finding feed on each other and create dissonance and where the source of the pronouncement information is trusted, and has an effective communication channel, the adoption of sealants is less likely to occur.

There is an interesting counter observation about practitioners finding more demineralization than anticipated in a pit or fissure. When discovered, these findings are conveyed to colleagues at lunch or society meetings. They help bias our views of pits and fissures and sealants placed therein. The other unanticipated finding is rarely discussed amongst even the closest of colleagues. Everyone who treats pit and fissure caries surgically has had the experience of operating on a surface that has clear "evidence" of significant demineralization, and when surgical repair is attempted, there is no demineralization to be found. This diagnostic "false positive" is at a minimum embarrassing and rarely discussed. It also generally changes our aggressiveness in treating dental caries for at least the next week.

These are only some of many reasons for the individual practitioner's do not adopt sealants. Others include a lack of information on sealant effectiveness (Fiset and

Grembowski, 1997), lack of public awareness and requests for services, the use of "minimally invasive dentistry" techniques that do not include sealants (Rossomando, 2007), and a myriad of dental societal factors. Clearly, sealants do not pass the temporal test of "observable results" for a surgically oriented practitioner.

The Healthy People 2010 goal is to have 50% of children receive sealants. Today, approximately 30–38% are the beneficiaries of sealants and the most "at-risk" groups have lower than the mean penetration of sealants (Statistics, 2007).

16.16   Periodontal maintenance

Virtually, all practitioners with periodontal patients with advancing disease advocate for the advantages of additional periodontal maintenance visits for their at-risk patients. This is a recognized "need" for the dental patient and the dental team. One of the major impediments in implementing a more frequent periodontal maintenance regimen is the remuneration system. Public and private insurance benefits designs have, in the past, limited the number of periodontal maintenance visits to two in a benefit period. This limitation was generally historically derived and was patterned after the dental prophylaxis benefit.

In 1996, Washington Dental Service, a Delta Dental Plan in Washington State, working with the Washington State Society of Periodontists, began a program wherein any covered patient with a then-current disease severity indices of 3 or greater was benefited four periodontal maintenance visits per year. As part of this agreement, if a subject's health improved to the point that they were no longer classified as a type 3 patient, they remained eligible for the added maintenance visits. The rationale for this was that no one wanted to continually cycle the patient between disease states when they had clinically shown a susceptibility to periodontal diseases.

Figures 16.2–16.4 demonstrate the adoption effects within the dental community and the outcomes as measured by scaling and root planing and the follow-up on surgical experiences. All the values are normalized to a per-thousand enrolled patient count. As can be seen, there was steady adoption of the periodontal maintenance during the 7-year study period. The majority of periodontal maintenance was performed in the office of the GP. The totals for each year are reflected in the total height of the bars showing the contribution to the total by GP and periodontal offices.

Figure 16.2 shows a slight decrease in the number of scaling and root planing events per 1,000 enrolled beneficiaries over the measured time. This small but clear decrease is attributed to the increased focus on those most at risk for advancing periodontal conditions and their increased maintenance as seen in Figure 16.3. The steady adoption of periodontal maintenance by the combined general practice and periodontal community had a temporally concomitant reduction in surgical periodontal services. While this outcome occurred at the same time as the increased incidence of periodontal maintenance, to ascribe cause and effect to this single event would be misleading. Many other social changes were underway in Washington State at the same time. Smoking was being banned in restaurants and the workplace making a significant influencer on periodontal disease progression less convenient as well as the national trend for less periodontal surgery.

This lack of clear cause and effect in no way diminishes the study of adoption of the practice of periodontal maintenance where the dental community leaders in periodontics advocated and taught the practice at dental society meetings all over the state. This

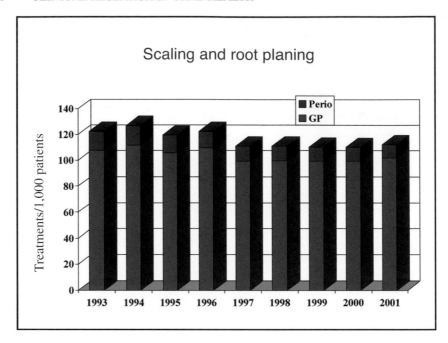

Figure 16.2 Effect of increased periodontal maintenance opportunity on scaling and root planing frequency. Data Analysis Center (2002).

innovation by both the periodontal and payment community provided a positive adoption experience that was consistent with the existing beliefs of most dentists and hygienists, thereby making adoption relatively simple.

Buried within these data for the same population was an interesting subset where adoption did not occur. At the time of this study, the American Academy of Periodontology recommended that those individuals receiving either osseous or flap periodontal surgical therapy receive four periodontal maintenance visits per year postsurgery. In this study, these maintenance visits were part of the benefit structure as previously described. Figure 16.5 shows the number of maintenance visits following surgery of either type for the first 4 years postsurgery. Most patients in both groups either did not receive follow-up maintenance visits or they were unreported. The latter seems unlikely because payment for these visits was benefited. Why there was a failure to adopt routine postoperative care remains an enigma.

16.17 Implant adoption

As implants have improved in predictability, they have been adopted by more and more dentists as a therapy option for patients with missing teeth.

A problem presented to dentists and patients alike is that in a number of situations, a fixed prosthesis can damage an abutment tooth (or teeth) and an implant is the preferred way of treating the missing tooth. Alternatives to limit the magnitude of this damage have been developed in the guise of a "Maryland bridge" or through the use of removable prosthetics to preclude or significantly reduce the surgical insult to the abutment teeth.

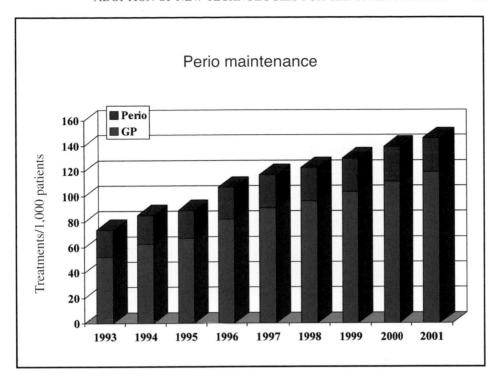

Figure 16.3 Periodontal maintenance frequency per 1,000 eligible patients. Beginning in 1996, four periodontal maintenance visits were benefited for patients with a disease severity index of 3 or greater. Data Analysis Center (2002).

Dentists and patients decisions on which intervention to employ are biased by the availability of funds for specific interventions. Where a full range of options are available, less bias is introduced.

The Data Analysis Center (DAC) studied the adoption of dental implants when these items became part of the covered benefits in 1998, thereby removing one of the selection biases. Figure 16.6 shows the use of fixed prostheses and implants in bounded tooth spaces from 1998 to 2005. The increasing use of implants is seen over the time period. The graph is designed with stacked bars to show the total number of bounded tooth spaces filled in each year per 1,000 eligible patients.

There is an interesting increase in the total number of spaces filled, all by the increasing frequency of implants. In an informal survey of dentists whose production of filled bounded tooth spaces increased, it was found that in most situations, they were filling a space that had abutment teeth with either no or minimal restorations and the opposing teeth had vertical stops that precluded either vertical supereruption or mesial drifting of the most distal tooth. Once the pent-up "need" to fill these spaces had been met, the total number of spaces filled trended below the third year numbers.

Here again is a practice that is highly desired by both dentists and patients where it has a perceived relative advantage over a fixed prosthesis; it is compatible with a surgical intervention behavior; once the techniques are mastered, they are not complex; the procedure

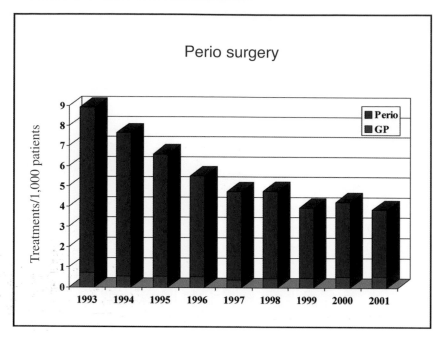

Figure 16.4 Periodontal surgery frequency during the time that increased periodontal maintenance visits were benefited. Data Analysis Center (2002).

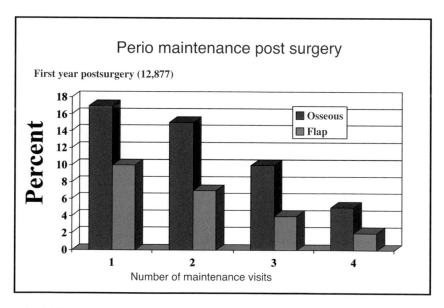

Figure 16.5 The percentage of individuals receiving periodontal maintenance visits in the first year postperiodontal surgery. Data Analysis Center (2002).

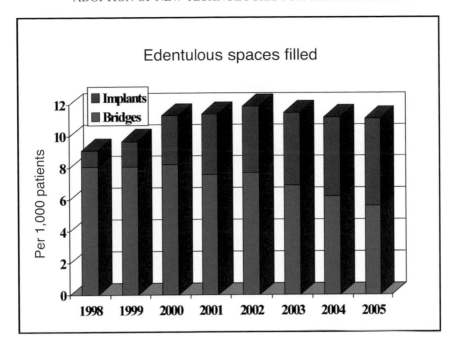

Figure 16.6 Adoption of implant services in bounded tooth spaces with a concomitant decrease in the placement of fixed partial dentures. Bar height reflects the total bounded spaces filled per 1,000 eligible subjects. Delta Data Analysis Center (2005).

is trialable in both training situations and in the clinic; and the results are observable. This latter category is increasingly strong as "immediately" loaded implants become more and more common.

There is a clear adoption curve for the implants, and at the same time, an extinction curve for fixed prostheses in these bounded tooth spaces.

16.18   Concluding remarks

Adopting new policies, practices, procedures, techniques, and materials remains a complex issue for heath care systems. Where innovations offer solutions to perceived problems, provide a relative advantage over current practices, are compatible with existing beliefs, lack complexity, are trialable, and have observable outcomes, they are more likely to be adopted. If a trusted source of external validation helps reduce the uncertainty about adoption of the new practice, there is also an increased chance of implementing the innovation.

Conversely, if these conditions are even partially reversed, adoption is less likely.

Awareness of these principles and their impact on the profession of dentistry is useful to policy makers, clinicians, and those who bring innovations to the community. It is hoped that understanding our own adoption behaviors may serve to shorten the adoption period and provide improved health outcomes to the populations we serve.

References

Ahovuo-Saloranta A, Hiiri A, Nordblad A, Mäkelä M, Worthington HV. 2004. Pit and fissure sealants for preventing dental decay in the permanent teeth of children and adolescents. *Cochrane Database Systematic Reviews* (3):CD001830.

Block MS, Jackson WC. 2006. Techniques for grafting the extraction site in preparation for dental implant placement. *Atlas of the Oral and Maxillofacial Surgery Clinics of North America* 14(1):1–25.

Bohannan HM, Disney JA, Graves RC, Bader JD, Klein SP, Bell RM. 1984. Indications for sealant use in a community-based preventive dentistry program. *Journal of Dental Education* 48(Suppl. 2):45–55.

Buonocore MG. 1973. Sealants: questions & answers. *Journal of the American Society for Preventive Dentistry* 3(1):44–50.

Chapko MK. 1991. Time to adoption of an innovation by dentists in private practice: sealant utilization. *Journal of Public Health Dentistry* 51(3):144–151.

Cohen L, Romberg E, LaBelle A. 1988. The use of pit and fissure sealants in private practice: a national survey. *Journal of Public Health Dentistry* 48(1):26–35.

Delta Dental Data Analysis Center. 2002. *Adoption effects within the dental community and the outcomes as measured by scaling and root planing and the follow-up on surgical experiences.* An internal Delta Dental Data Analysis Center report.

Delta Dental Data Analysis Center. 2005. *Use of Sealants by General Practice Dentists.* An internal Delta Dental Data Analysis Center report.

Eklund SA. 1986. Factors affecting the cost of fissure sealants: a dental insurer's perspective. *Journal of Public Health Dentistry* 46(3):133–140.

Fiset L, Grembowski D. 1997. Adoption of innovative caries-control services in dental practice: a survey of Washington State dentists. *Journal of American Dental Association* 128(3):337–345.

Frazier PJ. 1984. Use of sealants: societal and professional factors. *Journal of Dental Education* 48(Suppl. 2):80–95.

Griffin SO OE, Kohn W, Vidakovic B, Gooch BF, Bader J, Clarkson J, Fontana MR, Meyer DM, Rozier RG, Weintraub JA, Zero DT. 2008. The effectiveness of sealants in managing caries lesions. *Journal of Dental Research* 87(2):169–174.

Horowitz AM, Frazier PJ. 1982. Issues in the widespread adoption of pit-and-fissure sealants. *Journal of Public Health Dentistry* 42(4):312–323.

Nakata M, Kuriyama S, Mitsuyasu K, Morimoto M, Tomioka K. 1989. Transfer of innovation for advancement in dentistry: a case study on pit and fissure sealants' use in Japan. *International Dental Journal* 39(4):263–268.

Office of Science, U.D.O.E. 2008. *Office of Scientific and Technical Information.* Available online at http://www.osti.gov/cgi-bin/scsearch/explhcgi?qry1894414116;sc-03563. Accessed on September 21, 2009.

Quality AfHRa. 2008. Available online at http://www.ahrq.gov/. Accessed on September 21, 2009.

Rogers EM. 2002. Diffusion of preventive innovations. *Addictive Behaviors* 27(6):989–993.

Rogers EM. 2003. *Diffusion of Innovations.* New York: Free Press.

Rossomando EF. 2007. Minimally invasive dentistry and the dental enterprise. *Compendium of Continuing Education in Dentistry* 28(3):166, 168.

Statistics NCfH. 2007. *Oral Health Improving for Most Americans, But Tooth Decay Among Preschool Children on the Rise.* Available online at http://www.cdc.gov/nchs/pressroom/07newsreleases/oralhealth.htm. Accessed on September 21, 2009.

Wikipedia. 2008. *James Lancaster.* Concomitant. Available online at http://en.wikipedia.org/wiki/James_Lancaster. Accessed on October 28, 2009.

17

Publication of research findings

James Bader, DDS, MPH

Making the results of a research project available to others is an important requirement of any research endeavor. Without this final step in the scientific process, the efforts of everyone involved in the project, including investigators, research and administrative staff, and patients will have been wasted, as will the resources expended to perform the research. Dissemination is usually accomplished through the publication of one or more articles in peer-reviewed scientific journals. Although alternative means are possible, the journal article is the standard for reporting research results, and should represent the ultimate aim of every research effort. The unique circumstances of clinical research demand the special attention of author-investigators. Reports of the findings of clinical research will contain information related to patient outcomes, thus holding the potential for attracting the widest variety of audiences, including clinicians, patients, and payers, as well as other researchers interested in the same questions. Also, the various designs for clinical research, particularly clinical trials, demand that certain reporting conventions be met. For these reasons, it is imperative that publication be an integral part of project planning, starting when the research proposal is developed. This chapter provides a description of the steps in planning, preparation, submission, and revision of a publication describing clinical research findings.

17.1 Planning for publication

No matter how large or small the research study, paying some attention to the eventual publication of the results during the earliest phases of the project will help ensure that the process of writing the paper or papers proceeds smoothly and efficiently.

17.1.1   Setting the stage

The first opportunity to facilitate publication occurs during the writing of the research proposal. A well-stated and well-documented justification for the research project not only enhances the probability that the proposal will be funded, but also can serve as the basis for the introduction, or first section of the principal paper describing the findings of the study. At a minimum, the "Background" and "Significance" sections of a research proposal should contain a thorough review of the relevant literature, and a well-crafted argument for why the question the research project addresses is important to answer. Ideally, the literature review will represent the results of a recent systematic review that addresses the same clinical question the proposed research project is designed to answer. Such a systematic review could have been completed in preparation for the proposal, or it could have been written by others, but it sparked the investigator's interest in the clinical question. In either event, the presence of a relevant systematic review not only pays immediate benefits in providing both a strong background to the proposal and some insight into research design pitfalls associated with prior work on the topic, but it also will form the backbone of the introduction section of the principal research paper. The arguments for the importance of the research question will tap other literatures, including epidemiological studies that describe the distribution of the problem the study addresses, and economic analyses of the societal costs of the problem. Again, work during the preparation of the proposal will be repaid by a stronger application, possible additions to the outcomes assessed in the study, and the longer term benefit of a "prewritten" argument for the significance of the research question for the eventual journal paper.

17.1.2   Developing publication policies

Any research project with more than one investigator is at risk of disagreements between and among the investigators concerning publication of the results of the project. For that reason, the development of formal project policies on publication is a recommended step that should occur early in the study timeline. The policies can be developed during a meeting of the project investigators, or if the complexity of the project staffing warrants it, a publications committee can be constituted. Typically, such a committee will be chaired by the principal investigator, and will have representatives from each clinical site and from the analysis unit. In either event, policies should be developed under an arrangement where all investigators have a voice, either directly or through a representative. Policies should be promulgated for identifying manuscript topics and priorities, authorship responsibilities, approval of manuscripts, and miscellaneous other publication-related issues.

17.1.2.1   Manuscript topics and priorities

It is helpful if the major papers that are anticipated products of the research project are identified at the outset. This process will be useful in disclosing almost inevitable uncertainties or misunderstandings among the investigators concerning outcomes and analysis and publication strategies. For most clinical investigations, there will be a "main study paper" that describes the principal outcomes of the project. There may be other outcomes papers that present results of analyses of secondary outcomes, or such outcomes may be reported in the main paper. The decision concerning what to include in each paper should be made by the investigators at the outset of the study. For example, if a caries prevention study collects longitudinal data on both cavitated lesions and noncavitated enamel lesions, the investigators should decide whether they wish to report the efficacy of the intervention in separate papers for the classical D_2 caries initiation measure and for the more recently reported D_1 caries initiation and progression measure (Slade and Caplan, 2000). The decision may depend on whether the investigators anticipate any difference in the conclusions regarding efficacy based on the two outcome measures, and whether the comparison of these two outcomes is perceived to be of interest.

In addition to the outcomes paper or papers, other topics usually can be identified at the outset that hold promise for eventual development as separate papers, either full-length manuscript, as brief reports, or simply as abstracts. Use of a unique recruitment technique, special attention to and enhanced assessment strategies for adherence, or planned subset analyses might all be seen as meriting the emphasis gained through a focused report. In any event, these discussions among investigators should assist in reaching appropriate decisions about maintaining the balance between "including too much" in a single paper and "salami science" (cutting what could be a single paper into multiple publications). It is also a truism that whatever is decided regarding publication prior to collecting data is sure to change by the time data collection has been completed. Hence, "lessons learned" papers describing solutions to problems encountered during the course of the study will often suggest themselves to one or more of the investigators, and can be valuable resources to other researchers. Revision of publication plans is certainly acceptable, but should follow the same types of consideration that created the original plans.

It is also useful to determine the priority order for preparation for all anticipated papers. Establishing a priority order ensures that the papers are completed and submitted in a sequence that maximizes their impact, and will aid analysts in planning how the study data might be structured to expedite the initial analyses. Normally, the main study paper will be assigned the highest priority, followed by other outcomes papers, and then papers on other topics. However, it is quite possible, especially in longitudinal studies with multiple phases, that the data necessary for preparation of the manuscript for one or more of these other topics will be available before the main outcomes are known. In those instances, the publications committee will need to decide whether these publications should appear prior to the main study paper. In any event, both the list of planned manuscripts and their priority for publication should be considered as tentative and subject to change during the course of the study at the discretion of the investigators.

17.1.2.2 Authorship assignments

(See also Chapter 3 on institutional responsibilities related to authorship)

Issues concerning authorship can be among the most contentious that arise in research projects, and they are quite capable of generating extreme dissatisfaction, and in some instances, hostility, among investigators. For these reasons, it is imperative that discussion and decisions about authorship occur well before manuscripts are initiated. Ideally, first authorships will be assigned immediately after the planned manuscripts are identified. Prior to this process, it is recommended that investigators familiarize themselves with the criteria for authorship developed by the International Committee of Medical Journal

Editors (ICMJE, web). These criteria state that "byline authors" (those identified by name as authors) should have participated in preparing the manuscript by

- substantially contributing to conception and design, or acquisition of data, or analysis and interpretation of data;

- drafting the article or revising it critically for important intellectual content;

- approving the final version to be published.

Note that all three conditions have to be satisfied for authorship credit to be appropriate. The criteria also indicate that all those who meet the above conditions should be listed as authors, and that each listed author should have participated sufficiently in the work to take public responsibility for appropriate portions of the content. This basic set of authorship criteria should signal to interested investigators what level of contribution is expected in return for credit as an author. Also, as a majority of peer-reviewed journals in dentistry have accepted the ICMJE criteria, it is probable that the senior author will have to attest to these criteria as a part of the submission process.

For most papers reporting the results of clinical dental research studies, the first author listed is considered as the senior author. First authorship has both special prestige and responsibilities. The prestige is exemplified by the assumption of university promotion and tenure committees that first authors are due for the lion's share of the "publication credit." The responsibilities are manifold. The first author actually prepares the paper. He or she writes the bulk of each draft. The electronic file resides on the first author's computer. The first author determines the order of coauthorship on the paper, which is usually predicated on the amount and importance of contributions to the paper. The first author is also responsible for ensuring that coauthors fulfill their responsibilities, and for withdrawing coauthorship status if an individual's contributions do not live up to expectations. Finally, the first author is responsible for the content of the paper, with many journals asking that this individual attests that the content is original work, and is truthful.

As with the identification of manuscripts, the assignment of authorships should be considered as tentative. Essentially, all investigators who are interested in being an author on a specific paper should indicate their interest to the first author, with the understanding that authorship credit and order will be finalized as the manuscript is written. If the list of potential authors is a long one, it is prudent for the first author of each planned manuscript to circulate a list of investigators who have expressed an interest in participating as a coauthor, together with some indications of the potential contributions that the first author expects each interested investigator to make.

When multisite studies are reported, the temptation is to list the principal investigator at each site as an author. Many journals, as well as the ICMJE, discourage this practice. It is unlikely that each individual in a large group of investigators can satisfy all three authorship criteria, and reduced individual responsibility for content is the result. Rather, individuals crucial to the completion of the study, but not necessarily of the manuscript, should be listed as contributors, with their roles identified, in the Acknowledgment section.

17.1.2.3   Other publication policies

Regardless of whether publication policies are formulated by a publications committee, or are the decisions of the principal investigator, some additional policies should be formalized at an early stage in the research process. Policies are usually needed to address the following questions:

- Does the principal investigator have the right to disallow submission of a manuscript based on project data?

- Who decides who gets to submit abstracts?

- Are abstracts reviewed internally before submission?

- Is the number of authors on any one paper limited?

- Can students participate as authors?

- What is the mechanism for proposing additional papers?

- Can the study data be used by other investigators for analyses (and publication) unrelated to the principal aims of the study?

As with all policies, it is advantageous to have discussed and formulated project policies in advance of their need. Existing policy should help guide individuals, especially if they have been involved in its creation. Thus, even the smallest project can benefit from a discussion of these issues early on, with the subsequent circulation of minutes of the meeting serving as a written version of the project policies.

17.2   Selecting a target journal

Deciding where to submit a manuscript can be approached in two ways. The first is to write the best manuscript possible, and then decide what journal might be appropriate, given the topic and structure of what has been written. The advantage that this approach offers is that the opinions of a number of more experienced authors can be solicited by asking them to read the manuscript and then recommend one or more appropriate journals. The drawbacks are that this approach is inefficient with respect to producing a manuscript that meets the journal's submission requirements, and it precludes the opportunity to tailor the manuscript directly for the style of a specific journal that represents the best combination of audience, topic, impact factor, and other considerations in selecting a "target journal."

17.2.1   Reasons for publishing

Investigators may have one or several reasons for publishing a report of a clinical investigation. Identifying and taking these reasons into account may make selection of a target journal more straightforward. Consider the following reasons for publication:

- Inform fellow clinicians and influence clinical practice

- Add new knowledge to the literature

- Meet requirements for promotion and tenure

- Meet sponsor's expectations

- Provide documentation for next research proposal

- Personal satisfaction

Satisfying some of these reasons may demand publication in a different journal than would be selected for other reasons. For example, publication in a prestigious journal may make more of an impression on a promotion and tenure committee, but the greatest exposure to practitioners may come from journals with the widest distribution. A journal with a reputation for "quick turnaround" time of accepted manuscripts from submission to appearance may be an important consideration for a commercial sponsor, and thus have to be weighed against the principal investigator's desire to place the paper in another journal for any one of a number of other reasons. It is often useful to rank order these and any other considerations as an initial step in selecting a target journal.

17.2.2   Journal characteristics to consider

A competently prepared report of the results of a clinical dental study is usually a plausible candidate for acceptance in several journals. Certainly, there is no shortage of potential targets. Currently, more than 800 journals indexed in PubMed carry a primary subject term of "Dentistry" (NLM(a), web). Subject terms are assigned by National Library of Medicine to MEDLINE journals to describe the journal's overall scope (NLM(a), web). This subset includes non-English language journals as well as a variety of publications of purely local or regional interest and circulation. A reasonably comprehensive university dental library will probably carry between 150 and 400 titles (University of Southern California, web; University of Toronto, web), and most investigators will select a target journal from among this smaller, but still heterogeneous group of dental periodicals. Investigators should consider several characteristics of these possible journals as they attempt to identify the best match with their ranked reasons for publishing. Among the most important characteristics to consider are audience, topic mix, sponsorship and circulation, and impact factor.

17.2.2.1   Audience

The desired audience for the paper should be identified early in the selection process, as it will influence the pool of candidate journals. Journals that publish reports of clinical research generally fall into two categories; they tend to be regarded as either "practice oriented" or "research oriented." Practice-oriented journals usually offer a mix of clinical research reports, case reports, and opinion pieces, all intended primarily for practicing dentists. Most, if not all, of the content of such journals will have immediate application to dental practice. A subset of practice-oriented journals are "specialty-oriented journals" comprising publications that are typically sponsored by a specialty organization. These journals focus on a single area of dental practice and usually present a mixture of research and practice-related papers, but enjoy wide distribution among specialty clinicians due to their sponsorship. Research-oriented journals may also publish reports of clinical research, but such papers may not form a majority of the content, and may be placed in a special section of the journal. Research-oriented journals primarily publish papers reporting both basic and applied research results, literature reviews of specific topics, and occasional opinion pieces or editorials. The principal readers are educators and researchers working in the disciplines covered by the journal. The investigator should decide which of these two audiences is preferred. Of course, with electronic access to an increasing number of journals, with increasingly sophisticated content awareness software, and with a growing number of journals publishing abstracts and critical summaries of research originally appearing elsewhere, the audience for most journals is no longer limited essentially to subscribers and those with access to dental libraries. However, there is no evidence that most practitioners search for information beyond that in journals that cross their desks. Thus, careful selection based on desired audience may be more important if the investigator wishes to inform practicing dentists, than if researchers and/or educators are the principal audience.

17.2.2.2   Topic mix

Certainly, the topic of the research paper is a factor in selecting a journal to which to submit the manuscript. Journals typically exhibit a range of subjects for which manuscripts are considered for publication. There are two tried and true methods for identifying journals appropriate for a given clinical research paper. One is to be generally familiar with the literature associated with the topic of the research project. Presumably, this familiarity will be gained through preparation of the research protocol and/or proposal. The other, which should be used even when the investigator is familiar with the literature, is to enter the topic of the research project or relevant keywords or authors' names into a MEDLINE search and note the journals that have published related papers in the past few months. This list of journals will necessarily be incomplete, but may suggest possibilities not otherwise evident.

17.2.2.3   Sponsorship and circulation

Journals are expensive propositions, and must either make profits through advertising and subscriptions, or be sponsored by one or multiple societies. The advantages that sponsored journals enjoy are that the subscription list is the membership of the society, usually a larger number than would subscribe individually, and that the prestige of the society is transferred to some extent to the journal. In general, sponsored journals will have larger circulations than commercial journals. The circulation for a journal can usually be determined by examining the required "Statement of Ownership, Management, and Circulation" that appears in most journals toward the end of the year. Once audience and topic considerations have narrowed the field of target journals, maximization of circulation may be an important selection criterion.

17.2.2.4   Impact factor and acceptance rate

The "impact factor" for a journal may be a criterion for selection, particularly if the investigator or sponsor is ambitious. Impact factors are calculated annually for all journals in the Science Citation Index-Expanded managed by Thompson Scientific (Thompson Scientific (a), web) and are published in *Journal Citation Reports* (Thompson Scientific (b), web). The impact factor is a measure of the frequency with which papers appearing in the journal are subsequently cited by other papers. Although not without its detractors, the impact factor is a handy if inexact estimate of the extent to which scientists and scholars pay attention to a journal's content. The impact factor is not useful for estimating the impact that journal articles may have on practitioner behavior, only on researchers' selection of journal articles cited in their work, which is taken as an implicit measure of quality and importance of the journal, and by transference, the papers it publishes.

Journal acceptance rates for unsolicited manuscripts are generally thought to reflect the inverse of the impact factor. The higher the impact factor, the lower the acceptance rate. A compendium of acceptance rates is not available for dental journals. Rates for sponsored journals are usually accessible through the editor's annual report to the sponsoring association. While many investigators hope to present their findings in a high impact, prestigious journal, the likelihood that their manuscripts will be perceived by reviewers as important for the discipline, and, hence, worthy of acceptance in a journal with a 15% acceptance rate, needs to be weighed against the inevitable delay in publication if the manuscript is not accepted.

17.2.2.5   Information for Contributors

Once the field of potential journals has been narrowed through consideration of the audience, topic mix, circulation and sponsorship, and impact factors, the Information for Contributors sections of the remaining target journals should be collected and carefully scrutinized. These sections, also entitled "Instructions for Authors" or "Author Guidelines," provide information useful in making the final selection of the journal for submission. These sections are printed in the journal, although they may only appear one or two times per volume. In most instances, they are available more easily at the journal's website. Web-accessible compendia of these author guidelines have been created by health sciences libraries, with at least one such collection having an unusually complete list of dental journals (University of Toledo, web).

The information most useful in making a final selection of the target journal usually appears in the initial of the instructions, where the types of manuscripts considered by the journal are typically described. Quite often, specific descriptions of the types of manuscripts that will be considered are presented. Almost all journals encourage "original research reports" but the other types of manuscripts listed may afford some insights into the journals' desired readership. For example, the inclusion of case reports and technique descriptions on the list of appropriate manuscripts is a signal that the journal wants to appeal to clinicians. Often, the range of topics or scope of the journal is also delineated. This delineation may be presented in detail in the initial paragraphs, or the reader may be referred to a separate document describing the journal's aims and scope.

The investigators should now be prepared to select the target journal. The decision is made by the principal or first author of the manuscript, but consultation with other authors is recommended. If there is still some uncertainty about the "best journal" for the planned manuscript, the investigators can seek the opinions of other investigators who may have had direct experience with one or more journals on the final list, or who may have a broader perspective of the relevant disciplines. Also, if the investigators are unfamiliar with one or more of the journals still under consideration, they should read multiple recent issues to get familiar with the types of papers that appear. While there is no one "right" journal, it is important that the investigators feel that they have made a careful, rational selection from among the available alternatives.

17.3   Writing the draft manuscript

Once the target journal has been identified, manuscript preparation can begin. The actual writing of the majority of the first draft of the manuscript is the responsibility of the first author. In some instances, specific sections of the draft, such as a description of a statistical analysis or a calibration exercise, may be prepared by another investigator with greater expertise in the topic, but if possible, these contributions should be limited to ensure a uniform style. While the writing task may be intimidating to the novice author, it is in essence simply preparing responses to a series of fairly well-defined requests for information. Those information requests are the traditional major sections of the scientific paper, that is, the Introduction, Methods, Results, and Discussion, together with several ancillary parts such as the Abstract, Acknowledgments, and References.

17.3.1   Preliminary steps

Before starting to write, the first author is well advised to engage in some preparation designed to minimize the amount of revision necessary, as well as to maximize the chances of a favorable reception by the target journal. Three basic steps should always be taken. The first is reviewing the Information for Contributors and reading the reports of clinical studies appearing in several recent issues of the target journal. The second is reviewing reporting guidelines relevant to clinical reports, and the third is reflecting on what practitioners will want to know.

17.3.1.1   Information for Contributors

The first author should thoroughly review the Information for Contributors section. Unlike the review performed while trying to decide which journal to select, this review must be more exacting, because the information obtained will guide the development of the paper. The level of detail of the Information for Contributors sections will vary, but they will usually present at least some basic guidance concerning:

- types of manuscripts solicited,
- suggested length or maximum number of pages or words, or both,
- expected structure or organization, order, and general content of manuscript sections,
- page formatting, including margins, line spacing, page numbering,
- table and figure formatting,
- reference formatting.

In addition, the Information for Contributors section will describe manuscript submission procedures, and also summarize the journal's review process. The first author should become familiar with all the information that applies to the planned manuscript, perhaps even underlining pertinent passages on a printed copy and placing it in the manuscript folder. Although noncompliance with the instructions in the Information for Contributors section may not result in immediate rejection of a manuscript, it will signal the editor and reviewers that the author did not make an effort to follow the directions. That signal may suggest that the author is lazy or sloppy, or that the manuscript was prepared for another format, and only submitted to the target journal following rejection elsewhere. These are not signals that will enhance the likelihood of acceptance.

The first author should also read, or at least scan the papers in several recent issues of the target journal to become familiar with aspects of the journal's style that may not be described in the Information for Contributors section. Use or nonuse of the first person, active voice, and penultimate commas in a series are all examples of small style points that may help reviewers and editors feel that the manuscript seems to "fit" the target journal.

17.3.1.2   Submission guidelines

Many, but not all, biomedical journals have adopted the same set of guidelines for formatting the submission of manuscripts. If the journal has adopted the guidelines, that fact will be stated in the Information for Contributors section, usually by referring to "Uniform Requirements for Manuscripts Submitted to Biomedical Journals," or the "ICMJE guidelines" (ICMJE, web). Known informally as the Vancouver guidelines after the setting of the original conference of medical editors where they were developed, the guidelines have been broadened over the past 30 years, and they now address not only basic manuscript preparation and submission topics, but also ethical considerations in the conduct and reporting of research, in publishing and in editorial issues. If the journal has adopted the guidelines, authors should be certain to review them before writing the first draft of the manuscript, to avoid unnecessary revisions. Often, the details about formatting that appear in the Information for Contributors sections of journals that have adopted the Vancouver guidelines will be incomplete, describing only certain journal-specific requirements. In these instances, the bulk of the expected formatting information will be that contained in the Vancouver guidelines.

17.3.1.3   Reporting guidelines

There are several reporting guidelines that can prove useful as authors begin to prepare a manuscript, depending on the type of study being reported. Reporting guidelines focus on *what* information is to be reported, as opposed to *how* that information is to be reported. The principal guidelines are CONSORT (Altman et al., 2001; Moher et al., 2001), STROBE (Vandenbroucke et al., 2007; von Elm et al., 2007), and STARD (Bossuyt et al., 2003a, 2003b, web), which concern themselves with randomized trials, observational studies in epidemiology, and diagnostic studies, respectively. Each of these guidelines is the product of a panel of experts who in turn invited additional input from researchers, editors, methodologists, and clinicians for the purpose of identifying and describing a basic set of information items that are essential for a complete understanding of the research being reported. A frequent problem encountered when evaluating studies reported in the scientific literature is not having the necessary information to assess the internal and external validity of the study, that is, to identify the potential for bias in the study, or to make a judgment about the generalizability of the results. These guidelines describe information considered to be essential for such assessments. They also describe suggested flow diagrams designed to clearly convey essential information about participants and the study design. Authors should thoroughly review the relevant guidelines at the outset of manuscript to ensure that they are aware of and able to report all of the information that reviewers can legitimately expect to be present in the manuscript.

17.3.1.4   Additional guidance

The audience for a paper reporting the results of a clinical research project will consist of both clinical researchers and practitioners. These two types of readers may bring different expectations and may raise different questions as they peruse the report. While the reporting guidelines identify the information needed for validity assessments, they do not address *utility* assessments that may be of some interest to practitioners. Thus, it is often useful to briefly sketch out in layman's terms responses to the following questions as an additional guide to the task at hand:

- What is the clinical problem on which this research seeks to shed some light?

- What implications do the results have for practice?

- How can I know whether what has been reported is applicable to my patients?

Keeping answers to these seemingly simple questions in mind as the draft manuscript is written will help ensure that in focusing on inclusion of all of the essential information needed to assess the validity of the results, the usefulness of the report to clinicians is not forgotten.

17.3.2   Introduction

The introduction to a clinical research paper should put the research question in context, allowing a reader to understand the potential contribution of the study without referring to other materials. The section should identify the problem being addressed by the research, discuss why the situation is considered a problem, describe what is known about the problem, identify what is not known about the problem, and describe the purpose of the research project in terms of how what is learned will help advance a solution to the problem. This information must be conveyed in a brief section, usually no more than several paragraphs. If a full protocol for the research project has been prepared, nearly all of the information needed for the introduction is already at hand, although a literature search should be performed to identify all new relevant publications that have appeared since protocol was originally written.

The description of the problem and the accompanying explanation of what is problematic should be kept quite narrow. For example, if the study is a clinical trial of a new preventive agent for dental caries in caries active and high caries risk adults, the problem is not dental caries, it is not the prevention of dental caries, and it is not the prevention of dental caries in adults. But it might be the prevention of dental caries in high caries risk adults. Identifying this specific problem, defined by both the disease process and the population affected, allows a very focused presentation of the literature describing what is known about the effectiveness of available approaches for prevention in this population. It also permits a cogent description of the magnitude and consequences of the problem in terms of numbers of individuals involved and costs of treatment or prevention. What remains is to briefly describe the approach being investigated and advance the rationale for evaluating it in a high caries risk population. Obviously, what is not known about the problem is how effective the new treatment might be, and this becomes the purpose of the study.

It is appropriate to comment on deficiencies in the studies that address the problem. If relevant literature studies contain substantial threats to internal validity, these threats should be identified and linked in the methods section to the study design that minimizes those threats. Alternatively, heterogeneity among the results of extant studies of a specific question may be the problem, that is, the answer is not clear.

The literature that is cited must be the most recent, and most relevant available. The introduction to a clinical study usually is not the place for historical review, or for setting a broad context for the problem. Economy will help focus the review, and some journals suggest limits on the number of studies cited. Often if there is a substantial literature addressing a particular question, there will also be one or more reviews. These should also be included in the review and, where possible, cited in lieu of individual studies. In most instances, however, a good rule of thumb is to describe all recent studies that have addressed the same question, so that everything that is known about the question is described in the introduction. Describing a study usually means identifying the study design and summarizing the pertinent results, but can also include features of the study design that might represent threats to validity. An archaic style still evident in a few journals saves the description of pertinent studies addressing the same question for presentation in the discussion section. Such a style defeats the purpose of the introduction, informing the reader of what is already known about the problem.

17.3.3   Methods

The methods section is often thought to be the easiest section of the research paper to write because virtually all of the information to be conveyed is already present in the study protocol. But skill is still required, primarily for crafting clear descriptions and ensuring that all necessary information has been included. Traditionally, the purpose of the methods section was to describe how an experiment was performed so that a reader could repeat the experiment and confirm the reported results. Although it is unrealistic that many clinical studies will be repeated exactly, methods sections are still expected to describe experimental procedures in some detail because complete information is absolutely necessary for readers to assess the internal and external validity of the study, and for others who wish to perform systematic reviews to accurately categorize the study's participants and methods.

The reporting guidelines described previously are extremely useful organizers for writing a methods section. To the extent possible, all of the items identified in the relevant guideline as belonging in the methods section should be described and, where necessary, explained or justified. These items can be grouped into the following general categories:

- *Study design*: Description of the overall approach (clinical trial, case-control study, cohort study, etc.) and key features (type of control group(s), matching, etc.).
- *Participants*: Inclusion and exclusion criteria for participants, recruitment settings, and methods.
- *Intervention (if performed)*: What was done to whom, when, where, and how tracked.
- *Data*: All variables collected, measurement methods, examiner training, reliability assessment, and so on.
- *Sample size*: Explanation of how size was determined.
- *Bias control*: Methods used to minimize bias (randomization, masking, etc.).
- *Analysis*: Primary outcomes, statistical methods, subgroup analyses, missing data, etc.

A useful approach to ensure that a draft methods section does describe all of the elements of the study protocol that will be expected by the reviewers and, eventually, readers is to compare the draft section to the methods sections of several reports of similar studies published recently in the target journal. Consider whether each aspect of the study description in the published study has a parallel in the draft.

Most journals now state in their Information for Contributors that they require a statement to the effect that the relevant Institution Review Board or Boards have reviewed and approved the study being described in the paper. A logical place for this statement is at the beginning of the methods section. The remainder of the information can be presented in the order suggested by the preceding bulleted categories.

17.3.4   Results

The results section contains just what the name implies, the results of the study. These are presented as simply and economically as possible, with minimal duplication between text and tables or figures. A simple check for inclusion is that every outcome measure described in the methods section should be represented in the results section, and no outcomes should appear in the results section that have not been described in the methods.

Again, the appropriate reporting guideline should be consulted, as it will be the best summary of contemporary expectations for what should be reported. All of these guidelines suggest that if the study design is at all complex, authors consider use of a flow diagram to help readers understand the study design and the numbers of subjects in each study group at each stage of the study. Such diagrams are an efficient method for presenting information about noneligibles, refusals to participate, exclusions, allocation to study groups, loss to follow-up at each stage, and analytic exclusions.

The usual order in which to describe the results is to first present a patient flow diagram, or data describing the number of participants at each study stage, followed by characteristics of participants. These descriptive data are then followed by the primary study outcomes, and finally any secondary outcomes that were evaluated. Recent reports of similar studies in the target journal will serve as useful models. Inspection of these reports will also provide some guidance and examples for the use of tables and figures to present results.

Almost all results sections will use tables; often the only question is how many to use. Two criteria are the usual number of tables used in similar papers in recent issues of the target journal, and the number of principal outcomes for which the study has collected data. If the number of outcomes is equal or smaller than the usual number of tables, prepare a table for each outcome. If there are too many outcomes, then some combining of outcomes should be considered. Keep the tables as simple as possible, presenting only the most pertinent data, and ensure that the tables are fully interpretable. Use figures sparingly, and only for illustration of principal outcomes where tabular presentation is too complex for easy understanding. For example, figures are quite useful for identifying changes over time in several variables, but are absolutely unnecessary for reporting simple distributions. Most journals will have detailed instructions for the design and presentation of tables and figures in their Information for Contributors sections.

17.3.5   Discussion

The discussion section is perhaps the most fun to write, because it is least structured and the author is expected to express an opinion. This lack of structure also makes the discussion section among the more difficult sections to write, but knowing that there are some basic elements that need to appear in a discussion section makes the job easier. At the most general level, the discussion should answer the question "so what?" To do so, the section should contain the following:

- A brief restatement of key results

- A consideration of the limitations of the study

- A comparison with existing knowledge about the problem

- An interpretation of the results

The discussion should first briefly restate the study's principal result by relating the outcomes back to the study objectives. This is not a reiteration of the specific findings, but a more general statement that is stated in the same terms as the objectives of the study. For example, if the study is designed to test a hypothesis, then the statement should simply acknowledge whether the null hypothesis has been rejected in favor of the alternative hypothesis. If the study was descriptive in nature, then the statement should summarize the key observation(s) that were the objective(s) of the study, for example, stating that the proportion of women in the study population with gingival inflammation was significantly greater than the proportion of men.

Regardless of the principal results, it should be assumed that the evidence generated by the study is experimental, and is subject to confirmation. For that reason, two discussion topics follow. One is the limitations of the current study and the other is the "fit" or agreement of the study with what else is known about the subject. The limitations are those imposed by the study design as well as circumstances that occurred during the execution of the study. The former are theoretically evident to all readers with a knowledge of research design, but not all readers will have this knowledge; so noting design-imposed limitations is a useful approach to increasing readers' understanding of the results. The latter are the responsibility of the investigator to report if there is any chance that such circumstances could have compromised the internal validity of the study.

With respect to agreement with previous findings, the extent of agreement and the quality of the previous studies should be considered. More discussion will be necessary where there is less agreement, and should be directed at possible reasons for differences. The generalizability of the results to larger populations can be addressed as a part of this discussion, or this topic can be addressed as a part of a consideration of the clinical implications of the results.

The heart of the discussion section is the interpretation of the results, answering the "so what?" question, that is, stating what the results mean with respect to the problem or question described in the introduction. In essence, this is bringing the research process full circle—one revolution of the repetitive scientific process known as the scientific method. The paper started by describing a problem, that is, an observation and describing what was known about it. Based on this information, a hypothesis or a question was proposed, a study was designed to answer the question, the study was executed to the results determined, and now it is time to talk about what was learned with respect to the problem or question addressed.

Interpreting the results is the only opportunity in a research report for an investigator to speculate and to argue. Because the paper is reporting clinical research, there will usually be two forms of speculation and argumentation. One form focuses on learning still more about the problem being investigated. This discussion will consider reasons for the observed results and advance new hypotheses or new questions based on these results. The other form addresses the implications of the results for the clinical practice of dentistry. It is rare that a clinical study will not have clinical implications, even if the message is simply that current practice would seem to be appropriate, no changes are necessary. It is also rare that the results of a single study will be so persuasive that the investigator can state unequivocally that a clinical procedure *must* be adopted or rejected. Rather, discussing the clinical implications of a clinical research study allows the author to advance an *opinion* about how clinicians should change their behavior. The discussion of such implications should be somewhat cautious, and must be based on the results of the study.

17.3.6   Other components

Journals will usually describe in the Information for Contributors any other manuscript components that the author is expected to prepare. Some journals may refer authors to the Uniform Requirements (ICMJE, web) for details, while others will present highly individualized descriptions of what is wanted. Typically, five components are described: Title, Abstract, References, Keywords, and Acknowledgments. In addition, almost all journals will require all authors to complete conflict-of-interest statements (see also Chapter 3 on institutional issues related to conflict-of-interest issues).

17.3.6.1   Title

The title should be as short as possible, while still conveying a sense of what is being reported. The study design should be identified, as well as the problem being examined. Some journals limit the number of words or total character spaces used for the title, and in some instances where electronic submission is used, the limitation will not be evident until the title is entered into the form.

17.3.6.2   Abstract

The abstract, which appears first, should be written last. Preparing the abstract after the main sections of the paper have been written ensures that its contents summarize what the paper presents, rather than what the author anticipated the paper would present at the outset. Accuracy in the abstract is important because this is all that many will read, and all that is available on services such as MEDLINE. Most but not all journals request structured or formatted abstracts, generally with four headings (e.g., Objectives, Methods, Results, Conclusions). Most also limit the length of abstracts to between 200 and 300 words.

17.3.6.3   References

A growing number of journals have adopted the reference and citation styles described in the Uniform Guidelines, although a substantial minority still employ older, often archaic and occasionally unique styles. Although it may seem to be a minor issue to contributors, adherence to reference style guidelines and accuracy of those references anecdotally have long been considered as indicators of the overall quality of a manuscript by editors and reviewers. Thus, efforts made to comply with the requested style and to recheck the accuracy of the references are advisable. Use of reference management software greatly simplifies both of these tasks.

17.3.6.4   Keywords

Most journals will request that a group of keywords be listed that describe the content of the manuscript. These keywords may be used by the journal publisher as index terms for an in-house search engine, and they may also appear in publisher-supplied citations to MEDLINE, but they are principally important as suggestions for the National Library of Medicine indexing process. For that reason, the keywords supplied should be MeSH (Medical Subject Headings) terms. A complete list of the MeSH tree structure can be reviewed online, and a browser is available to access descriptors, qualifiers, or supplementary concepts of interest (NLM(b), web).

17.3.6.5   Acknowledgments

(See also Chapter 3 on institutional policies regarding manuscript and study acknowledgment)

Acknowledgments remain a relatively unstandardized component of research papers. Acknowledgments are used to recognize individuals who contributed to the research project in important ways that do not merit authorship credit. Acknowledgments are also used to thank research participants and employees of institutions where the research was conducted. The former use is generally appropriate while the latter may be superfluous. All acknowledgments should indicate the contributions of the persons being acknowledged, and any person acknowledged by name should have previously agreed to that recognition. A special form of acknowledgment is indication of any financial support for the study. All such support should be identified and described. In particular, any involvement of the sponsor in study design, data collection, analysis, interpretation of the results, or preparation of the manuscript must be disclosed. Journals may or may not indicate where general acknowledgments and statements of financial support should be placed in the manuscript. If no location is described, these components should appear following the References section.

17.3.6.6   Conflict-of-interest statement

Authors are expected to disclose all financial and personal relationships that might conceivably bias their study and its report. Usually, the journal will have a form that is to be completed by each author as a part of the submission process. Financial arrangements are the most obvious conflicts and may include employment or consultantships supported by the study's sponsor, or a financial interest in the company whose product is evaluated.

17.4   Manuscript submission and revision

Once an initial draft of the manuscript has been prepared, authors may feel the urge to "get if off their desk" and submit it to the target journal as soon as possible. Giving in to this urge is a mistake, as the first draft of any manuscript is seldom ready for submission.

For that reason, critical review by all authors should be considered as the first step in the submission process.

17.4.1   Review at home

The draft manuscript should be circulated to all authors for comment. The first author should request how comments are to be made, for example, marginal annotations on a paper copy or tracking of suggested revisions on an electronic copy, and specify a due date for receipt of the comments. Authors should be aware that a careful, thoughtful evaluation of the entirety of the manuscript is an important responsibility, and one that must be fulfilled if the requirements for authorship are to be met. The first author then incorporates those comments into a revised draft. Where there is disagreement between contributing authors' suggestions, or where the first author disagrees with a contributing author's suggestion, discussion should precede any decision, although the final authority remains with the first author. In extreme instances where disagreement cannot be resolved, it is appropriate to suggest or accept an offer to renounce authorship. The review cycle may involve several drafts before there is agreement among authors that the draft is ready for submission.

Concomitant with this internal review, the manuscript should also be read by one or more external reviewers, that is, colleagues who were not involved in manuscript preparation, and likely not involved in the study being reported. The primary purpose of this review is to obtain a fresh perspective on the report by readers who cannot "fill in the blanks" from local knowledge. These are essentially "prereviews," offering scrutiny similar to that expected by the journal's reviewers. Because these reviewers would not be familiar with the research study, they will be better positioned to identify needed explanations, justifications, and rationales. In addition to these external reviewers, the manuscript should also be proofread by one or more persons, who will focus on punctuation, usage, repetition, redundancy, spelling, and "stile" (spell checkers do not think). The first author should check the references to ensure that they are accurate and correctly linked to the citations in the text.

17.4.2   Manuscript submission

When the manuscript has been revised to address the comments of the authors, external reviewers, and proofreaders, it is prepared for submission. Most likely, a title page, and if requested, an author page will need to be prepared. The requirements for these pages will be described in the journal's Information for Contributors section. More broadly, for every criterion, instruction, or requirement described in the target journal's Information for Contributors, the manuscript must be checked for adherence. As noted, these sections will vary in the level of detail described, and if a question arises that is not answered by the journal's instructions, the Uniform Requirements should be consulted (ICMJE, web). If the manuscript cannot be made to adhere to one or more of the journal's stated requirements, that fact should be noted and the reason for the deviation explained in the cover letter.

The cover letter itself should contain the information requested in the Information for Contributors section, or failing that, the Uniform Requirements. If the contents of the manuscript have been or will be presented orally or as an abstract, that presentation should be identified. The letter should not be used as an opportunity to inform the editor of the importance of the manuscript, as that quality will be assessed by the journal's reviewers. However, the cover letter may provide brief relevant background not described in the manuscript itself, such as pointing out that the contents represent the first publication of results from a large multisite trial, or that the manuscript addresses a secondary outcome from a previously reported study.

17.4.3   Manuscript revision

The possible outcomes of a manuscript submission are three: outright acceptance, request for submission of a revised manuscript, or outright rejection. Chances are slim that a manuscript will be accepted outright upon its first submission, and even if it is, there are usually requests for revision based on reviewers' comments. Outright rejections are rare for some journals, and common for others, but they are usually unequivocal, the manuscript will "not be considered further." It is most likely that the principal or corresponding author will receive a message from the editor conveying the comments of two or more reviewers, and requesting that the author prepare and resubmit a revised version of the manuscript that responds to these comments.

Deciding how to respond to the reviewers' comments depends very much on the authors' opinion of those comments, as well as their ability to respond. In any event, each comment should be considered separately, discussed with coauthors if the first author deems it necessary, and a response decided upon. As a general rule, if a reviewer's suggestion does not detract from the manuscript, it should be followed if for no other reason than to improve the chances of eventual acceptance. However, there will be instances where the authors believe the reviewer is wrong, either in fact or in interpretation. In these instances, it is appropriate to indicate disagreement with the comment. If the problem is, in the authors' opinion, a result of the reviewer misunderstanding some aspect of the manuscript, the "evidence" for that misunderstanding should be identified, and consideration should be given to revisions to clarify the authors' meaning. If the problem is a difference in interpretation, the authors might consider acknowledging differing interpretations in the manuscript.

Responses to all of the comments should be compiled in a "authors' response," either as a part of a cover letter for the resubmission or, as more frequently requested, in a separate document. The responses should identify each comment, either by number or by quoting part or all of it, then describe what was done in response to the comment, and then if needed, present a rationale for this response. In instances where the manuscript was changed to incorporate the reviewer's comment or suggestion, this and the location of the change in the manuscript are all that need be specified in the authors' response. If, however, the reviewer's comment was not acted upon, or was only partially adopted, the authors' response should present a concise and dispassionate rebuttal of the reviewer's comment, together with any revisions made to lessen the chances of other readers laboring under the same misapprehension.

References

Altman DG, Schulz KF, Moher D, Egger M, Davidoff F, Elbourne D, Gøtzsche PC, Lang T; CONSORT GROUP (Consolidated Standards of Reporting Trials). 2001. The revised CONSORT statement for reporting randomized trials: explanation and elaboration. *Annals of Internal Medicine* 134(8):663–694.

Bossuyt PM, Reitsma JB, Bruns DE, Gatsonis CA, Glasziou PP, Irwig LM, Moher D, Rennie D, de Vet HC, Lijmer JG; Standards for Reporting of Diagnostic Accuracy. 2003a. The STARD statement for reporting studies of diagnostic accuracy: explanation and elaboration. *Annals of Internal Medicine*. 138(1):W1–W12.

Bossuyt PM, Reitsma JB, Bruns DE, Gatsonis CC, Glasziou PP, Irwig LM, Moher D, Rennie D, de Vet HC, Lijmer JG; Standards for Reporting of Diagnostic Accuracy. 2003b. Towards complete and accurate reporting of studies of diagnostic accuracy: the STARD initiative. *Annals of Internal Medicine* 138: 40–44. Available online at http://www.stard-statement.org/website%20stard/. Accessed on September 23, 2009.

International Committee of Medical Journal Editors. web. *Uniform Requirements for Manuscripts Submitted to Biomedical Journals: Writing and Editing for Biomedical Publication*. Available online at http://www.icmje.org. Accessed on September 23, 2009.

Moher D, Schulz KF, Altman DG; CONSORT GROUP (Consolidated Standards of Reporting Trials). 2001. The CONSORT statement: revised recommendations for improving the quality of reports of parallel-group randomized trials. *Annals of Internal Medicine* 34(8):657–662. Available online at http://www.consort-statement.org/?o=1001. Accessed on September 23, 2009.

National Library of Medicine (a). web. *Journal Subject Terms*. Available online at http://www.nlm.nih.gov/bsd/journals/subjects.html. Accessed on September 23, 2009.

National Library of Medicine (b). web. *Medical Subject Headings*. Available online at http://www.nlm.nih.gov/mesh/meshhome.html. Accessed on September 23, 2009.

Slade GD, Caplan DJ. 2000. Impact of analytic conventions on outcome measures in two longitudinal studies of dental caries. *Community Dentistry and Oral Epidemiology* 28: 202–210.

Thompson Scientific (a). web. *Science Citation Index Expanded*. Available online at http://thomsonreuters.com/products_services/science/science_products/a-z/science_citation_index_expanded. Accessed on September 23, 2009.

Thompson Scientific (b). web. *Journal Citation Reports*. Available online at http://thomsonreuters.com/products_services/science/science_products/scholarly_research_analysis/research_evaluation/journal_citation_reports. Accessed on September 23, 2009.

University of Southern California. web. *Jennifer Ann Wilson Dental Library and Learning Center*. Available online at http://www.usc.edu/hsc/dental/library/. Accessed on September 23, 2009.

University of Toledo, Raymon H. web. *Mulford Library. Instructions to Authors in the Health Sciences*. Available online at http://mulford.meduohio.edu/instr/. Accessed on September 23, 2009.

University of Toronto, Faculty of Dentistry. web. *Dental Library, Journals*. Available online at http://www.utoronto.ca/dentistry/newsresources/library/Journals.html. Accessed on September 23, 2009.

Vandenbroucke JP, von Elm E, Altman DG, Gotzsche PC, Mulrow CD, Pocock SJ, Poole C, Schlesselman JJ, Egger M; STROBE initiative. 2007. Strengthening the Reporting of Observational Studies in Epidemiology (STROBE): explanation and elaboration. *Annals of Internal Medicine* 147(8):W163–W194.

von Elm E, Altman DG, Egger M, Pocock SJ, Gøtzsche PC, Vandenbroucke JP. 2007. The Strengthening the Reporting of Observational Studies in Epidemiology (STROBE) statement: guidelines for reporting observational studies. *Annals of Internal Medicine* 146: 573–577. Available online at http://www.strobe-statement.org/index.html. Accessed on September 23, 2009.

18

The evidence base for oral health

Helen Worthington, CStat, PhD**, Ian Needleman,** BDS, MSc, PhD, MRDRCS(Eng), FDSRCS(Eng), FFPH, FHEA, **and Anne-Marie Glenny,** PhD

David Sackett's definition of evidence-based medicine (EBM) is the one most generally quoted: "Evidence-based medicine is the conscientious, explicit, and judicious use of current best evidence in making decisions about the care of the individual patient. It means integrating individual clinical expertise with the best available external clinical evidence from systematic research" (Sackett, 1996). These two aspects should be further integrated with the choices and preferences of the patient. It is clear from this that evidence-based medicine requires new skills of the clinician, including being able to search the literature efficiently and being able to critically evaluate the literature using formal rules. The steps involved in the EBM process are taking a clinical problem or question that has developed from the care of a patient, constructing an appropriate clinical question, searching the literature, appraising the evidence, and finally, reassessing the care of the patient integrating this evidence with clinical expertise and the patient's preferences.

Evidence-based health care (EMHC) has a wider definition as decisions that affect the care of patients are not only taken by clinicians, but managers and health policy makers may also be involved. From this, it is clear that clinicians, managers, and health policy makers need clear summaries of the evidence provided in a form that they can understand and interpret easily. The medical or dental journals publish an overwhelming number of randomized controlled trials (RCT) annually that usually form the evidence base for determining the relative effectiveness of different therapies including drugs, procedures, and treatments for the management of different diseases or conditions. Depending on the volume of literature for a particular topic, it is often not sensible for the health care professionals to undertake this searching and appraising of the evidence and researchers have developed a methodology for summarizing the evidence in the form of systematic reviews. Systematic reviews are not just for answering questions relating to therapies but

Table 18.1   Types of questions, study designs, and examples.

Type of question addressed	Study design	Example
Therapy	Randomized controlled trial	Is ibuprofen better or worse than diclofenac at reducing postoperative pain?
Diagnosis/screening	Cross-sectional	Is the electric caries monitor (ECM) more or less accurate than x-rays for the diagnosis of enamel caries?
Prognosis	Cohort	Does brushing a child's teeth before the age of 2 years lead to less caries at 5 years?
	Case-control	Is fluoride tablet use in young children a risk factor for severe fluorosis?
Occurrence	Cross-sectional/cohort	What proportions of adults have orofacial pain?

may be used to answer other sorts of questions relating to diagnosis, screening, prognosis, and frequency of occurrence, which may require alternative research designs from RCT. Some examples of these are shown in Table 18.1.

There has been some confusion about the terms "systematic review" and "meta-analysis." Some researchers have used the two terms synonymously but perhaps the more widely accepted definition is that a systematic review is the whole process of locating the studies to be included, appraising their quality, and summarizing the results, including a summary of the data from different studies if appropriate. The specific statistical pooling of the data is known as meta-analysis.

Systematic reviews differ from traditional reviews of the literature in several ways. They are based on a focused question and are undertaken in a systematic manner according to predetermined criteria, specifying which databases are searched, what the inclusion criteria are, and how the study quality will be assessed and the data will be synthesized. Traditional reviews of the literature were frequently undertaken in a haphazard manner and tended to be prone to bias often reflecting the views of the authors. Systematic reviews are important as they reduce large amounts of information into manageable portions. They are used to formulate guidelines and policy and are therefore an efficient use of resources. Systematic reviews may increase the power or precision of the effect estimate of the relative effectiveness between the interventions being assessed and if well conducted should be used to limit bias and improve accuracy.

Systematic reviews, such as primary research studies, may be well or poorly conducted and there are guidelines for assessing the quality of systematic reviews. PRISMA provides a checklist and flowchart for the reporting of systematic reviews that include randomized controlled trials (http://www.equator-network.org). MOOSE is a similar checklist and flowchart, also available through this website, for assessing reviews of observational studies.

18.1   The Cochrane Collaboration

The Cochrane Collaboration was established in Oxford in 1993 led by Sir Iain Chalmers. The ideas behind the initial aims of the Cochrane Collaboration collecting together and summarizing data from randomized controlled trials were put forward by Archie Cochrane in his book "Effectiveness and Efficiency" (Cochrane, 1972) that was the original textbook on evidence-based medicine. In 1979, Archie Cochrane had issued a call to assemble "a critical summary, adapted periodically, of all . . . relevant randomized controlled trials" (Cochrane, 1979). The Cochrane Collaboration website (http://www.cochrane.org/index.htm) is very helpful and summarizes its function as follows:

> The Cochrane Collaboration is an international not-for-profit and independent organization, dedicated to making up-to-date, accurate information about the effects of healthcare readily available worldwide. It produces and disseminates systematic reviews of healthcare interventions and promotes the search for evidence in the form of clinical trials and other studies of interventions.

The major product of the collaboration is the Cochrane Database of Systematic Reviews (CDSR) that is published quarterly as part of The Cochrane Library, a regularly updated collection of evidence-based health care databases available on CD-ROM and on the internet. In October 2009, there were 4,027 Cochrane reviews and 1,906 protocols published in CDSR.

Additional databases in The Cochrane Library include the following:

- The Database of Abstracts of Reviews of Effects (structured abstracts of 11,000 non-Cochrane systematic reviews from around the world. The reviews have been appraised by reviewers at the Centre for Reviews and Dissemination in the United Kingdom).

- The Cochrane Central Register of Controlled Trials (CENTRAL) (the Cochrane Collaboration's register of controlled trials, providing bibliographic information on over 600,000 reports of trials identified by contributors to the Cochrane Collaboration).

Databases of methodological issues relating to systematic reviews, economic evaluations, and health technology assessments are also available.

The Cochrane Library has free access in many countries with free or nearly free access for all developing economies appearing in the World Bank's list of "low-income economies."

Those who prepare the reviews are mostly health care professionals who volunteer to work in one of the many Cochrane Review Groups, with editorial teams overseeing the preparation and maintenance of the reviews, as well as application of the rigorous quality standards for which Cochrane reviews have become known. There are 52 review groups, 24 currently based in the United Kingdom, one of which is the Cochrane Oral Health Group (COHG).

18.2   The Cochrane Oral Health Group (COHG)

Go to website http://www.ohg.cochrane.org/.

The Cochrane Oral Health Review Group comprises an international network of health care professionals, researchers, and consumers preparing, maintaining, and disseminating systematic reviews of randomized controlled trials in oral health. Oral health is broadly conceived to include the prevention, treatment, and rehabilitation of oral, dental, and craniofacial diseases and disorders.

The COHG was registered with the Cochrane Collaboration in June 1994. The editorial base was initially set up in the United States under the coordinating editorship of Alexia Antczak Bouckoms. In August 1996, the editorial base was transferred to Manchester within the University's School of Dentistry, with Bill Shaw and Helen Worthington as coordinating editors.

The COHG aims to produce systematic reviews that primarily include all RCT of oral health.

Oral Health Group protocols (details of planned reviews) and reviews are published in the CDSR on The Cochrane Library. In October 2009, the COHG had published 96 systematic reviews and 77 protocols with a further 16 reviews and 21 protocols in preparation and 23 registered titles. The progress of the group can be seen in Figure 18.1. There has been a steady increase in the number of reviews and protocols since 1998. One of the challenges faced by the editorial base of the COHG is encouraging authors to update their reviews every 2 years or so as appropriate. This updating process is one of the strengths of Cochrane reviews compared with systematic reviews published in other journals.

The Group also maintains a Trials Register that is submitted every quarter for publication in the CENTRAL on The Cochrane Library. There is a process within Cochrane where the

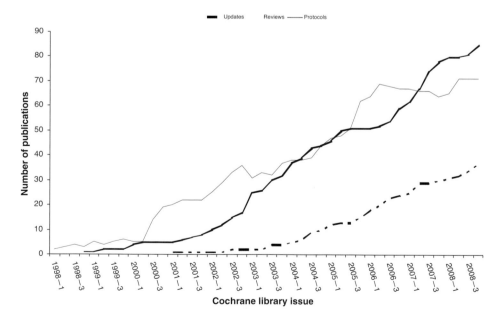

Figure 18.1 Progress of Cochrane Oral Health Group.

new trials in CENTRAL are fed back to MEDLINE to ensure that trials have been correctly indexed in MEDLINE.

The work of the COHG is carried out by over 624 members from 40 different countries around the world. Members contribute to the Group in many different ways: preparing systematic reviews, peer reviewing, manually searching journals, translating articles, and offering consumer input. The activities of the COHG are coordinated and supported by the editorial team located at the editorial base at the School of Dentistry, The University of Manchester, United Kingdom. The COHG has an editorial process as outlined below:

- Register title

- Prepare protocol

- Editorial and external review of protocol

- Protocol published on The Cochrane Library

- Identify trials

- Complete systematic review

- Peer review of systematic review

- Systematic review published on The Cochrane Library

- Regularly updated

To ensure the quality of the reviews, the COHG undertake editorial and external peer review at both the protocol and completed systematic review stage, and the COHG have methodological experts who work with the review teams. The structure of a Cochrane review is outlined in Table 18.2 (taken from http://www.cochrane.org/index.htm).

Randomized controlled trials, which satisfy the inclusion criteria, are usually included in Cochrane reviews of interventions. Some reviews will also include quasi-randomized trials when methods such as alternate allocation have been used to allocate patients to groups. The inclusion criteria for trials relate to the objectives of the review and use a PICO format, which includes specific criteria defining the type of patients to be included, the intervention, what it is to be compared with, and the outcomes measures to be included in the review. Randomized trials may therefore be excluded if they include a patient group different to the one specified, different interventions, or do not include any of the outcomes of interest. The trials included in the Cochrane review of interventions for preventing oral candidiasis (Clarkson et al., 2007a) included patients who were receiving treatment for cancer, did not have candidiasis at the baseline examination, were comparing interventions for preventing candidiasis with control/placebo or another interventions, and included candidiasis as an outcome measurement.

The evaluation of the validity of the included studies is an essential component of a Cochrane review, and this evaluation should also influence the analysis, interpretation, and conclusions of the review. One of the key dimensions in considering whether a study is valid relates to whether it answers its research question "correctly," that is, in a manner free from bias. This is often described as "internal validity," or "quality." Therefore, it is appropriate to consider risk of bias when assessing studies. This is done by addressing six specific domains: sequence generation, allocation concealment, blinding, incomplete outcome data, selective outcome reporting, and other sources of bias.

Table 18.2   Structure of Cochrane review.

1. Plain-language summary	A brief statement summarizing the review, specifically aimed at lay people
2. Structured abstract	A structured summary of the review, subdivided into sections similar to the main review. This may be published independently from the review and appears on the medical bibliographic database MEDLINE
3. Background	This gives an introduction to the question considered, including, for example, details on causes and incidence of a given problem, the possible mechanism of action of a proposed treatment, uncertainties about management options
4. Objectives	A short statement of the aim of the review
5. Selection criteria	A brief description of the main elements of the question under consideration. This is subdivided into the following: • Types of studies—often randomized controlled trials • Types of participants—the population of interest • Types of interventions—the main intervention under consideration and any comparison treatments • Types of outcome measures—considered important by the author, defined in advance; not necessarily outcome measures actually used in trials
6. Search strategy for identification of studies	Details of how an exhaustive identification of relevant studies was attempted, including details of searches of electronic databases, searches for unpublished information, handsearching of journals or conference proceedings, searching of reference lists of relevant articles
7. Methods of the review	Includes a description of how studies eligible for inclusion in the review were selected, how their risk of bias was assessed, how data were extracted from the studies, and how data were analyzed
8. Description of studies	Information on how many studies were found, with specific information for each study such as study size and where it was conducted
9. Methodological quality of included studies	The assessment of the risk of bias of each study, which is then considered in the results and discussion sections
10. Results	Detailed presentation of the results. This section may be accompanied by a graph to show a meta-analysis, if this was carried out
11. Discussion	Interpretation and assessment of results
12. Authors' conclusions	This is subdivided into "Implications for practice" and "Implications for research"

18.3   Statistical methods

Statistical methods have been developed for the meta-analysis or pooling of binary, continuous, and time to event (survival) outcomes from trials. For binary data, often the odds ratio or risk ratio is calculated for each trial and the summary of these presented as the summary statistic for the meta-analysis.

Figure 18.2 shows an example of a forest plot of seven trials included in the Cochrane review of interventions for preventing oral candidiasis (Clarkson et al., 2007a). The interventions were divided into three groups: those absorbed, partially absorbed, and not absorbed from the gastrointestinal tract. The trials included here classed as absorbed from the gastrointestinal tract and were compared to placebo or no-treatment control groups. In the Bodey et al. (1990) trial, 1 out of 58 patients in the absorbed drug group experienced oral candidiasis over the trial period compared with 15 out of 54 in the control group. The risk ratio for this trial was 0.06 with a 95% confidence interval from 0.01 to 0.45, indicating that there was a statistically significant difference between the two groups, in favor of the absorbed drug, as the confidence interval did not include 1. Most of the other trials had confidence intervals including 1 and were not indicating a statistically significant benefit for the drug. The meta-analysis pools together the risk ratios for the trials, weighting them according to how much information each trial gives, to produce the overall risk ratio. The overall risk ratio in Figure 18.2 is 0.47 (95% CI 0.29–0.78), with a p value for overall effect of 0.004. The risk of getting candidiasis is 53% less when taking a drug absorbed from gastrointestinal tract than not doing so.

When undertaking a meta-analysis, it is important to examine the variability in the treatment effects being evaluated in the different trials, which is known as heterogeneity, and is a consequence of clinical and/or methodological differences. This can be examined by consideration of the difference in the observed treatment effects for the trials. Heterogeneity exists if these differences are above what we would expect by chance. Heterogeneity is examined here by the chi-square test and by using the I^2 statistic. Due to the chi-square test's lack of power, a p value of 0.10 is sometimes used to determine statistical significance. In the example given here, there does not appear to be substantial heterogeneity, and this is supported by the I^2 value indicating 41% of the variability is due to heterogeneity rather than chance.

For continuous data, the mean difference for each trial is calculated and the meta-analysis calculates the pooled mean difference across trials weighting each according to the information provided. In this example, the three trials were of approximately the same size and so the weights are similar (Figure 18.3). In this orthodontic review, early orthodontic treatment with a functional appliance was compared to no treatment for the reduction of overjet in children with prominent upper front teeth (Harrison et al., 2007). Three trials were included, each trial showing statistically significant reductions in overjet when the functional appliance was applied. The overall mean difference was a 4.04 mm reduction in overjet (95% CI 0.6 to 7.5), which was statistically significant; however, there was also substantial heterogeneity. Although it is important to consider possible reasons for the heterogeneity, as all the results are in the same direction, there does appear to be a reduction in overjet when the functional appliance is fitted.

There is no restriction on the number of trials included in a meta-analysis. This may be conducted on two trials and provided that they are similar, have no heterogeneity, and are both assessed as at low risk of bias, then a meta-analysis producing a statistically significant effect would be strong evidence of a benefit. The reason for considering

Study	Treatment n/N	Control n/N	Relative risk (random) 95% CI	Weight (%)	Relative risk (random) 95% CI
01 drugs absorbed from GI tract					
Bodey 1990	1/58	15/54		5.5	0.06 [0.01, 0.45]
Brincker 1983	2/19	8/19		9.6	0.25 [0.06, 1.03]
Caselli 1990	7/20	6/10		19.8	0.58 [0.27, 1.28]
Menichetti 1999	10/201	11/204		18.6	0.92 [0.40, 2.12]
Nucci 2000	1/104	6/106		5.0	0.17 [0.02, 1.39]
Palmblad 1992	12/50	19/53		24.4	0.67 [0.36, 1.23]
Winston 1993	6/123	16/132		17.1	0.40 [0.16, 1.00]
Subtotal (95% CI)	575	578		100.0	0.47 [0.29, 0.78]

Total events: 39 (treatment), 81 (control)
Test for heterogeneity chi-square=10.18 df=6 p=0.12 I^2=41.1 %
Test for overall effect z=2.91 p=0.004

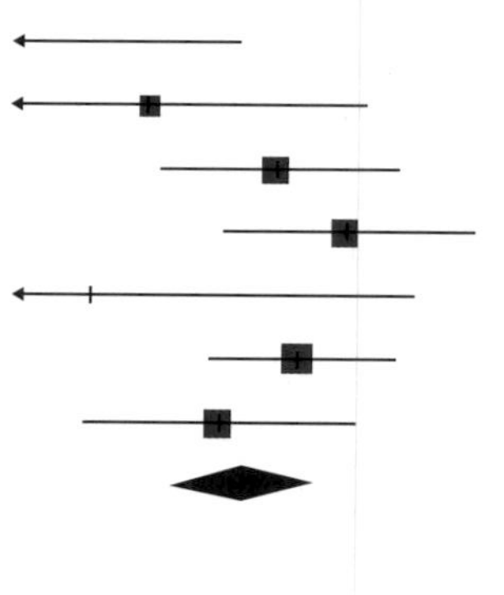

Figure 18.2 Comparisons of interventions absorbed in the gastrointestinal tract with placebo/no treatment for the outcome, the presence of oral candidiasis. Taken from the Cochrane review, Clarkson et al. (2007a).

Review: Orthodontic treatment for prominent upper front teeth in children.
Comparison: 01 Early treatment at the end of phase I: functional versus control
Outcome: 01 Final overjet

Study or subcategory	Functional N	mean (SD)	Control N	mean (SD)	WMD (random) 95% CI	Weight %	WMD (random) 95% CI	Order
Florida	85	3.38 (1.90)	79	5.42 (2.67)		33.45	−1.54 [−2.25, −0.83]	0
North Carolina	41	5.38 (2.67)	54	8.94 (1.84)		33.08	−3.56 [−4.51, −2.61]	0
United Kingdom (Mixed)	89	3.70 (2.27)	84	10.70 (2.40)		33.47	−7.00 [−7.70, −6.30]	3
Total (95% CI)	215		217			100.00	−4.04 [−7.47, −0.60]	

Total for heterogeneity: chi^2 = 117.02, df = 2 (p < 0.00001), I^2 = 98.3%
Test for overall effect: z = 2.30 (p = 0.02)

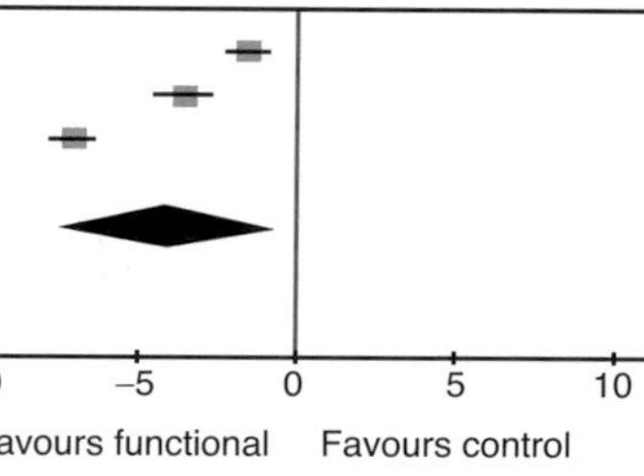

Favours functional   Favours control

Figure 18.3 Comparisons of functional treatment versus no treatment for the reduction of overjet at the end of phase 1. Taken from the Cochrane review, Harrison et al. (2007).

meta-analysis of only a few studies of potential value for health care decision making is related to original rationale for the meta-analysis. The prime reason for conducting meta-analysis is to overcome the problems of inadequate study power in small studies. It is possible that combining only two studies will reveal a statistically significant effect to be demonstrated, where the component studies alone lacked power to show this (type II error). Whether such a result is clinically meaningful is a separate issue and will be dependent on the size of the benefit and the chances of achieving it.

What is more important than numbers of studies is their quality and that there is no heterogeneity between them. There is debate over whether it is "better" to have one large well-conducted trial showing a benefit or a meta-analysis consisting of several smaller trials also showing a benefit (Egger et al., 2001).

18.4   COHG reviews

Ninety-six reviews have been published on The Cochrane Library (October 2009). Putting these into broad categories, the main areas are orthodontics, caries, and intervention for replacing missing teeth (Table 18.3). Many of these reviews have already been incorporated into clinical guidelines and form the evidence base on specific topics.

Some of the more influential reviews are highlighted below:

- The series of topical fluoride reviews for preventing caries in children and adolescents form the basis of the international evidence base for fluorides and are used in many guidelines such as SIGN (Marinho et al., 2002a, 2002b, 2003a, 2003b, 2003c, 2004a, 2004b).

- The review on using penicillins for the prophylaxis of bacterial endocarditis in dentistry has led to a change in the international guidelines for prophylactic cover (Gould et al., 2006; Wilson et al., 2007; Oliver et al., 2008).

- The ozone review investigating whether ozone treatment is effective in arresting or reversing the progression of dental caries was followed by an HTA report and

Table 18.3   Oral Health Group reviews published on The Cochrane Library, October 2009.

Area	Number of published reviews (%)
Orthodontics	11 (11)
Caries—fluoride	9 (9)
Caries—other	10 (10)
Endodontics	5 (5)
Interventions for replacing missing teeth	13 (14)
Periodontal disease	9 (9)
TMJ/TMD	4 (4)
Cancer: screening, mouthcare, treatment	7 (7)
Oral medicine	5 (5)
Other reviews	23 (24)
Total	**96 (100)**

NICE guideline that also concluded that there was insufficient evidence to claim or refute such a benefit for ozone (Rickard et al., 2004; Brazzelli et al., 2006; http://www.nice.org.uk/).

- The manual versus powered toothbrush review compared the ability of these brushes to remove plaque, maintain healthy gingivae, staining, and calculus (Robinson et al., 2005). The results were widely reported internationally and appeared on the front page of the Observer Newspaper in April 2005. The results of this review are sometimes misreported as "head-to-head" comparisons of powered toothbrushes, rather then comparing powered brushes to manual toothbrushes.

- The review on hyperbaric oxygen therapy for irradiated patients who require dental implants concluded that there were no trials and therefore there is insufficient evidence to either claim or refute a benefit from the hyperbaric oxygen therapy treatment (Esposito et al., 2008).

- Frequency of dental recall and scale and polish reviews informed the NICE guideline on dental recall, which is now a contractual requirement of NHS dentists in England (Beirne et al., 2007a, 2007b; Pitts et al., 2004).

- The benefit of fissure sealants has been established firmly and is the core for many international guidelines (e.g., SIGN). This has led to change in policy and practice in Scotland (Ahovuo-Saloranta et al., 2008).

- Four reviews of oral mucositis and candidiasis (Clarkson et al., 2007a, 2007b; Worthington et al., 2007a, 2007b) have influenced international guidelines and the new UCCUK guidelines for children (Glenny, 2006).

- A series of 12 Cochrane reviews on dental implants have established a comprehensive international evidence base for dental implants (Coulthard et al., 2002, 2003; Esposito et al., 2005b, 2006a, 2006b, 2006c, 2007a, 2007b, 2007c, 2007d, 2008; Grusovin et al., 2008).

- Two reviews on periodontal regeneration treatments have quantified the predictability of achieving clinically significant benefits (Esposito et al., 2005a; Needleman et al., 2006).

18.5   Non-RCT reviews

Obviously, not all systematic reviews are reviews of RCT. Systematic reviews of other study designs are undertaken for a number of reasons. For example, systematic reviews do not necessarily address questions relating to the effectiveness of an intervention. While RCT are recognized as the gold standard for assessing such questions, they are not suitable for all types of research questions (see Table 18.1). It would be inappropriate for a review focusing on the potential risks of artherosclerosis associated with periodontal disease to include RCT; in such circumstances, observational studies (e.g., case-control studies) would be required. Several reviews have previously investigated whether there is an association between heart disease and periodontal disease, and between low birth weight babies and periodontal disease in mothers (Madianos et al., 2002; Khader et al., 2004; Vettore et al., 2006; Xiong et al., 2006; Vergnes and Sixou, 2007). All of these reviews focus on observational studies, namely, cohort, case-control, and cross-sectional surveys. The Cochrane Collaboration has recently decided to take forward the methodology for reviews looking at the accuracy of diagnostic tests, and the COHG will be considering taking on these types of reviews from 2010.

Sometimes an RCT may not be feasible or ethical. Therefore, even though the systematic review focuses on the effectiveness of an intervention, it may need to include other types of evidence if it has any chance of answering the research question. For example, in the Cochrane review looking at the effectiveness of penicillins for the prevention of bacterial endocarditis in dentistry (Oliver et al., 2004), it was necessary to include cohort and case-control studies. This was due to the fact that the low incidence of bacterial endocarditis is likely to prohibit an RCT being undertaken in this area. Similarly, it is logistically difficult if not impossible to undertake an RCT on water fluoridation to prevent caries. The Centre for Reviews and Dissemination at the University of York undertook a systematic review with the primary objective "What are the effects of fluoridation of drinking water supplies on the incidence of caries?" (CRD, 2000). The review included prospective studies with quite explicit inclusion criteria as outlined in Table 18.4. The results stated, "The best available evidence suggests that fluoridation of drinking water supplies does reduce caries prevalence, both as measured by the proportion of children who are caries free and by the mean change in dmft/DMFT score. The studies were of moderate quality (level B), but of limited quantity."

In some circumstances, evidences from observational studies are used to supplement data from RCT. For example, in reviews that encompass both effectiveness and safety, it may be necessary to look further than evidence from RCT. Certain harmful events are unlikely to be addressed adequately in RCT (McIntosh et al., 2004). Events that are rare, or those that emerge in the long term, may again require evaluation through observational data.

Finally, systematic reviews of nonrandomized evidence are sometimes undertaken simply because there are no, or limited, RCT available (even if they are feasible and appropriate for the research question being addressed by the review). It is perhaps harder to justify the use of such evidence in this situation. By including other types of evidence, the need for future RCT may be overlooked.

Whatever the reason for including nonrandomized evidence in a systematic review, the process of conducting the review is similar to that of reviews of RCT. The review should follow well-defined protocol that includes the following:

- A well-formulated question
- Comprehensive data search
- Unbiased selection and abstraction process
- Validity assessment of papers
- Synthesis of data

Particular areas of difficulty in the conduct of reviews of nonrandomized data arise in the identification of studies and their validity assessment. While there are highly sensitive search strategies available for identifying RCT, the often unclear description of observational studies, and their subsequent inaccurate coding in bibliographic databases such as MEDLINE, make their identification problematic. With regard to the most appropriate methods of assessing the validity of observational data, empirical evidence is, as yet, lacking.

Table 18.4   Studies considered for the water fluoridation review conducted by CRD, New York (CRD, 2000).

Level A (highest quality of evidence, minimal risk of bias)
- Prospective studies that started within 1 year of either initiation or discontinuation of water fluoridation and have a follow-up of at least 2 years for positive effects and at least 5 years for negative effects
- Studies either randomized or address at least three possible confounding factors and adjust for these in the analysis where appropriate
- Studies where fluoridation status of participants is unknown to those assessing outcomes

Level B (evidence of moderate quality, moderate risk of bias)
- Studies that started within 3 years of the initiation or discontinuation of water fluoridation, with a prospective follow-up for outcomes
- Studies that measured and adjusted for less than three but at least one confounding factor
- Studies in which fluoridation status of participants was known to those assessing primary outcomes, but other provisions were made to prevent measurement bias

Level C (lowest quality of evidence, high risk of bias)
- Studies of other designs (e.g., cross-sectional), prospective or retrospective, using concurrent or historical controls that meet other inclusion criteria
- Studies that failed to adjust for confounding factors
- Studies that did not prevent measurement bias

Studies meeting two of the three criteria for a given evidence level were assigned the next level down
Evidence rated below level B was not considered in our assessment of positive effects

---

18.6 Summary

As health care practitioners, it is important to offer the best possible care for patients. Evidence-based dentistry aims to achieve this by integrating current best evidence, clinical expertise, and patient preference (Sackett, 1996). It encourages the practitioner to look for, appraise, and make sense of the available research evidence in order to apply it to everyday clinical problems. However, the constant development of new dental materials and techniques, changing sociodemographic patterns, and the abundance of emerging research evidence all place greater demands on the clinical decision-making process. It can be argued that summaries of research evidence, such as those provided by systematic reviews, provide a more realistic opportunity for practitioners to implement evidence-based dentistry in their everyday practice.

The Cochrane Library and its databases of Cochrane reviews (CDSR) and other systematic reviews (DARE) offer an excellent starting point in identifying research evidence. Other resources that provide access to evidence-based dentistry material include the Oral Health Specialist Library (part of the NHS Library for Health http://www.library.nhs.uk/oralhealth/), the Centre for Evidence Based Dentistry (http://www.cebd.org/), the International Centre for Evidence-Based Oral Health (http://www.eastman.ucl.ac.uk/iceboh/), and Evidentista (http://www.evidentista.org/). While these resources may not currently provide the answer to all questions that arise through dental clinical practice, it is clear that evidence base for oral health is increasing. It is important that those involved in promoting evidence-based dentistry continually strive to improve the quantity and quality of the research evidence and present it in a way that assists practitioners in their clinical decision making.

References

Ahovuo-Saloranta A, Hiiri A, Nordblad A, Mäkelä M, Worthington HV. 2008. Pit and fissure sealants for preventing dental decay in the permanent teeth of children and adolescents. *Cochrane Database of Systematic Reviews* (4). Art. No.: CD001830. DOI: 10.1002/14651858.CD001830.pub3.

Beirne P, Clarkson JE, Worthington HV. 2007a. Recall intervals for oral health in primary care patients. *Cochrane Database of Systematic Reviews* (4). Art. No.: CD004346. DOI: 10.1002/14651858.CD004346.pub3.

Beirne P, Worthington HV, Clarkson JE. 2007b. Routine scale and polish for periodontal health in adults. *Cochrane Database of Systematic Reviews* (4). Art. No.: CD004625. DOI: 10.1002/14651858.CD004625.pub3.

Bodey GP, Samonis G, Rolston K. 1990. Prophylaxis of candidiasis in cancer patients. *Seminars in Oncology* 17(3):24–28.

Brazzelli M, McKenzie L, Fielding S, Fraser C, Clarkson JE, Kilonzo M, Waugh N. 2006. Systematic review of the effectiveness and cost-effectiveness of HealOzone® for the treatment of occlusal pit/fissure caries and root caries. *Health Technology Assessment* 10(16):1–96. Available online at http://www.ncchta.org/fullmono/mon1016.pdf.

Brincker H. 1983. Prevention of mycosis in granulocytopenic patients with prophylactic ketoconazole treatment. *Mykosen* 26(5):242–247.

Caselli D, Arico M, Michelone G, Cavanna C, Nespoli L, Burgio GR. 1990. Antifungal chemoprophylaxis in cancer children: a prospective randomized controlled study. *Microbiologica* 13(4):347–351.

Clarkson JE, Worthington HV, Eden OB. 2007a. Interventions for preventing oral candidiasis for patients with cancer receiving treatment. *Cochrane Database of Systematic Reviews* (1). Art. No.: CD003807. DOI: 10.1002/14651858.CD003807.pub3.

Clarkson JE, Worthington HV, Eden OB. 2007b. Interventions for treating oral mucositis for patients with cancer receiving treatment. *Cochrane Database of Systematic Reviews* (2). Art. No.: CD001973. DOI: 10.1002/14651858.CD001973.pub3.

Cochrane AL. 1972. *Effectiveness and Efficiency. Random Reflections on Health Services*. London: Nuffield Provincial Hospitals Trust.

Cochrane AL. 1979. *1931–1971: A Critical Review, with Particular Reference to the Medical Profession. In: Medicines for the Year 2000*. London: Office of Health Economics, pp. 1–11.

Coulthard P, Esposito M, Worthington HV, Jokstad A. 2002. Interventions for replacing missing teeth: preprosthetic surgery versus dental implants. *Cochrane Database of Systematic Reviews* (4). Art. No.: CD003604. DOI: 10.1002/14651858.CD003604.

Coulthard P, Esposito M, Jokstad A, Worthington HV. 2003. Interventions for replacing missing teeth: surgical techniques for placing dental implants. *Cochrane Database of Systematic Reviews* (1). Art. No.: CD003606. DOI: 10.1002/14651858.CD003606.

CRD Report 18. 2000. Systematic review of the efficacy and safety of the fluoridation of drinking water. Available online at http://www.york.ac.uk/inst/crd/CRD_Reports/crdreport18.pdf.

Egger M, Davey Smith G, Altman DG. 2001. *Systematic Reviews in Health Care: Meta-Analysis in Context*, 2nd edn. London: BMJ Books.

Esposito M, Grusovin MG, Coulthard P, Worthington HV. 2006a. Interventions for replacing missing teeth: treatment of perimplantitis. *Cochrane Database of Systematic Reviews* (3). Art. No.: CD004970. DOI: 10.1002/14651858.CD004970.pub2.

Esposito M, Grusovin MG, Maghaireh H, Coulthard P, Worthington HV. 2007a. Interventions for replacing missing teeth: management of soft tissues for dental implants. *Cochrane Database of Systematic Reviews* (3). Art. No.: CD006697. DOI: 10.1002/14651858.CD006697.

Esposito M, Grusovin MG, Martinis E, Coulthard P, Worthington HV. 2007b. Interventions for replacing missing teeth: 1- versus 2-stage implant placement. *Cochrane Database of Systematic Reviews* (3). Art. No.: CD006698. DOI: 10.1002/14651858.CD006698.

Esposito M, Grusovin MG, Patel S, Worthington HV, Coulthard P. 2008. Interventions for replacing missing teeth: hyperbaric oxygen therapy for irradiated patients who require dental implants. *Cochrane Database of Systematic Reviews* (1). Art. No.: CD003603. DOI: 10.1002/14651858.CD003603.pub2.

Esposito M, Grusovin MG, Willings M, Coulthard P, Worthington HV. 2007c. Interventions for replacing missing teeth: different times for loading dental implants. *Cochrane Database of Systematic Reviews* (2). Art. No.: CD003878. DOI: 10.1002/14651858.CD003878.pub3.

Esposito M, Grusovin MG, Worthington HV, Coulthard P. 2005a. Enamel matrix derivative (Emdogain®) for periodontal tissue regeneration in intrabony defects. *Cochrane Database of Systematic Reviews* (4). Art. No.: CD003875. DOI: 10.1002/14651858.CD003875.pub2.

Esposito M, Grusovin MG, Worthington HV, Coulthard P. 2006b. Interventions for replacing missing teeth: bone augmentation techniques for dental implant treatment. *Cochrane Database of Systematic Reviews* (1). Art. No.: CD003607. DOI: 10.1002/14651858.CD003607.pub2.

Esposito M, Murray-Curtis L, Grusovin, MG; Coulthard P, Worthington HV. 2007d. Interventions for replacing missing teeth: different types of dental implants. *Cochrane Database of Systematic Reviews* (4). Art. No.: CD003815. DOI: 10.1002/14651858.CD003815.pub3.

Esposito M, Worthington HV, Coulthard P. 2005b. Interventions for replacing missing teeth: dental implants in zygomatic bone for the rehabilitation of the severely deficient edentulous maxilla. *Cochrane Database of Systematic Reviews* (4). Art. No.: CD004151. DOI: 10.1002/14651858.CD004151.pub2.

Esposito MAB, Koukoulopoulou A, Coulthard P, Worthington HV. 2006c. Interventions for replacing missing teeth: dental implants in fresh extraction sockets (immediate, immediate-delayed and delayed implants). *Cochrane Database of Systematic Reviews* (4). Art. No.: CD005968. DOI: 10.1002/14651858.CD005968.pub2.

Glenny A-M. 2006. *Mouth Care for Children, Teenagers and Young Adults Treated for Cancer.* Guideline Report. UKCCSG UK Childhood Cancer Support Group.

Gould FK, Elliott TSJ, Foweraker J, Fulford M, Perry JD, Roberts GJ, Sandoe JAT, Watkin RW. 2006. Guidelines for the prevention of endocarditis: report of the Working Party of the British Society for Antimicrobial Chemotherapy. *Journal of Antimicrobial Chemotherapy* 57(6):1035–1042.

Grusovin, MG, Coulthard P, Jourabchian E, Worthington HV, Esposito MAB. 2008. Interventions for replacing missing teeth: maintaining and recovering soft tissue health around dental implants. *Cochrane Database of Systematic Reviews* (1). Art. No.: CD003069. DOI: 10.1002/14651858.CD003069.pub3.

Harrison JE, O'Brien KD, Worthington HV. 2007. Orthodontic treatment for prominent upper front teeth in children. *Cochrane Database of Systematic Reviews* (3). Art. No.: CD003452. DOI: 10.1002/14651858.CD003452.pub2.

Khader YS, Albashaireh ZS, Alomari MA. 2004. Periodontal diseases and the risk of coronary heart and cerebrovascular diseases: a meta-analysis. *Journal of Periodontology* 75(8):1046–1053.

Madianos PN, Bobetsis GA, Kinane DF. 2002. Is periodontitis associated with an increased risk of coronary heart disease and preterm and/or low birth weight births? *Journal of Clinical Periodontology* 29(Suppl. 3):22–36; discussion 37–38.

Marinho VCC, Higgins JPT, Logan S, Sheiham A. 2002a. Fluoride gels for preventing dental caries in children and adolescents. *Cochrane Database of Systematic Reviews* (1). Art. No.: CD002280. DOI: 10.1002/14651858.CD002280.

Marinho VCC, Higgins JPT, Logan S, Sheiham A. 2003a. Fluoride mouthrinses for preventing dental caries in children and adolescents. *Cochrane Database of Systematic Reviews* (3). Art. No.: CD002284. DOI: 10.1002/14651858.CD002284.

Marinho VCC, Higgins JPT, Logan S, Sheiham A. 2002b. Fluoride varnishes for preventing dental caries in children and adolescents. *Cochrane Database of Systematic Reviews* (1). Art. No.: CD002279. DOI: 10.1002/14651858.CD002279.

Marinho VCC, Higgins JPT, Logan S, Sheiham A. 2003b. Fluoride toothpastes for preventing dental caries in children and adolescents. *Cochrane Database of Systematic Reviews* (1). Art. No.: CD002278. DOI: 10.1002/14651858.CD002278.

Marinho VCC, Higgins JPT, Logan S, Sheiham A. 2003c. Topical fluoride (toothpastes, mouthrinses, gels or varnishes) for preventing dental caries in children and adolescents. *Cochrane Database of Systematic Reviews* (4). Art. No.: CD002782. DOI: 10.1002/14651858.CD002782.

Marinho VCC, Higgins JPT, Sheiham A, Logan S. 2004a. Combinations of topical fluoride (toothpastes, mouthrinses, gels, varnishes) versus single topical fluoride for preventing dental caries in children and adolescents. *Cochrane Database of Systematic Reviews* (1). Art. No.: CD002781. DOI: 10.1002/14651858.CD002781.pub2.

Marinho VCC, Higgins JPT, Sheiham A, Logan S. 2004b. One topical fluoride (toothpastes, or mouthrinses, or gels, or varnishes) versus another for preventing dental caries in children and adolescents. *Cochrane Database of Systematic Reviews* (1). Art. No.: CD002780. DOI: 10.1002/14651858.CD002780.pub2.

McIntosh HM, Woolacott NF, Bagnall A-M. 2004. Assessing harmful effects in systematic Reviews. *BMC Medical Research Methodology*. 4: 19. DOI: 10.1186/1471-2288-4-19.

Menichetti F, Del Favero A, Martino P, Bucaneve G, Micozzi A, Girmenia C, Barbabietola G, Pagaño L, Leoni P, Specchia G, Caiozzo A, Raimondi R, Mandelli F. 1999. Intraconazole oral solution as prophylaxis for fungal infections in neutropenic patients with hematologic malignancies: a randomized, placebo-controlled, double-blind, multicenter trial. *Clinical Infectious Diseases* 28(2):250–255.

Needleman IG, Worthington HV, Giedrys-Leeper E, Tucker RJ. 2006. Guided tissue regeneration for periodontal infra-bony defects. *Cochrane Database of Systematic Reviews* (2). Art. No.: CD001724. DOI: 10.1002/14651858.CD001724.pub2.

Nucci M, Biasoli I, Akiti T, Silveira F, Solza C, Barreiros G, Spector N, Derossi A, Pulcheri W. 2000. A double-blind, randomized, placebo-controlled trial of itraconazole capsules as antifungal prophylaxis for neutropenic patients. *Clinical Infectious Diseases* 30(2):300–305.

Oliver R, Roberts GJ, Hooper L. 2004. Penicillins for the prophylaxis of bacterial endocarditis in dentistry. *Cochrane Database of Systematic Reviews* (2). Art. No.: CD003813. DOI: 10.1002/14651858.CD003813.pub2.

Oliver R, Roberts GJ, Hooper L, Worthington HV. 2008. Antibiotics for the prophylaxis of bacterial endocarditis in dentistry. *Cochrane Database of Systematic Reviews* (4). Art. No.: CD003813. DOI: 10.1002/14651858.CD003813.pub3.

Palmblad J, Lönnqvist B, Carlsson B, Grimfors G, Järnmark M, Lerner R, Ljungman P, Nyström-Rosander C, Petrini B, Oberg G. 1992. Oral ketoconazole prophylaxis for Candida infections during induction therapy for acute leukaemia in adults: more bacteraemias. *Journal of Internal Medicine* 231(4):363–370.

Pitts N, Batchelor P, Clarkson J, Davenport C, Davies R, Elley K, Fayle S, Grey E, Harley K, Hawksworth S, Lewis M, Lowndes P, Mulcahy M, Richards D, Seppings R, Smart G, Tilling E, Wilkins P, Worthington H, Beirne P, Dutchak J, Needleman IG, Okem G, Sharpin C, Thomas L, Wonderling D, Robb P, Struthers J, Duncan P, Williams A. 2004. *Dental Recall. Recall Interval between Routine Dental Examinations, Clinical Guidelines Series*. London: National Institute for Clinical Excellence (NICE). ISBN: 1842578014. pp. 38.

Rickard GD, Richardson R, Johnson T, McColl D, Hooper L. 2004. Ozone therapy for the treatment of dental caries. *Cochrane Database of Systematic Reviews* (3). Art. No.: CD004153. DOI: 10.1002/14651858.CD004153.pub2.

Robinson PG, Deacon SA, Deery C, Heanue M, Walmsley AD, Worthington HV, Glenny A-M, Shaw WC. 2005. Manual versus powered toothbrushing for oral health. *Cochrane Database of Systematic Reviews* (2). Art. No.: CD002281. DOI: 10.1002/14651858.CD002281.pub2.

Sackett D. 1996. Evidence based medicine: what it is and what it isn't. *British Medical Association* 312: 71–72.

Vergnes JN, Sixou M. 2007. Preterm low birth weight and maternal periodontal status: a meta-analysis. *American Journal of Obstetrics and Gynecology* 196(2):135.e1–e7.

Vettore MV, Lamarca Gde A, Leão AT, Thomaz FB, Sheiham A, Leal Mdo C. 2006. Periodontal infection and adverse pregnancy outcomes: a systematic review of epidemiological studies. *Cadernos De Saude Publica*. 22(10):2041–2053.

Wilson W, Taubert KA, Gewitz M, Lockhart PB, Baddour Larry M, Levison M, Bolger A, Cabell CH, Takahashi M, Baltimore RS, Newburger JW, Strom BL, Tani Lloyd Y, Michael G, Bonow RO, Pallasch T, Shulman ST, Rowley AH, Burns JC, Ferrieri P, Gardner T, Goff D, Durack David T; American Heart Association Rheumatic Fever, Endocarditis and Kawasaki Disease Committee; Council on Cardiovascular Disease in the Young; Council on Clinical Cardiology; Council on Cardiovascular Surgery and Anesthesia; Quality of Care and Outcomes Research Interdisciplinary Working Group; American Dental Association. 2007. Prevention of infective endocarditis: guidelines from the American Heart Association: a guideline from the American Heart Association Rheumatic Fever, Endocarditis and Kawasaki Disease Committee, Council on Cardiovascular Disease in the Young, and the Council on Clinical Cardiology, Council on Cardiovascular Surgery and Anesthesia, and the Quality of Care and Outcomes Research Interdisciplinary Working Group. *Journal of American Dental Association* 138(6):739–745, 747–760. Review. PMID: 17545263 [PubMed—indexed for MEDLINE].

Winston DJ, Maziarz RT, Chandrasekar PH, Lazarus HM, Goldman M, Blumer JL, Leitz GJ, Territo MC. 1993. Fluconazole prophylaxis of fungal infections in patients with acute leukemia. Results from a randomised placebo-controlled, double-blind, multicentre trial. *Annals of Internal Medicine* 118(7):495–503.

Worthington HV, Clarkson JE, Eden OB. 2007a. Interventions for preventing oral mucositis for patients with cancer receiving treatment. *Cochrane Database of Systematic Reviews* (4). Art. No.: CD000978. DOI: 10.1002/14651858.CD000978.pub3.

Worthington HV, Clarkson JE, Eden OB. 2007b. Interventions for treating oral candidiasis for patients with cancer receiving treatment. *Cochrane Database of Systematic Reviews* (2). Art. No.: CD001972. DOI: 10.1002/14651858.CD001972.pub3.

Xiong X, Buekens P, Fraser WD, Beck J, Offenbacher S. 2006. Periodontal disease and adverse pregnancy outcomes: a systematic review. *BJOG: An International Journal of Obstetrics and Gynaecology*. 113(2):135–143.

Index